The Biomechanics of Back Pain

For Churchill Livingstone:

Editorial Director (Health Professions): Mary Law
Project Manager: Derek Robertson
Design Direction: Judith Wright

The Biomechanics of Back Pain

Michael A. Adams BSc PhD
Senior Research Fellow, Department of Anatomy, University of Bristol, Bristol, UK

Nikolai Bogduk BSc(Med) MB BS MD PhD DSc DipAnat DipPainMed FAFRM(RACP) FFPM(ANZCA)
Professor of Anatomy and Musculoskeletal Medicine, University of Newcastle, and
Director, Newcastle Bone and Joint Institute, Royal Newcastle Hospital, Newcastle, New South Wales, Australia

Kim Burton DO PhD
Director, Spinal Research Unit, University of Huddersfield, Huddersfield, UK

Patricia Dolan BSc PhD
Senior Lecturer, Department of Anatomy, University of Bristol, Bristol, UK

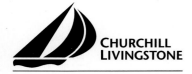
CHURCHILL
LIVINGSTONE

EDINBURGH LONDON NEW YORK PHILADELPHIA ST LOUIS SYDNEY TORONTO 2002

CHURCHILL LIVINGSTONE
An imprint of Elsevier Science Limited

First published 2002
Reprinted 2002

ISBN 0 443 06207 2

British Library Cataloguing in Publication Data
A catalogue record for this book is available from the British
Library

Library of Congress Cataloging in Publication Data
A catalog record for this book is available from the Library of
Congress

Note
Medical knowledge is constantly changing. As new information becomes available, changes in treatment, procedures,
equipment and the use of drugs become necessary. The
authors and the publishers have taken care to ensure that the
information given in this text is accurate and up-to-date.
However, readers are strongly advised to confirm that the
information, especially with regard to drug usage, complies
with the latest legislation and standards of practice.

 ELSEVIER SCIENCE your source for books,
journals and multimedia
in the health sciences

www.elsevierhealth.com

The
publisher's
policy is to use
**paper manufactured
from sustainable forests**

Printed in China by RDC Group Limited

Contents

Acknowledgement

The authors would like to thank Bob Coyne of the Department of Anatomy, Bristol University, for digital enhancement of the colour photographs included in this book.

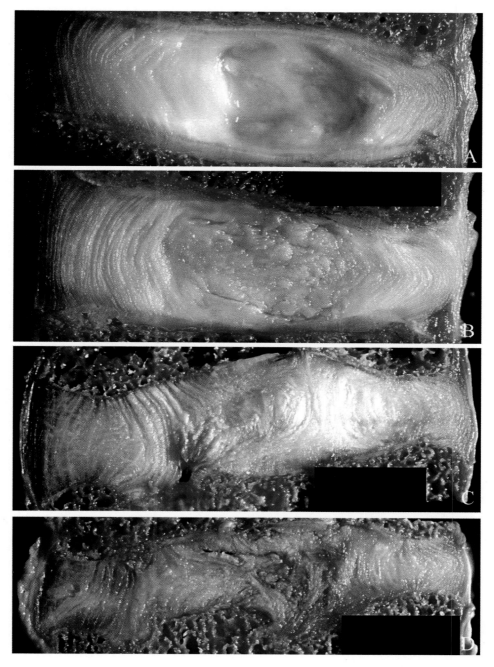

Plate 1 Lumbar intervertebral discs sectioned in the mid-sagittal plane, anterior on left. These discs, which were not subjected to any post-mortem loading, represent the first four stages of disc degeneration described on p. 126. (A) Grade 1 disc, typical of ages 15–40 years. (Male, 35 years.) (B) Grade 2 disc, typical of ages 35–70 years. The nucleus appears fibrous, and there is some brown pigmentation typical of ageing. However, the disc's structure is intact, and the disc is not 'degenerated'. (Male, 47 years, L2–3.) (C) Grade 3 disc, showing moderate degenerative changes. Note the anulus bulging into the nucleus, damage to the inferior endplate, and the lack of pigmentation in some regions of the disc. (Male, 31 years, L2–3.) (D) Grade 4 disc, showing severe degeneration. Note the brown pigmentation, the disruption to both endplates, and internal collapse of the anulus, with corresponding reduction in disc height. (Male, 31 years, L4–5.)

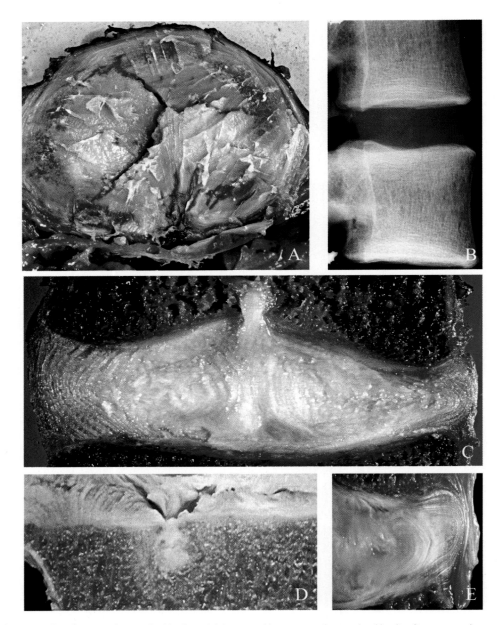

Plate 2 (A) Large stellate fracture of a vertebral body endplate caused by compressive overload in-vitro (transverse plane, anterior on top). The disc has been cut away to reveal the underlying bone, covered centrally by the hyaline cartilage endplate. (B) Radiograph of a lumbar motion segment following compressive overload in-vitro. One of the endplates adjacent to the disc was found to be damaged, but this is not apparent from the radiograph. (Male, 21 years, L2–3.) (C) Lumbar disc sectioned in the mid-sagittal plane following mechanical loading in-vitro (anterior on left). The disc was subjected to a minor compressive overload injury (which damaged the upper endplate and decompressed the nucleus) followed by cyclic loading in compression. Some nucleus pulposus has herniated vertically into the vertebral body and the inner lamellae appear to be collapsing into the nucleus. Note the marked concavity of the damaged (upper) endplate, and the hairpin bending of the outer posterior anulus. (Male, 42 years, L4–5.) (D) Lumbar disc and vertebral body sectioned in the mid-sagittal plane (anterior on left). There is a vertical herniation of nucleus pulposus through the lower endplate, apparently of long standing. Note the degenerative changes in the disc. Adjacent discs were not degenerated, and their endplates were intact. (E) Detail of lumbar disc sectioned in the mid-sagittal plane following mechanical loading in-vitro in compression and backwards bending (posterior on right). Note the hair-pin bending of the outermost lamellae, causing the anulus to protrude beyond the posterior margin of the vertebral body.

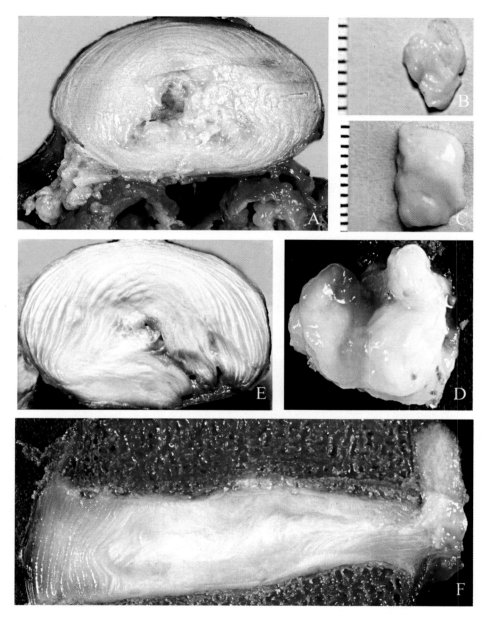

Plate 3 (A) Lumbar intervertebral disc sectioned in the horizontal plane, following mechanical loading in-vitro (anterior on top). Note the large postero-lateral herniation of nucleus pulposus (bottom left) which occurred suddenly following severe loading in bending and compression (details on p. 148). Bending was applied about an oblique axis so that the left postero-lateral region of outer anulus was stretched the most. (Male, 43 years, L4–5.) (B) Herniated material collected from in-vitro experiments (as in A). (C) The same material as in B), following 4 h of swelling in physiological saline at 37°C. The tissue has increased its weight by approximately 150%. Data from Dolan et al.[213] (D) Close-up view of herniated nucleus pulposus obtained as in (A). (Male 40 years, L2–3.) (E) Lumbar disc sectioned in the transverse plane, following cyclic mechanical loading in bending and compression in-vitro (anterior on top). Details on p. 150. Note the 'bell'-shaped deformation of the anular lamellae, and the large postero-lateral radial fissure. The endplate was fractured, allowing blood to pass down the fissure. (F) Lumbar disc sectioned in the mid-sagittal plane following mechanical loading in-vitro (anterior on left). The disc was compressed to failure (9.8 kN) while positioned in 6° of flexion. Note the radial fissure and the herniated nucleus pulposus trapped behind the posterior longitudinal ligament. (Male 40 years, L2–3.)

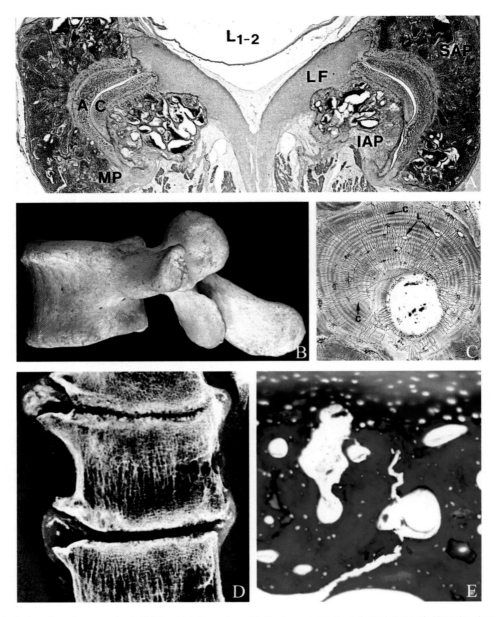

Plate 4 (A) Histological section of zygapophysial joints at L1–2, sectioned in the transverse plane (anterior at top). Note the shape of the joint surfaces covered in articular cartilage (stained purple) and the thick amorphous ligamentum flavum (LF) which blends in with the anterior margin of the joint capsule. IAP/SAP: inferior/superior articular process. From: Singer KP 1994 Anatomy and biomechanics of the thoracolumbar junction. In: Boyling JD, Palastanga N (eds) Grieve's Modern Manual Therapy, 2nd edn, with permission of Churchill Livingstone, Edinburgh. (B) Lumbar vertebra viewed in the sagittal plane, following removal of all soft tissue (anterior on left). Note the long, wide spinous process, and the oblique orientation of the inferior articular processes. (C) Histological section of bone showing a large osteon (explained in Figure 4.8). The contents of the central Haversian canal are indistinct, but osteocytes in their lacunae (L) and their radiating cytoplasmic extensions which lie in canaliculi (C) are clearly visible. Reproduced, with permission, from Young B, Heath JW 2000 Wheater's Functional Histology, Churchill Livingstone, Edinburgh. (D) Radiograph of old and degenerated lumbar spine (anterior on left). Disc space height has collapsed, and large marginal osteophytes effectively increase the surface area of the vertebral body. Note the bony sclerosis adjacent to the endplates, and the preferential loss of horizontal trabeculae in the vertebral body, which is typical of osteopaenia (p. 58). The calcification of the anterior margin of the disc may indicate an early stage in the formation of 'bridging' osteophytes, as shown posteriorly at the upper level. (E) Histological section of the junction between articular cartilage (stained blue) and subchondral bone (red) in young bovine tissue. Calcified cartilage is dark blue. Note the marrow spaces in the subchondral bone, some of which are in direct contact with cartilage. Compare with Figure 4.13 of the vertebral endplate. Mechanical loading of the articular cartilage surface has created two large cracks in the subchondral bone.

1

Introduction

MECHANICAL LOADING AND BACK PAIN

Mechanical loading is good for your back. The bones, muscles, ligaments and discs of the spine are all capable of adapting to physical exercise by becoming stronger, and this makes them less vulnerable to injury. Old notions concerning the harmful effects of physical exercise are gradually being discredited, as is the use of bed-rest as a treatment for back pain. Instead, current research emphasises the importance of exercise in maintaining the health of the musculoskeletal system. The new 'enemies' of spinal health are considered to be genetic inheritance, which exerts a dominant influence on the risk of intervertebral disc degeneration, and the human personality, which influences all aspects of back pain behaviour, including the decision to report it. The 'Back Pain Revolution' is how one leading expert has summarised these recent changes in attitudes.[840]

However, it would be wrong to assume that genetic influences on spinal pathology somehow reduce the importance of mechanical or biochemical factors: on the contrary, genes exert their influence by affecting the mechanical, biochemical and metabolic properties of spinal tissues. Likewise it is a mistake to assume that psychosocial factors such as depressive tendencies and work dissatisfaction are important causes of back pain; in fact they have less influence than certain physical and metabolic factors in explaining first-time back pain. Psychosocial factors explain people's responses to pain rather than the pain itself.

1

Recent pain-provocation studies have not only located the anatomical origins of severe back pain, they have also confirmed that patients' characteristic back pain is often reproduced when the affected tissue is mechanically stimulated. These considerations have been acknowledged previously[840]: 'The balance of back pain research has perhaps swung too far towards these psychosocial issues, to the neglect of the physical. … Hopefully, the pendulum will swing back over the next 10 years.'

PURPOSE OF THIS BOOK

The purpose of this book is not just to push the pendulum back again, but to bring it to rest in a balanced position where all of the factors which influence back pain are given due attention. The title 'The biomechanics of back pain' does not imply a bias towards mechanical explanations of back pain; it merely reflects the fact that mechanical factors are the most obvious and preventable influences in a complex natural history which involves biological and psychological processes as well as mechanical ones (hence 'biomechanics'). The title is also intended to imply a mechanistic approach to back pain, in which our knowledge of the biological and physical sciences is applied to explaining the various chains of events which lead to back pain. Back pain is certainly a difficult and multifaceted problem, but it is not so difficult that we must abandon the normal scientific method in favour of some vague holistic approach. Back pain should be explained, not explained away. The varied background of the authors of this book reflects a desire by them, and by the publishers, to produce a balanced and integrated text which incorporates all of the recent scientific advances in our understanding of back pain.

THE AUTHORS

Mike Adams graduated in natural philosophy (physics) before studying for a PhD in spinal mechanics. Much of his research has involved mechanical testing of cadaveric spines and articular cartilage, but this strong biomechanics influence has been moderated by more than 10 years of teaching musculoskeletal biology to science students. His primary interest in back pain is to explain the interactions between mechanical and biological (cell mediated) events which lead to degenerative changes within spinal tissues.

Nik Bogduk began studies into back pain while still an undergraduate medical student. He investigated the nerve supply of the lumbar spine with the view to establishing the possible sources of back pain. After graduating in Medicine, he pursued a PhD in Neurology in which he developed diagnostic procedures for back pain and for neck pain, based on his anatomical studies. His work subsequently progressed to apply those diagnostic procedures and others to determine the relative prevalence of different sources of back pain and neck pain, and to evaluate neuro-ablative, surgical procedures for the treatment of pain. In the course of these clinical studies he continued to contribute to basic sciences on the anatomy of spinal muscles and the kinematics of spinal movement.

Kim Burton graduated as an osteopath before moving into research and undertaking a PhD in the biomechanics and epidemiology of back pain. Subsequent research involved epidemiological studies of different occupational groups, with a focus on the relative influence of psychosocial and ergonomic factors on disability due to back pain. More recently his research has been in the clinical environment, developing and testing interventions addressing psychosocial factors as obstacles to recovery. He has been involved in the development of the UK primary care and occupational health guidelines for the management of low back pain, and is the Editor-in-Chief of *Clinical Biomechanics*.

Trish Dolan graduated in biological sciences before concentrating on exercise and muscle physiology for her PhD. This was followed by post-doctoral experience in a biomechanics tissue-testing laboratory, and her subsequent research has continued to straddle the boundaries of physiology and biomechanics. Her primary research interests include the measurement of forces that muscles apply to the spine, and the quantification and analysis of function in patients with spinal disorders.

WHO SHOULD READ THIS BOOK?

The book has evolved from seminars in musculoskeletal tissues given by two of the authors (MA and PD) to final year undergraduate students in Anatomical Science, and to post-graduate students of physiotherapy, orthopaedic surgery and ergonomics. This knowledge base has been augmented by the anatomical and clinical expertise of the other two authors. The book is intended primarily for those who treat back pain, including physiotherapists, osteopaths, chiropractors, general practitioners, occupational health professionals, and nurses. It may also interest advanced undergraduate science students, surgeons, ergonomists, and those involved in personal injury litigation.

Very little previous knowledge of musculoskeletal tissue biology or biomechanics is required, because introductory chapters are included to explain the concepts and terminology used later in the book. However, in order to do justice to the many controversies regarding back pain, certain areas of the research literature have been analysed in more detail, and with more rigour, than is customary in undergraduate texts.

INTRODUCTION TO INDIVIDUAL CHAPTERS

Chapters 2 and 3 describe the functional anatomy of the lumbosacral spine and the overlying muscles and fascia. All terms used later in the book are defined, and in most cases illustrated with line diagrams. Structure and function are conveniently described together, but where a particular function is considered to be controversial, reference is made to the relevant sections later in the book.

The biology of spinal tissues is dealt with in detail in Chapter 4, because some knowledge of the interactions between cell metabolism, tissue integrity and mechanical loading are required to understand the clinical relevance of later sections on spine mechanics. An attempt is made to distinguish between the ageing and degeneration of spinal tissues, because this is of fundamental clinical importance.

The provocative question 'where does back pain come from?' is tackled in Chapter 5. A satisfactory answer could be offered on the basis of pain provocation and pain-blocking studies alone, but additional sections in this and the previous chapter attempt to link back pain to the underlying neuroanatomy, and to common diagnostic syndromes. The evidence from this chapter justifies the emphasis placed on intervertebral discs in subsequent sections of the book.

Chapter 6 reviews the epidemiological evidence concerning the causes of spinal pathology and back pain. This information is essential to understand the relative importance of mechanical and other influences in the aetiology of back pain. It is a key chapter, which justifies the title and scope of the entire book.

Before considering how the spine responds to mechanical loading, it is necessary to consider the origins and magnitude of the forces applied to it during the activities of daily living. Spinal loading is analysed in Chapter 7.

The normal response of the spine to non-damaging forces is described in Chapter 8. This indicates how each spinal structure has a specific job to do, and it is a prerequisite to understanding mechanical dysfunction and failure. Wherever possible, qualitative descriptions are supported by experimental measurements, because it is generally true to say that you do not really understand a mechanism until you have measured it. To give an example, the observation that intervertebral discs bulge radially outwards when compressed may seem to be of some clinical interest – until, that is, you learn that the bulge is generally a small fraction of 1 mm, even when the compressive force is several times bodyweight!

Chapter 9 describes mechanisms of injury and fatigue failure in each spinal structure. It is the largest chapter, and the primary focus of the book. Intervertebral disc failure is treated in particular detail, and numerous colour plates are presented to give the reader a 'feel' for normal and dysfunctional discs. The final section of this chapter attempts to reconcile the results of mechanical experiments on cadaveric tissues with the evidence from previous chapters concerning spinal loading in life, and the response of living tissues to changes in their mechanical environment.

Many clinicians will require little convincing that back pain can arise in the apparent absence of injury or degenerative changes. Chapter 10 suggests that 'functional pathology' can arise from high localised stress concentrations within innervated tissues, and it shows how stress concentrations might be generated by small changes in posture, spinal loading, and loading history.

This leads directly to possibilities for preventing and treating back pain. The suggestions given in Chapter 11 arise from recent clinical and epidemiological research, and are shown to be consistent with the evidence presented in previous chapters. The view that mechanical loading is necessarily bad for the back and must be minimised following back pain is exposed as a fallacy, and the positive benefits of certain types of physical and mental treatments are emphasised.

Financial compensation and personal injury litigation are considered by some experts to be a natural consequence of chronic back pain coupled with ineffective treatment. Others view them as an important cause of back pain reporting, and subsequent disability. Chapter 12 shows that there is some truth in both points of view, but concludes nevertheless that certain spinal disorders, including disc prolapse, can often be attributed to mechanical loading of vulnerable tissues. The nature of tissue 'vulnerability', and its medicolegal implications, is a key issue in this chapter.

The concluding Chapter 13 attempts to 'pull together' the main themes of the book. It suggests that cell-mediated degenerative changes are a consequence rather than a cause of tissue failure, and it attempts to explain why the links between spinal pathology and pain are so complex.

BIOMECHANICAL TERMS AND CONCEPTS

Certain words and concepts used later in the book are explained here for ease of reference. These notes are intended to provide helpful explanations for likely readers of the book, rather than rigorous definitions to satisfy the specialist.

Force. Force is an action exerted on a body which causes it to deform or to move. It is a **vector** quantity which has a magnitude (the size of the force) and a direction. The unit of force is the Newton (N). Approximately, $9.81\,N = 1\,kg = 2.2\,lb$.

A force is **compressive** if it compacts an object, **tensile** if it pulls it apart, and **shear** if it acts to deform the object without compacting or stretching it (Fig. 1.1).

A force can be represented (in two dimensions) by two **components** which act in convenient directions, usually at right angles to each other, as shown in Figure 1.2. 'Resolving' forces into components is a useful means of adding together two

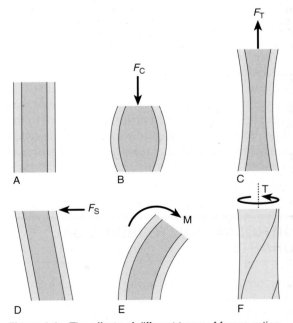

Figure 1.1 The effects of different types of forces acting on a solid object. (A) No forces acting; (B) compressive force F_C; (C) tensile force F_T, (D) shear force F_S, (E) bending moment B; (F) torsional moment, or torque T.

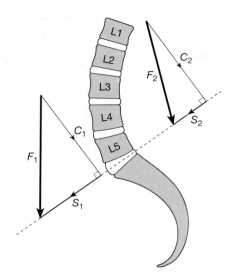

Figure 1.2 F_1 and F_2 represent the abdominal and back muscle forces acting on the lumbar spine. Because F_1 and F_2 act in slightly different directions, they can not simply be added together to give the overall 'resultant' force on the spine. To calculate the resultant, it is necessary to represent each force by two 'components', C and S, which act in two directions at 90° to each other. The components are added up to give the total force acting in these two directions (i.e. $C_1 + C_2$, and $S_1 + S_2$). Then the overall resultant force, R (not shown), acting on the L5–S1 disc is given by: $R^2 = (C_1 + C_2)^2 + (S_1 + S_2)^2$. When adding forces in this manner, it is useful to calculate components in two meaningful directions, in this case, perpendicular to and parallel to the L5–S1 intervertebral disc.

(or more) forces which act in different directions: the component forces can easily be summed, and then used to reconstruct the 'resultant' of the two original forces.

Mass. The mass of an object is the quantity of matter it contains, and represents the resistance of that body to being moved quickly (i.e. being accelerated). Mass simply has a magnitude, and so is a **scalar** quantity. The unit of mass is the kilogramme (kg).

Weight. The weight of an object is the force exerted on it by the gravitational pull of the Earth. According to Newton's 2nd Law of motion:

Force = mass × acceleration   [1]

so the weight of an object is given by ($m \times g$), where m is its mass, and g the acceleration due to gravity. g depends on the height above sea level, falling to zero in outer space. Therefore, the

weight of an object also diminishes with height above sea level. For this reason, weight should not be confused with mass. Equation [1] enables the unit of force (N) to be expressed in terms of the more familiar unit of mass (kg): 9.81 N = 1 kg = 2.2 lb. This is approximate only, because the acceleration due to gravity is not exactly 9.81 m/s².

Stress. This is the intensity of loading, equal to the force exerted divided by the area over which it is applied. The unit of stress is the Mega-Pascal (MPa): 1 MPa = 1 N/mm². 1 MPa is equivalent to a 10 kg weight being applied to an area the size of a fingernail. A **shear stress** is equal to the shear force divided by the area over which it is applied.

Fluid. A fluid is a substance with such little rigidity that it deforms to take the shape of its container. In a fluid, shear stresses are very small, so there is little resistance to the substance spreading out to equalise the pressure within it. In a static fluid, pressure does not vary with direction (e.g. vertically or horizontally) or with location.

Pressure (or hydrostatic pressure). This is the intensity of loading within a fluid. It has the same units (MPa) as stress and so the two are often confused; but they should not be, because stress refers to solids, and pressure to fluids. In a healthy intervertebral disc, the nucleus behaves like a fluid whereas most of the anulus behaves like a fibrous solid. Therefore the intensity of loading throughout the nucleus can be given by a single scalar quantity, the intradiscal pressure (IDP), whereas the intensity of loading within the anulus must be described by stresses which vary with location and direction.

Displacement. Displacement defines the location of one point relative to another. It is a vector quantity which has a magnitude (the **distance** between the two points) and a direction. Units: metres (m), millimetres (mm), micrometres (μm) or nanometres (nm). 1000 nm = 1 μm; 1000 μm = 1 mm; 1000 mm = 1 m. Approximately, 25.4 mm = 1 inch.

Velocity. This is the rate of change of displacement with time. Again, it is a vector quantity with a magnitude (the **speed**) and a direction. Units are metres/second (m/s).

Acceleration. This is the rate of change of velocity with time. It is another vector quantity with magnitude (acceleration) and a direction. Units are metres/second/second (m/s^2).

Strain. This is the amount an object deforms when a force is applied to it.

Strain = change in length/original length   [2]

Strain can be expressed as a fraction or as a percentage, so if the length of an object was increased by half, the strain would be 0.5 or 50%. Small deformations of stiff materials can be expressed in micro-strains, where 10 000 micro-strains is equivalent to a strain of 1%.

Energy. Energy and **work** are essentially the same thing. If a force f is applied to an object in order to move it a distance d, then the work done is equal to $f \times d$. If the object is raised vertically against gravity, then it gains energy (in this case 'potential energy') equal to the work done in moving it. If the object is allowed to fall, its potential energy is converted to energy of movement, or 'kinetic energy'. (In fact, the kinetic energy of an object of mass m moving at a velocity v is equal to $\frac{1}{2} mv^2$.) Energy can transform itself into many other forms, including heat, and the unit of energy (the Joule) is defined in terms of heat rather than forces and distances.

Momentum. Momentum is the mass of an object multiplied by its velocity. Bodies with a lot of momentum require a lot of stopping!

Bending moment. This is a measure of the turning or bending effect of a force which is applied to an object. It is equal to the size of the force (in Newtons) multiplied by the lever arm (in metres) between the force and the chosen centre of rotation, so its units are Newton metres (Nm). Note that any location can be chosen as the 'centre of rotation', and that the bending moment of a given force about each centre of rotation will be different (Fig. 1.3). For example, when a person bends forwards, as shown on page 95, the weight of their upper body (a force!) exerts a different bending moment about the centre of each of the intervertebral discs. A bending moment can be specified relative to the centre of rotation of the disc, or relative to its geometric centre, or indeed relative to any other point.

Torque. This is the equivalent to a bending moment except that the applied force acts to twist

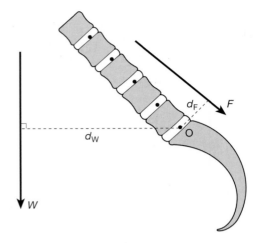

Figure 1.3 The 'moment' generated by a force is equal to the magnitude of that force multiplied by the length of its lever arm. In this example, body weight W exerts a flexor moment of $W \times d_W$ about the centre of rotation 'O'. No movement occurs if this is balanced by the extensor moment $F \times d_F$, generated by the back muscle force F. Moments can be calculated relative to any point whatsoever, but it is usual to select a point which coincides with a physical pivot, such as the centre of rotation within each intervertebral disc.

a body (Fig. 1.1) rather than to bend it. Its units are also Newton metres (Nm).

Stiffness and strength. Stiffness is a measure of how strongly an object resists being deformed. It is normally measured as the deforming force (in Newtons) divided by the deformation it causes (in millimetres) so a convenient unit of stiffness is the Newton/millimetre (N/mm). If a biological tissue is referred to as being 'non-linear' it means that its stiffness increases as the applied load increases, so that a graph of deformation against applied force is curved as shown in Figure 1.4. Stiffness is then measured as the gradient of the graph at any specified level of force (or deformation). Strength is the force (or stress) at which an object is damaged. Because the stiffness of most biological tissues depends on the force applied (Fig. 1.4), it can not be used to predict strength, and stiffness and strength should not be confused.

Damage. Damage can be defined as a permanently impaired resistance to deformation, and is indicated on a force–deformation graph by the first fall in stiffness (reduction in gradient). The point on the graph at which this occurs is the

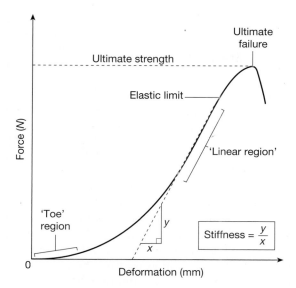

Figure 1.4 Typical force–deformation graph obtained when stretching or compressing a biological tissue. In the 'toe region', deformation increases rapidly with increasing force, indicating that the stiffness of the specimen is low. (In some tissues, this region of low stiffness is attributable to straightening out the crimp structure of collagen fibres.) At higher loads, there is often a 'linear' region in which the stiffness is approximately constant. The 'elastic limit' marks the point where stiffness begins to fall, and this usually indicates that the specimen is starting to be damaged. Ultimate failure occurs when the stiffness falls to zero, and the force at this point is the (ultimate) strength of the specimen.

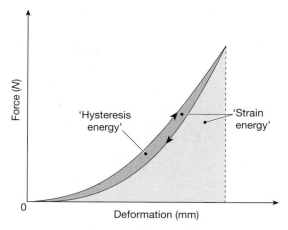

Figure 1.5 Typical force–deformation graph for a biological tissue which is subjected to a non-damaging loading cycle. The unloading part of the curve (indicated by the downwards pointing arrow) is below the loading curve, indicating that specimen deformation is greater for the same applied load. The area under the loading curve has units of energy (force × distance moved) and in fact this area represents the work done in deforming the specimen, or 'strain energy'. Most of the strain energy is returned when the specimen is unloaded, but a small proportion is lost as heat. This small fraction is the 'hysteresis energy' and is indicated by the hatched area between the loading and unloading curves.

'elastic limit' (Fig. 1.4). Any deformation occurring beyond the elastic limit is 'plastic' (non-recoverable) deformation which remains as a 'permanent set' when the object is unloaded. Sometimes, an 'ultimate strength' is defined as the force (or stress) at which the stiffness (gradient) not only reduces, but falls to zero. Warning! These concepts were developed to explain engineering materials, and 'permanent' changes can sometimes be reversed in living tissues.

Modulus. Young's modulus is a measure of how stiff a material is, and is given by applied stress divided by strain. Unlike stiffness, which describes an object, modulus is independent of specimen size.

Strain energy, hysteresis and toughness. The work done in deforming an object is indicated by the area under a force–deformation graph (Fig. 1.5). This work is stored by the object as 'strain energy', and any body which can absorb a lot of strain energy before it is damaged is called 'tough'. A tin can is tough because it is strong and deformable, whereas a wine glass is the opposite ('brittle') because it can not deform sufficiently to absorb much strain energy. When the deforming force is released, the object returns towards its original shape, and the strain energy is released. If the object is perfectly 'elastic', then the original shape is exactly regained, and all of the strain energy is recovered. However, many biological tissues exhibit a certain amount of inelastic deformation, in which some of the stored strain energy is lost as heat, and the original shape is not regained immediately. The non-recovered strain energy is referred to as 'hysteresis energy', and can be measured as the area between the loading and unloading curves (Fig. 1.5). Hysteresis energy is responsible for warming up any object that is repeatedly deformed and released: think of a squash ball after a hard game, or a small packet of butter after being squeezed repeatedly.

Creep. Creep is time-dependent deformation (or strain) under constant load (Fig. 1.6). In most biological materials, creep occurs because water is slowly expelled from the loaded tissue. However, other mechanisms of creep exist, and the lead on a church roof creeps over many years because of gradual relative slipping of adjacent atoms within the material. Creep arising from fluid flow can usually be reversed: when the loading is reduced, the expelled fluid simply flows back in again, rapidly at first, but then slowing down later.

Tissues such as anulus fibrosus and articular cartilage are termed **poroelastic** because they can behave rather like an elastic body if they are loaded quickly (i.e. they spring back to shape as soon as the load is removed) but when loaded slowly, they creep, as fluid is expelled through tiny pores in the tissue. The term **biphasic** is also used to describe these tissues, because their fluid phase (water) is capable of moving relative to its solid phase (collagen and proteoglycans). Note, however, that articular cartilage and anulus fibrosus do not contain any macroscopic pores

filled with fluid: the solid and liquid phases are mixed at the molecular level to form a fibrous solid, and the intensity of loading within these tissues must be characterised by stresses, not a pressure.

Fatigue failure. A structure can be damaged by applying a high force to it once, or a smaller force to it many times. Small forces can create microscopic damage, perhaps in the form of tiny cracks, or a small plastic deformation, which would pass unnoticed if the force was applied and removed only once. However, after a large number of loading cycles, the microscopic damage can accumulate until the entire weakened structure fails, even though the applied loading remains relatively low. This is 'fatigue failure', and the process is often referred to as 'fatigue'. Fatigue failure can occur after only a few loading cycles if the applied load is greater than 60% of the strength of the structure, or it may require millions of loading cycles if the load is below 30% (Fig. 1.7). Sometimes a structure or material has a 'fatigue limit': a force below which fatigue failure never occurs, no matter how many loading cycles are applied. Fatigue explains how engine

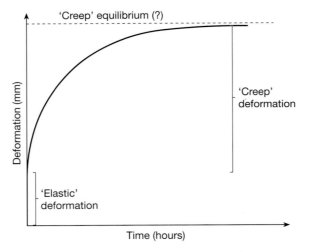

Figure 1.6 'Creep' curve for a typical biological specimen. When a constant force is initially applied, there is an immediate 'elastic' deformation. If the force is not removed, then further 'creep' deformation occurs as water is expelled from the specimen. Creep is rapid at first, but usually approaches an equilibrium as the water expulsion slows down. The word 'creep' can be used to denote the time-dependent deformation itself, or the process which causes it.

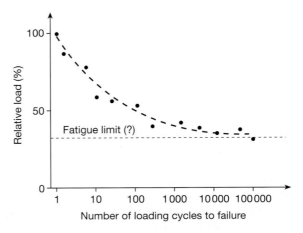

Figure 1.7 Typical 'fatigue' curve showing how the strength of biological specimens decreases markedly with the number of loading cycles applied. The relative load (or stress) is the percentage of the load required to cause failure in a single loading cycle. In some (but not all) specimens there is a 'fatigue limit', which defines a threshold load below which fatigue failure never occurs, no matter how many loading cycles are applied.

vibrations can eventually cause aeroplane wings to fall off, and why athletes can suffer so-called 'stress fractures' of bones during intense training or competition.

Cube-square Law. If a solid object is scaled up in size, its volume (and therefore its weight) will increase approximately in proportion to its length cubed. However, its area or 'footprint' will increase in proportion to its length squared, so the compressive stress (weight per unit area) acting on the base of the object will steadily increase.

If the scaling up continues, the object will eventually crush itself. This general principle of scaling-up explains why polystyrene can be used to make a model bridge, but not a real bridge, and why an elephant can not fall as far as a mouse without hurting itself. The 'cube-square law' is far from accurate, but it is often useful when attempting to interpret the significance of animal experiments to human beings. In general, large structures must be made from stronger materials than small structures.

2

The lumbar vertebral column and sacrum

The lumbar vertebral column is that section of the vertebral column between the thorax cranially and the sacrum and pelvis caudally. When endowed with muscles and other surrounding tissues the lumbar vertebral column is converted into a structure known as the lumbar spine. The lumbar vertebral column, therefore, constitutes the skeleton of the lumbar spine.

DESIGN FEATURES

In mechanical terms, the lumbar vertebral column is a device that:

- provides axial rigidity to the abdominal portion of the trunk
- separates the thorax from the pelvis
- enables certain movements between the thorax and pelvis.

Secondarily, the lumbar vertebral column:

- affords an origin for parts of the abdominal muscles
- offers points of attachment for the latissimus dorsi.

The individual components of the lumbar vertebral column, in one way or another, are designed to contribute to one or other of these functions. Conversely, disorders of the lumbar spine may present with impairment of one or other of these functions. It is, therefore, pertinent to appreciate how the elements of the lumbar spine are designed to subserve their functions, not only to understand normal anatomy but also to understand the effects of pathology.

RIGIDITY

Axial rigidity is the cardinal feature that distinguishes vertebrates from soft-bodied molluscs. In biomechanical terms, rigidity means stiffness, or resistance to bending or collapse. This property is essential for the ability of humans to walk upright in the earth's gravitational field.

In order to provide rigidity, the lumbar vertebral column consists largely of bone, in the form of five lumbar vertebrae, named by number, from above downwards, as L1 to L5. If rigidity was its sole function, a single bone would suffice, acting as a strut between the thorax and pelvis. A single bone, however, would not allow mobility. For that reason multiple bones form the skeleton of the lumbar spine.

The notion of a single bone is, however, not totally absurd, because for a variety of reasons some individuals undergo surgical fusion of their lumbar spine, usually at one or two levels, but in some instances at up to all five levels. Such patients effectively have their lumbar vertebral column converted to a single bone. Rigidity is maintained and, indeed, increased, but the cost is loss of mobility.

SEPARATION

The essential component of each lumbar vertebra is its vertebral body. This is a block of bone, rectangular in profile in a side view, with flat superior and inferior surfaces (Fig. 2.1A), and semi-columnar in top view, with curved anterior and lateral surfaces but a flat posterior surface (Fig. 2.1B). Because of the height of each vertebral body, the lumbar vertebral column is endowed with length, and thereby achieves separation of the thorax from the pelvis. Separation is essential in order to provide space through which the thorax can move relative to the pelvis. Without separation, the thoracic cage would clash against the pelvic brim and movement would be obstructed. The taller the vertebral bodies the greater the

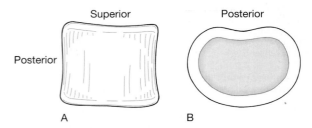

Figure 2.1 Side view (A) and top view (B) of a lumbar vertebral body.

length of the lumbar spine, and the greater the possible range of movement between the thorax and pelvis. Conversely, if the lumbar spine is shorter, the available range of movement is less.

Although the lumbar vertebral column most commonly consists of five vertebrae, variations do occur. Some individuals have four lumbar vertebrae; others have six. Changing the number of vertebrae changes the length of the lumbar spine and the potential mobility of the thorax. The clinical relevance of vertebral number lies in the naming of the last lumbar vertebra. Normally this is L5, but in a shorter lumbar spine it will be L4; in a longer lumbar spine it will be L6. In individuals with an abnormal number of lumbar vertebrae, disorders that normally befall L5 will affect L4 or L6 accordingly.

COMPRESSION

In fish, which live in a buoyant environment and are oblivious to the earth's gravitational field, rigidity, separation and mobility are the only mechanical design requirements of the lumbar spine. However, any animal that ventures to be upright in the earth's gravitational field inherits a liability resulting from the separation of the thorax from the pelvis. Under the influence of gravity, the weight of the thorax, and of any load carried in the upper limbs, will exert a compression load on the lumbar vertebral column. Moreover, these loads are amplified by the contraction of the back muscles that control the position of the upright lumbar spine (see Chs 3 and 7). Consequently, the lumbar vertebrae are designed to sustain axial compression loads.

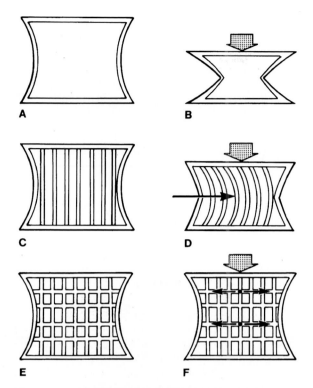

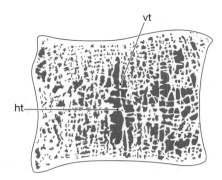

Figure 2.3 A sketch of a sagittal section through a lumbar vertebral body showing the appearance of its vertical (vt) and horizontal (ht) trabeculae.

Figure 2.2 Reconstruction of the internal architecture of the vertebral body. (A) With just a shell of cortical bone, a vertebral body is like a box, and collapses when a load is applied (B). (C) Internal vertical struts brace the box (D). (E) Transverse connections prevent the vertical struts from bowing, and increase the load-bearing capacity of the box. Loads are resisted by tension in the transverse connections (F). (From Bogduk N 1997 Clinical Anatomy of the Lumbar Spine and Sacrum, 3rd edn, with permission of Churchill Livingstone, Edinburgh.)

Each lumbar vertebral body consists of an outer shell of cortical bone, much like a box (Fig. 2.2). Although strong, this shell is not strong enough to sustain the axial loads that are habitually exerted on the lumbar spine. Therefore, the vertebral bodies are reinforced internally by narrow struts of bone called trabeculae (Fig. 2.2). Basically, these are arranged in vertical and horizontal arrays (Fig. 2.3). The vertical trabeculae act like columns that transmit compression loads from the upper surface of the vertebral body to its lower surface. The horizontal trabeculae serve to reinforce the vertical trabeculae by preventing them from buckling sideways under large compression loads.

Absence of horizontal trabeculae weakens the vertebral body. Under load, the vertical trabeculae buckle and can fracture. Lacking the support of the vertical trabeculae, the cortical shell and, therefore, the entire vertebral body can subsequently be easily crushed. This phenomenon is of particular relevance to the condition of spinal osteoporosis (page 58).

MOBILITY

In order to be mobile, the lumbar spine requires joints. The principal joints occur between the vertebral bodies. These joints have no formal name (other than 'the intervertebral amphiarthroses', which few people use), but they can be conveniently referred to as the interbody joints. They occur between the inferior surface of one vertebral body and the superior surface of the next. Each is a secondary cartilaginous joint, in which the vertebral bodies are separated by an intervertebral disc. The structure of these joints is such that they allow bending, twisting and sliding movements between vertebral bodies, and the total mobility of the lumbar spine is the sum of the mobilities of its five joints.

INTERVERTEBRAL DISCS

The intervertebral discs are designed to separate consecutive lumbar vertebrae, thereby producing a potential space between them into which the vertebral bodies can dip and execute bending movements. In order to separate the vertebral bodies, each intervertebral disc must have height, but in order to allow movement, the tissue of the disc must be pliable. Meanwhile, the tissue must also be stiff and strong in order to sustain the compression loads between the vertebral bodies.

The essential component of the intervertebral disc is the anulus fibrosus. This consists of some 10–20 sheets of collagen, called lamellae, tightly packed together in a circumferential fashion around the periphery of the disc (Fig. 2.4). While packed tightly together, these lamellae are stiff, and can sustain considerable compression loads. A suitable analogy is the stiffness of a telephone directory that is wrapped into a cylindrical shape and stood end-on. Nevertheless, being collagenous, the anulus fibrosus is sufficiently pliable that it can deform and thereby enable bending movements between vertebral bodies. However, herein lies the liability of the anulus fibrosus. If it buckles it loses its stiffness, and is less able to sustain compression loads. To prevent this, the anulus fibrosus requires the second component of the intervertebral disc – the nucleus pulposus.

The nucleus pulposus is a hydrated gel located in the centre of each disc (Fig. 2.4). When compressed, this semi-fluid mass expands in a radial fashion. On the one hand this radial expansion is resisted by the surrounding anulus fibrosus, but on the other hand, the expansion braces the anulus fibrosus from the inside, thereby preventing it from buckling inwards and losing its stiffness. Co-operatively, the nucleus pulposus and anulus fibrosus maintain the stiffness of the disc against compression loading, but both tissues are sufficiently compliant that they allow some degree of movement between vertebral bodies.

The third component of the intervertebral disc are the superior and inferior vertebral endplates. These are plates of cartilage that cover the superior and inferior aspects of the disc, and bind the disc to their respective vertebral bodies (Fig. 2.4). Each endplate covers almost the entire surface of the adjacent vertebral body; only a narrow rim of bone, called the ring apophysis, around the perimeter of the vertebral body is left uncovered by cartilage.

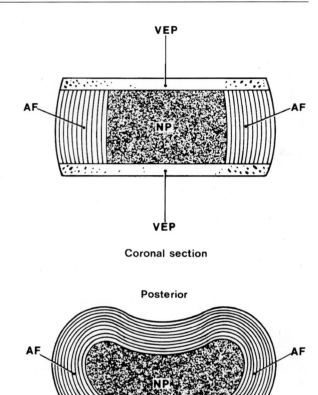

Figure 2.4 The basic structure of a lumbar intervertebral disc. The disc consists of a nucleus pulposus (NP) surrounded by an anulus fibrosus (AF), both sandwiched between two cartilaginous vertebral endplates (VEP). (From Bogduk N 1997 Clinical Anatomy of the Lumbar Spine and Sacrum, 3rd edn, with permission of Churchill Livingstone, Edinburgh.)

That portion of the vertebral body to which the cartilaginous vertebral endplate is applied lacks a formal name, but can be referred to as the subchondral bone (of the vertebral body) or the bony vertebral endplate. It is, however, a component of the vertebral body and not a component of the disc, as is the cartilaginous vertebral endplate. Notwithstanding this distinction in nomenclature, mechanical disorders that affect the region of the endplate, typically involve both the osseous and cartilaginous endplates simultaneously.

In addition to enabling bending movements between vertebral bodies, the intervertebral disc allows for twisting and sliding movements of small amplitude. These are resisted by tension developed in the collagen fibres of the anulus fibrosus, and their amplitude is a function of the elasticity and tensile stiffness of the anulus.

MICROSTRUCTURE

The anulus fibrosus consists of type I and type II collagen. The concentration of type I collagen is greater towards the periphery of the anulus, while that of type II collagen is reciprocally greater towards the centre of the disc. This distribution of type I collagen matches the greater tensile role of the outer anulus fibrosus.

Within each lamella of the anulus fibrosus, the collagen fibres are arranged in parallel. They pass obliquely from one vertebral body to the next, at an angle of about 65° to the sagittal plane. However, as a rule, the fibres in each successive lamellae are orientated in an opposite sense, with one layer inclined to the left, the next layer inclined to the right, and so on (Fig. 2.5). This alternating arrangement precludes any cleavage plane through the anulus, through which nuclear material might seep or burst, and is critical to the integrity of the disc. Moreover, the alternating orientation allows the anulus to resist tension in a variety of directions.

Sliding movements between the vertebral bodies will be resisted by all those collagen fibres that are inclined in the direction of movement (Fig. 2.6A). Similarly, twisting movements will be resisted by those fibres inclined in the direction of movement (Fig. 2.6B). All fibres will contribute to resisting separation of the vertebral bodies (Fig. 2.6C).

In this regard, it is the outermost fibres of the anulus fibrosus that contribute most to resisting these movements. To that end, they are attached directly to bone, around the ring apophysis, and for that reason they are referred to as the ligamentous portion of the anulus fibrosus (Fig. 2.7). The inner fibres of the anulus do not attach to

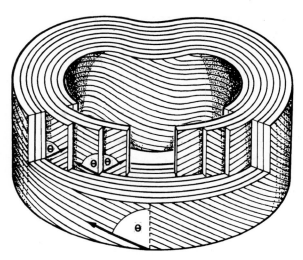

Figure 2.5   The architecture of the anulus fibrosus. Collagen fibres are arranged in 10–20 concentric, circumferential lamellae. The orientation of fibres alternates in successive lamellae, but their orientation with respect to the vertical (θ) is approximately the same, and measures about 65°. (From Bogduk N 1997 Clinical Anatomy of the Lumbar Spine and Sacrum, 3rd edn, with permission of Churchill Livingstone, Edinburgh.)

bone but insert into the vertebral endplate. Within the endplate they can be traced forming a continuous envelope around the nucleus pulposus. For this reason they are, at times, referred to as the capsular portion of the anulus fibrosus.

The nucleus pulposus consists largely of proteoglycans, which are large molecules consisting of complex sugars and protein (p. 60). They have the valuable property of being able to imbibe and retain large amounts of water. It is this property that endows the nucleus pulposus with its hydrodynamic properties. If the nucleus loses its proteoglycans, it can no longer hold its water, and the nucleus can no longer properly brace the anulus fibrosus. If that function is lost, the disc can no longer resist compression loads, and will be progressively compressed and narrowed under the loads of daily living.

DISC HEIGHT

Each lumbar intervertebral disc is about 10 mm in height. Collectively, the five lumbar intervertebral discs add 5 cm to the length of the lumbar spine.

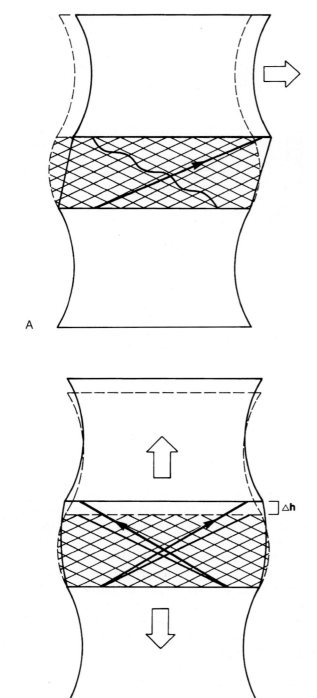

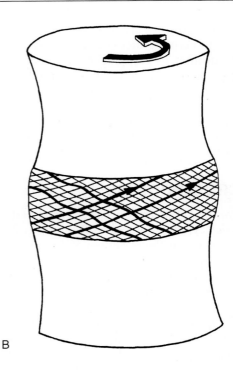

Figure 2.6 Mechanics of the anulus fibrosus. (A) Sliding movements between vertebral bodies are resisted by tension developing in those fibres of the anulus that are inclined in the direction of movement. Other fibres are relaxed by the displacement. (B) Twisting movements are resisted by those fibres lengthened by the movement. Other fibres are relaxed. (C) Separation of the vertebral bodies is resisted by all fibres regardless of their orientation. (From Bogduk N 1997 Clinical Anatomy of the Lumbar Spine and Sacrum, 3rd edn, with permission of Churchill Livingstone, Edinburgh.)

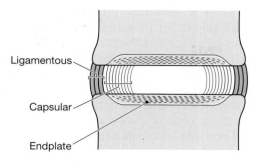

Figure 2.7 Detailed structure of the anulus fibrosus. The peripheral fibres attach to the ring apophysis and constitute the tensile, ligamentous portion of the anulus. The inner fibres surround the nucleus pulposus and constitute the capsular portion. They can be traced into the cartilage of the vertebral endplate, thereby forming a complete envelope around the nucleus. Because of these fibres the superficial parts of the endplate are fibrocartilage. The deeper parts are hyaline cartilage.

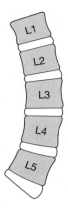

Figure 2.8 The essential lumbar vertebral column consists of the five lumbar vertebral bodies and their intervertebral discs.

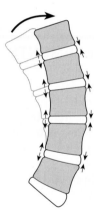

Figure 2.9 Forward bending of the vertebral column is achieved by compression of the anterior ends of the intervertebral discs, and resisted by tension in the posterior anulus fibrosus.

During activities of daily living, when an individual is upright, water is squeezed out of the lumbar discs, and they each lose height. After rest in a recumbent position this height is restored, as water is re-imbibed (p. 169). Disc height is fully restored at night, during sleep.

Disc height is preserved with age. Discs do not narrow because of age. Indeed, if anything, the discs of the elderly are slightly taller on the average.[811] However, disc narrowing can occur in certain disorders of the disc. Any disorder that disrupts or degrades the proteoglycans of the nucleus pulposus will impair their water-binding capacity, and compromise the ability of the disc to restore and maintain its height.

THE ESSENTIAL LUMBAR VERTEBRAL COLUMN

The five vertebral bodies and their respective discs constitute the essential components of the lumbar vertebral column (Fig. 2.8). From above downwards, the five vertebral bodies are named numerically as lumbar one to five, i.e. L1, L2, L3, L4 and L5. The intervertebral discs are numbered according to the vertebral bodies that each separates, i.e. L1–2, L2–3, L3–4, L4–5, and the last disc is known as the lumbosacral disc, or L5–S1.

Collectively the vertebral bodies and discs form a column that provides rigidity and length, and permits movements. The vertebral bodies and intervertebral discs strongly resist compression, and easily bear the loads of the thorax and upper limbs. Forward bending is achieved by each intervertebral disc being compressed slightly, anteriorly, and is resisted by tension developed in the posterior anulus fibrosus (Fig. 2.9). Extension and lateral flexion are achieved by corresponding events in the opposite direction and in the coronal plane, respectively. Rotation of the lumbar spine is achieved by each disc allowing a small degree of twist, and is resisted by tension developed in the anulus fibrosus.

However, the vertebral bodies and discs are not the complete structure of the lumbar vertebral column. Alone these structures are relatively unstable and susceptible to injury. The anulus fibrosus is not strong enough, on its own, to resist excessive torsion of the lumbar spine without being damaged. Nor can the vertebral bodies and discs alone maintain a straight, or upright, posture; the discs are sufficiently compliant that the slightest axial load will tend to bend the column. In order to maintain stability, and to afford control of movements, the essential lumbar vertebral column requires additional elements. These are the posterior elements of the lumbar vertebrae.

POSTERIOR ELEMENTS

The posterior elements of the lumbar vertebrae are designed to control the position of the vertebral bodies. Forces may be exerted directly by muscles acting on the posterior elements, or indirectly by loads on the thorax trying to bend or twist the lumbar spine.

Towards the upper end of its posterior surface, each lumbar vertebral body is endowed with a pair of stout pillars of bone called the pedicles (Fig. 2.10). These support the posterior elements, and transmit forces from them to the vertebral body, and vice-versa.

From each pedicle, a plate of bone, called the lamina, projects towards the midline, in a manner like a sloping roof (Fig. 2.10). At the midline, the two laminae fuse seamlessly. In a top view, the pedicles and laminae can be perceived as forming an arch, known as the neural arch, which together with the posterior surface of the vertebral body encloses a space and channel, behind the vertebral body, known as the vertebral foramen (Fig. 2.10). By convention, the laminae are perceived to form the roof of the foramen, and the vertebral body to form the floor.

At the junction of its two laminae in the midline, each lumbar vertebra bears a spinous process which projects dorsally in the shape of the blade of an axe (Fig. 2.10). Projecting laterally from the junction of the pedicle with its lamina on each side, is a long, rectangular, flattened bar of bone called the transverse process (Fig. 2.10). On its posterior surface, near its root, each transverse process bears a thick but narrow spike of bone called the accessory process (Fig. 2.10). These several processes serve as sites of attachment for muscles that control the lumbar vertebral column, and endow these muscles with lever-arms.

From its superior, lateral corner, the lamina gives rise to an extension of bone called the superior articular process (Fig. 2.10). On its medial surface, the superior articular process presents an articular facet that is covered by articular cartilage. On its dorsal surface, each superior articular process bears a small bump, known as the mamillary process, which serves as a site for muscle attachments.

From its inferior, lateral corner, the lamina gives rise to an inferior articular process that bears an articular facet on its lateral surface (Fig. 2.10). The superior articular processes of one vertebra receive the inferior articular processes of the vertebra above to form synovial joints known as the zygapophysial joints. These joints serve to enable certain movements of the lumbar vertebral column but to limit or prevent others.

THE COMPLETE LUMBAR VERTEBRAL COLUMN

When the posterior elements of the lumbar vertebrae are added to the essential vertebral column, they provide a series of interlocking bony elements behind the vertebral bodies and discs (Fig. 2.11). The laminae of consecutive vertebrae are separated from one another by a short interval, but consecutive vertebrae are articulated through the zygapophysial joints. The complete lumbar vertebral column sits on the sacrum, articulating with it anteriorly through the L5–S1 intervertebral discs, and posteriorly through the lumbosacral (L5–S1) zygapophysial joints.

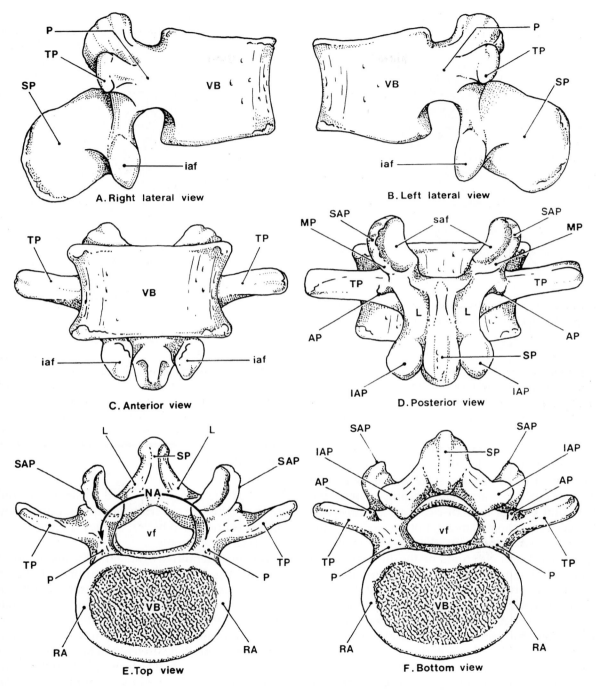

Figure 2.10   The parts of a typical lumbar vertebra. VB: vertebral body; P: pedicle; TP: transverse process; SP: spinous process; L: lamina; SAP: superior articular process; IAP: inferior articular process; saf: superior articular facet; iaf: inferior articular facet; MP: mamillary process; AP: accessory process; vf: vertebral foramen; RA: ring apophysis; NA: neural arch. (From Bogduk N 1997 Clinical Anatomy of the Lumbar Spine and Sacrum, 3rd edn, with permission of Churchill Livingstone, Edinburgh.)

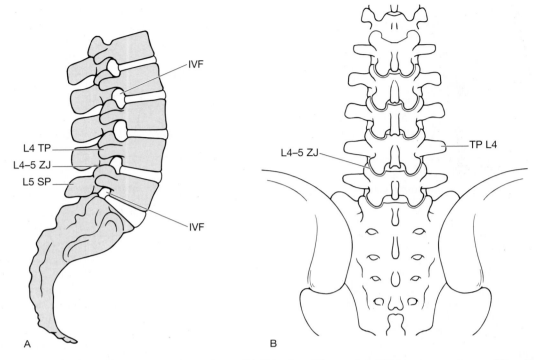

Figure 2.11 The complete lumbar vertebral column. (A) Side view; (B) rear view. TP: transverse process; SP: spinous process; ZJ: zygapophysial joint; IVF: intervertebral foramen.

When the vertebral foramina of the five lumbar vertebrae are longitudinally aligned, they form a series of arcades surrounding what can be perceived as a canal running behind the vertebral bodies and discs. This is known as the vertebral canal. Amongst other elements, the vertebral canal transmits the lower end of the spinal cord and the roots of the lumbar, sacral and coccygial nerves (see Ch. 3). Routes of access to the vertebral canal occur in the form of passages between consecutive pedicles, behind each intervertebral disc and in front of the zygapophysial joints at each level. These passages are called the intervertebral foramina (Fig. 2.11).

The resting shape of the intact lumbar vertebral column is a curve concave posteriorly. The basis for this curve is tension in the joints of the vertebral column and the ligaments that bind the lumbar vertebrae together.

LIGAMENTS

Many of the structures called ligaments in the lumbar spine are not truly ligaments. Either they do not connect two bones, or they are too feeble to serves as ligaments.

The most definitive ligament is the ligamentum flavum (Fig. 2.12). It consists of fibres of elastin that connect the lower end of the internal surface of one lamina to the upper end of the external surface of the lamina below, and closes the gap between consecutive laminae. This is a very extensible ligament that stretches when the lumbar vertebral column bends forwards. It consists of elastin in order that, upon resumption of the neutral posture of the lumbar spine after flexion, the fibres of the ligamentum flavum can recoil and shorten but without buckling. A ligament made of collagen could just as well resist flexion

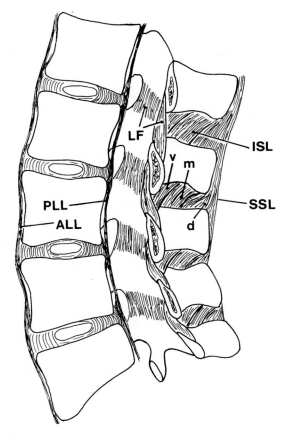

Figure 2.12 A median sagittal section of the lumbar spine to show its various ligaments. ALL: anterior longitudinal ligament; PLL: posterior longitudinal ligament; SSL: supraspinous ligament; ISL: interspinous ligament; v: ventral part; m: middle part; d: dorsal part; LF: ligamentum flavum, viewed from within the vertebral canal, and in sagittal section at the midline. (From Bogduk N 1997 Clinical Anatomy of the Lumbar Spine and Sacrum, 3rd edn, with permission of Churchill Livingstone, Edinburgh.)

they constitute membranes that separate the ventral muscle compartment of the lumbar spine from its dorsal muscle compartment (see Ch. 3).

The opposing edges of spinous processes are connected by collagen fibres referred to as the interspinous ligaments (Fig. 2.12). Although the ventral portions of these ligaments are distinctly ligamentous, their dorsal portions actually constitute tendinous fibres of the erector spinae muscle (see Ch. 3).

A supraspinous ligament has traditionally been recognised, but this structure is not a ligament. It consists of tendinous fibres of various muscles (see Ch. 3), and is lacking below L3.

In addition to the ligaments of the posterior elements, the lumbar vertebral column is reinforced by ligaments that connect the vertebral bodies. The posterior longitudinal ligament covers the floor of the vertebral canal (Fig. 2.12). Its fibres are attached to the posterior aspects of the lumbar vertebral bodies and to the intervertebral discs. It has short fibres that span consecutive vertebra, and longer fibres that span several vertebrae. The anterior longitudinal ligament covers the anterior aspects of the vertebral bodies and discs (Fig. 2.12). Its fibres are attached to the edges of the vertebral bodies. Many of its fibres, however, are not truly ligamentous, but constitute the prolonged tendons of the crura of the diaphragm.

The strongest ligament attached to the lumbar vertebral column is the iliolumbar ligament. Its fibres arise from the tip and borders of the transverse process of the fifth lumbar vertebra, and pass backwards and laterally to the ilium. They serve to anchor the L5 vertebra on the pelvic girdle, to prevent it from sliding forwards and from rotating.

as does the ligamentum flavum, but it could not shorten. As a result it would buckle inwards towards the neural elements within the vertebral canal, with the risk of compressing them. The virtue of an elastic ligamentum flavum is that it ensures that the neural elements are always presented with a smooth flat surface.

The transverse processes are connected by thin sheets of collagen fibres. Although called the intertransverse ligaments, these structures are too insubstantive to function as ligaments. Rather,

ZYGAPOPHYSIAL JOINTS

The zygapophysial joints provide an important locking mechanism between consecutive lumbar vertebrae. They are designed to block axial rotation and forward sliding of the lumbar vertebrae. By blocking axial rotation the joints protect the intervertebral discs from excessive torsion.

By blocking forward slide they prevent the vertebral bodies from dislocating under the weight of the trunk when the spine is flexed forwards.

Axial rotation of the lumbar vertebrae occurs around a longitudinal axis that passes through the posterior third or so of the vertebral bodies and intervertebral discs. When rotation occurs about this axis, the posterior elements of the moving vertebra swing laterally, in a direction opposite to that of the rotation. To block this rotation, the zygapophysial joints are arranged in such a way as to block the lateral displacement of the posterior elements.

Each pair of superior articular processes clasps the inferior articular processes of the vertebra above (Fig. 2.13A). The flat, medially facing facet of each superior articular process apposes the laterally facing facet of the inferior articular process. If the upper vertebra attempts to rotate

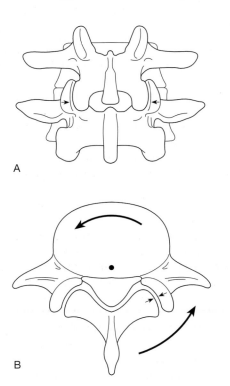

Figure 2.13 (A) A sketch of a posterior view of a lumbar zygapophysial joint showing how the superior articular processes clasp the inferior articular processes laterally. (B) A top view showing how the superior articular processes block rotation of the inferior articular processes.

to the left, its right inferior articular process will ram into the apposing superior articular process (Fig. 2.13B). This locking mechanism limits axial rotation at each intervertebral joint, and protects the intervertebral disc from torsion (p. 139).

In order to prevent forward slide, the inferior articular processes act as hooks. Projecting downwards from the pedicles, the inferior articular processes extend below the bottom of the vertebral body and engage the superior articular processes of the vertebra below, from behind (Fig. 2.14A).

Consequently, if the upper vertebra attempts to slide forwards, its inferior articular processes hook onto the superior articular processes which oppose the motion and thereby prevent forward sliding. In order to exert resistance to the inferior articular processes, the superior articular processes have to face backwards to some extent. This is achieved in one of several ways.

When examined in a top view, the superior articular processes exhibit one of three basic shapes. Their articular facets may be flat, C-shaped, or J-shaped. Flat facets afford resistance to axial rotation and to forward sliding by being obliquely orientated, such that they face backwards as well as medially (Fig. 2.14B). C-shaped and J-shaped facets offer a posterior end that faces medially and opposes axial rotation, and an anterior end that faces posteriorly and opposes forward slide (Fig. 2.14C and 2.14D).

Notwithstanding their shape in top view, the superior articular facets are flat in a longitudinal sense, as are the apposing inferior articular facets. This shape allows for unrestricted gliding movement between the facets in a supero-inferior direction. This gliding allows the inferior articular processes freely to lift upwards as its vertebral body flexes on the one below (Fig. 2.15). Thus, whereas the zygapophysial joints restrict axial rotation and forward slide, they permit flexion between their vertebrae. Extension is permitted in the same way but is limited in range as the tips of the inferior articular processes impact the lamina of the vertebra below (Fig. 2.15).

To facilitate the gliding movement between the articular processes, the facets of the zygapophysial joints are covered by articular cartilage, which in turn is lubricated by a film of synovial fluid.

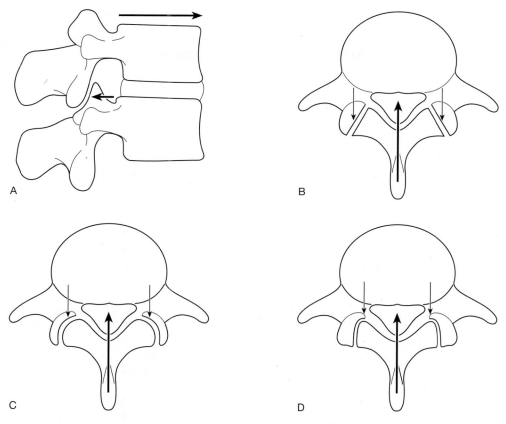

Figure 2.14 (A) A sketch of a lateral view of a lumbar zygapophysial joint showing how the inferior articular processes hook behind the superior articular processes. The external surface of the superior articular process has been cut away in order to reveal the internal features of the joint. (B) A top view of a flat zygapophysial joint showing how it resists forward sliding of the inferior articular processes. (C) A top view of a C-shaped zygapophysial joint showing how its anterior end resists forward sliding of the inferior articular processes. (D) A top view of a J-shaped zygapophysial joint showing how its narrow anterior end resists forward sliding of the inferior articular processes.

The fluid is retained by a synovial membrane that attaches to the edges of the articular cartilage, and the membrane is supported by a joint capsule (Fig. 2.16). Posteriorly the joint capsule is fibrous, with short, tight fibres running transversely between the articular processes. Superiorly and inferiorly the fibrous capsule is lax in order to accommodate the displacement of the articular processes during flexion and extension movements. Anteriorly the fibrous capsule is replaced by the most lateral fibres of the ligamentum flavum.

As the inferior articular process in a zygapophysial joint slides across the apposing superior articular facet during flexion, it subluxates, i.e. while the lower half of its articular facet remains in contact with the facet of the superior articular process, its upper half loses contact, and is effectively 'exposed'. Similarly the lower half of the superior articular facet is exposed. In order to protect these exposed surfaces, and to maintain a film of synovial fluid over their articular cartilages, the zygapophysial joints are endowed with intra-articular meniscoids. These fibroadipose structures are crescentic wedges, located at the superior and inferior poles of the joint, with a base attached to the joint capsule, and a tapering apex that projects into the joint cavity (Fig. 2.16).

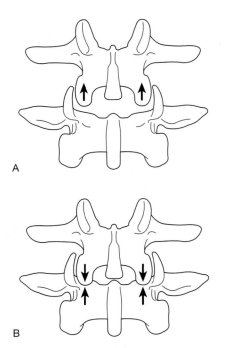

A

B

Figure 2.15   Posterior views of a lumbar zygapophysial joint. (A) During flexion the inferior articular processes are free to glide upwards across the superior articular processes. (B) During extension the inferior articular processes glide downwards across the superior articular processes but are arrested by impaction against the lamina below.

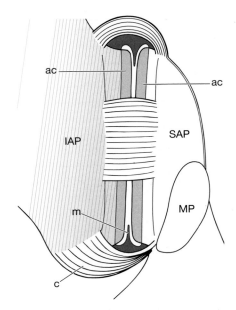

Figure 2.16   A posterior view of the components of a right, lumbar zygapophysial joint. The facets of the superior articular process (SAP) and inferior articular process (IAP) are covered by articular cartilage (ac). The capsule (c) is loose and abundant at the superior and inferior poles of the joint. Dorsally it consists of transverse fibres. These have been resected superiorly and inferiorly to reveal the fibroadipose meniscoids (m) that lie between the articular cartilages at the superior and inferior poles.

In the neutral position of the joint, the meniscoids project between the articular cartilages. As the inferior articular process slides upwards across the superior articular process, it leaves the inferior meniscoid applied to the exposed surface of the superior articular facet, and takes the superior meniscoid with it to protect its own exposed surface.

THE SACRUM

The sacrum is a block of bone that supports the lumbar vertebral column. However, it is also an integral component of the pelvic girdle, and thereby serves to transmit forces between the vertebral column and the lower limbs.

In front and rear views the sacrum is triangular in shape, with a broad upper end tapering to a blunt point inferiorly (Figs 2.17 and 2.18). In profile the sacrum is curved, with a smooth, concave anterior surface and a rough, convex posterior surface (Fig. 2.19). Superiorly it presents features designed to receive the lumbar vertebral column. Laterally, it is designed to articulate with the ilium on each side.

Intrinsically the sacrum consists of five segments that are fused together, each representing a rudimentary vertebra. On the anterior surface of the sacrum the superior and inferior edges of the vertebral bodies are represented as transverse ridges (Fig. 2.17). Between these ridges a narrow block of bone replaces what might have been an intervertebral disc. In longitudinal sections of the sacrum (Fig. 2.19), rudimentary discs may be found deep within the substance of the bone, particularly between the first and second sacral segments.

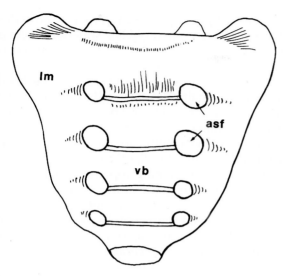

Figure 2.17   An anterior view of the sacrum vb: vertebral body; lm: lateral mass; asf: anterior sacral foramina. (From Bogduk N 1997 Clinical Anatomy of the Lumbar Spine and Sacrum, 3rd edn, with permission of Churchill Livingstone, Edinburgh.)

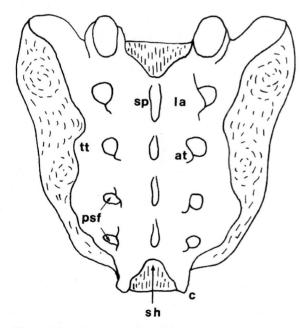

Figure 2.18   A posterior view of the sacrum. sp: spinous process; la: lamina; tt: transverse tubercle; psf: posterior sacral foramen; at: articular tubercle; sh: sacral hiatus; c: cornu. (From Bogduk N 1997 Clinical Anatomy of the Lumbar Spine and Sacrum, 3rd edn, with permission of Churchill Livingstone, Edinburgh.)

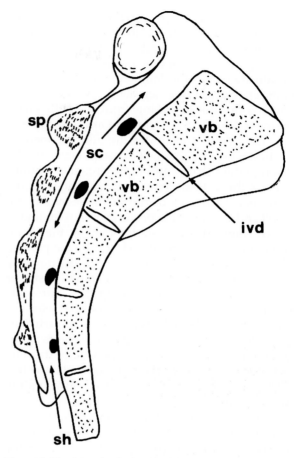

Figure 2.19   A longitudinal section through the sacrum. sc: sacral canal; sh: sacral hiatus; sp: spinous process; vb: vertebral bodies; ivd: remnant of an intervertebral disc. (From Bogduk N 1997 Clinical Anatomy of the Lumbar Spine and Sacrum, 3rd edn, with permission of Churchill Livingstone, Edinburgh.)

Projecting laterally from the vertebral bodies are the lateral masses of the sacral segments (Fig. 2.17). These represent the transverse processes, but instead of remaining separate, the tips of these transverse processes are fused together laterally to form a single mass of bone. However, fusion does not occur more medially where between consecutive transverse processes foramina are formed. The foramina seen on the anterior surface of the sacrum transmit the anterior rami of the sacral spinal nerves, and are known as the anterior sacral foramina.

Posteriorly, each of the sacral segments exhibits components homologous to the posterior elements of the lumbar vertebrae. Prominent in the midline are the spinous processes (Fig. 2.18). Beside these are the laminae, which are fused between consecutive segments. A lamina and spinous process is lacking from the fifth sacral segment, leaving a hole, known as the sacral hiatus. This hiatus constitutes the inferior opening of the sacral canal, which passes longitudinally through the sacrum, and represents the continuation of the lumbar vertebral canal. Laterally, the transverse processes of the sacral segments are fused and surround the posterior sacral foramina, which transmit the posterior rami of the sacral spinal nerves. The tip of each transverse process is marked by a small prominence, each known as a transverse tubercle. Medial to each posterior sacral foramen, is a small bump that represents what might have been a zygapophysial joint, for which reason the bump is known as the articular tubercle. The fifth sacral segment presents a pair of definitive articular processes which articulate with the coccyx. They flank the sacral hiatus like horns, for which reason they are known as the sacral cornua.

The superior end of the sacrum presents a central surface that resembles the superior surface of a lumbar vertebral body (Fig. 2.20). It receives the L5–S1 intervertebral disc. Laterally, the transverse process is long and thick, and is known as the ala (wing) of the sacrum. From its posterior surface on each side projects a superior articular process which receives the inferior articular process of the L5 vertebra.

In the upright position, the sacrum is inclined forwards, such that its upper surface slopes below horizontal at an angle of about 50° (Fig. 2.21). This orientation compromises the base for the lumbar vertebral column, for it invites the lumbar vertebral column to slip forwards and downwards across the sloping superior surface of the sacrum. Three design features mitigate against this tendency. First, the L5–S1 intervertebral disc is wedge-shaped, by about 16°, so as to lessen the angle between the top of the sacrum and the bottom of the L5 vertebral boy. Secondly, the superior articular processes of the sacrum face backwards, at between 45° and 90° to the sagittal plane. As a result, the inferior articular processes of L5 hook securely onto the sacrum, and prevent

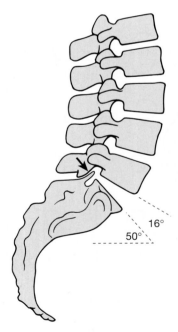

Figure 2.21 A side view of the lumbosacral junction in the upright standing position. The superior surface of the sacrum slopes downwards at about 50° below horizontal. The L5–S1 intervertebral disc is wedge-shaped. The inferior articular processes of L5 hook behind the superior articular processes of the sacrum, so as to prevent slipping of the L5 vertebra on the sloping surface of the sacrum.

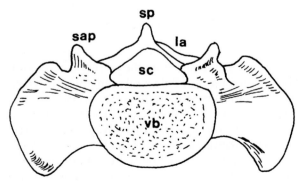

Figure 2.20 A superior view of the sacrum. vb: vertebral body; sap: superior articular process; sp: spinous process; la: lamina; sc: sacral canal. (From Bogduk N 1997 Clinical Anatomy of the Lumbar Spine and Sacrum, 3rd edn, with permission of Churchill Livingstone, Edinburgh.)

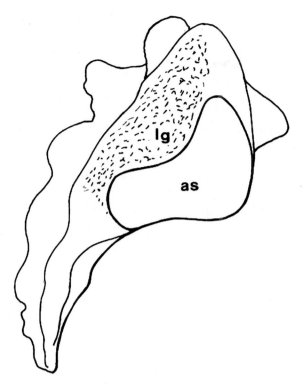

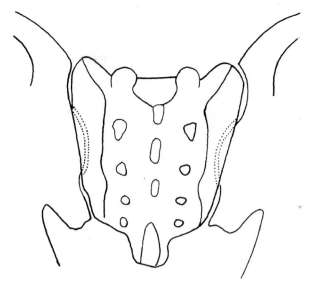

Figure 2.23   A posterior view of the sacroiliac joints, showing the sinuous shape of the joint space, and how the undulating surface of the sacrum locks into reciprocal surfaces of the ilium. (From Bogduk N 1997 Clinical Anatomy of the Lumbar Spine and Sacrum, 3rd edn, with permission of Churchill Livingstone, Edinburgh.)

Figure 2.22   A lateral view of the sacrum. as: auricular surface; lg: ligamentous surface. (From Bogduk N 1997 Clinical Anatomy of the Lumbar Spine and Sacrum, 3rd edn, with permission of Churchill Livingstone, Edinburgh.)

the lumbar vertebral column from sliding forwards. Finally, the L5 transverse processes are strongly secured to the ilium on each side by the iliolumbar ligaments. These large ligaments prevent forward displacement of the L5 vertebra in relation to the sacrum and pelvis.

The lateral surface of the sacrum presents a large, ear-shaped, articular surface, known either as the articular surface or the auricular surface, and a roughened ligamentous area behind it (Fig. 2.22). These are designed to lock the sacrum into the pelvic ring through the sacroiliac joint.

SACROILIAC JOINT

Unlike the typical joints of the limbs, or even those of the lumbar vertebral column, the sacroiliac joint is not designed to accommodate substantial ranges of movement. Indeed, its mobility is limited to about 2°. Moreover, there are no muscles that act to produce active, physiological movements of this joint. Rather, the sacroiliac joint is designed to act as a stress-relieving joint in the pelvic girdle.

During gait, the pelvic girdle is subjected to complex, twisting forces, the nature of which can be likened to the effect of taking a ring and twisting it towards a figure of eight. The stresses applied to the pelvic girdle are such that if it were a solid ring of bone, it would crack. Intriguingly, this phenomenon occurs in elderly individuals in whom the sacroiliac joints are fused as a result of age changes or disease. If they remain mobile, their pelvic girdle fails by fractures that develop parallel to the line of the sacroiliac joints. By having sacroiliac joints, the pelvic girdle avoids cracking. For this purpose the sacroiliac joint is endowed with strong ligaments that absorb the stresses applied to the pelvic girdle during gait.

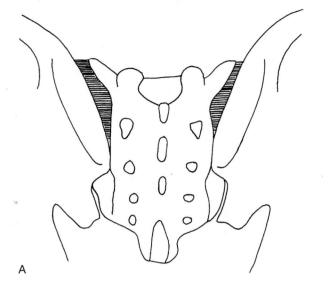

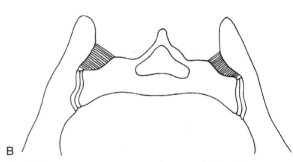

A

B

Figure 2.24 The interosseous sacroiliac ligament. (A) Posterior view. (B) Axial view. (From Bogduk N 1997 Clinical Anatomy of the Lumbar Spine and Sacrum, 3rd edn, with permission of Churchill Livingstone, Edinburgh.)

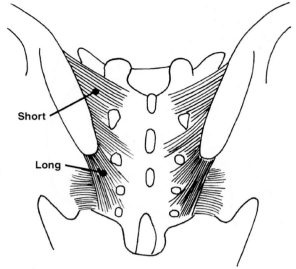

Short

Long

Figure 2.25 The posterior sacroiliac ligaments. (From Bogduk N 1997 Clinical Anatomy of the Lumbar Spine and Sacrum, 3rd edn, with permission of Churchill Livingstone, Edinburgh.)

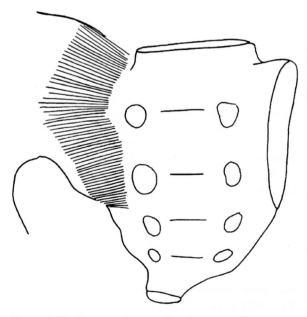

Figure 2.26 The anterior sacroiliac ligaments. (From Bogduk N 1997 Clinical Anatomy of the Lumbar Spine and Sacrum, 3rd edn, with permission of Churchill Livingstone, Edinburgh.)

The sacroiliac joint is a synovial joint between the auricular surface of the sacrum and the articular surface of the ilium. The auricular surface of the sacrum is not flat, but presents a depression opposite the second sacral segment, and prominences opposite the first and third segments. These undulations articulate with reciprocal surfaces on the ilium, such that the sacrum is locked between the two ilia of the pelvic girdle (Fig. 2.23). Provided the ilia are kept pressed against the sacrum, the sacrum is prevented by the locking mechanism from being driven downwards by the weight of the trunk, or from rotating forwards.

The ilia are attached to the sacrum by the inter-osseous sacroiliac ligament.

This ligament is short but thick. It arises from the ligamentous area of the sacrum and inserts into an opposing area of the ilium (Fig. 2.24). Tension within the ligaments on both sides keeps the ilia pressed against the sacrum. Injuries that tear this ligament, or conditions that slacken it, such as pregnancy, can compromise the integrity of the sacroiliac joint by relaxing the pressure of the ilium against the sacrum.

Additional ligaments reinforce the sacroiliac joint. Posteriorly, the long and short posterior sacroiliac ligaments connect the ilium to the posterior surface of the sacrum (Fig. 2.25). Anteriorly, the capsule of the joint is thickened to form the anterior sacroiliac ligament (Fig. 2.26). It serves to prevent the anterior edges of the sacrum and ilium from separating. Remote from the sacroiliac joint, the sacrospinous and sacrotuberous ligaments anchor the sacrum to the spine of the ischium and the tuberosity of the ischium, respectively. They serve to prevent forward rotation of the sacrum.

FURTHER READING

Bogduk N 1997 Clinical Anatomy of the Lumbar Spine and Sacrum, 3rd edn. Churchill Livingstone, Edinburgh.

3

The lumbar spine

Whereas the joints and ligaments of the lumbar vertebral column endow it with a certain amount of intrinsic stability, they protect it only passively from excessive movement. For the control of movement, the column is endowed with muscles. Muscles are the principal tissues that surround the lumbar vertebral column. Its other adnexae are the nerves and vessels that supply these muscles, and the neural structures contained within the vertebral canal. The lumbar vertebral column and its adnexae become the lumbar spine.

MUSCLES

Topographically, the muscles of the lumbar spine are located in three distinct groups: the tiny muscles that connect the transverse processes, the anterolateral muscles, and the posterior muscles. Within and between groups, individual muscles differ with respect to their functions in relation to the lumbar vertebral column.

INTERTRANSVERSE MUSCLES

Several, distinct, small muscles are attached to the transverse processes of the lumbar vertebrae (Fig. 3.1). The intertransversarii mediales are tiny slips that pass essentially from an accessory process to the mamillary process below. The intertransversarii laterales dorsales are similar slips that pass from an accessory process to the

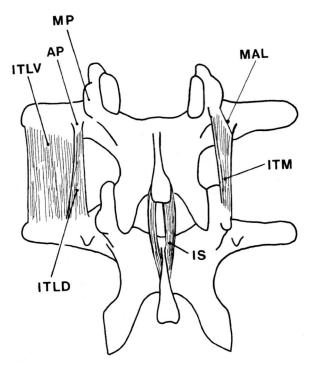

Figure 3.1 The short, intersegmental muscles. ITLV: intertransversarii laterales ventrales; ITLD: inter-transversarii laterales dorsales; ITM: intertransversarii mediales; IS: interspinales; AP: accessory process; MP: mamillary process; MAL: mamillo-accessory ligament. (From Bogduk N 1997 Clinical Anatomy of the Lumbar Spine and Sacrum, 3rd edn, with permission of Churchill Livingstone, Edinburgh.)

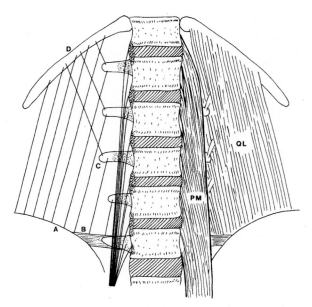

Figure 3.2 Psoas major (PM) and quadratus lumborum (QL). At each segmental level psoas major attaches to the transverse process, the intervertebral disc and adjacent vertebral margins. The attachments of quadratus lumborum are to the iliac crest (A), the iliolumbar ligament (B), the transverse processes (C), and the 12th rib (D). (From Bogduk N 1997 Clinical Anatomy of the Lumbar Spine and Sacrum, 3rd edn, with permission of Churchill Livingstone, Edinburgh.)

transverse process below. The intertransversarii lateral ventrales are fibres that pass from the lower edge of one transverse process to the superior edge of the transverse process below.

These muscles are too small to be responsible for the execution of movements of the lumbar vertebrae. However, they are densely endowed with muscle spindles. For this reason they are believed to play an important role in proprioception from the lumbar spine.

ANTEROLATERAL MUSCLES

Two muscles cover the lumbar vertebral column anterior to the transverse processes and lateral to the vertebral bodies. The first is a muscle that takes an adventitious origin from the lumbar

vertebral column in order to act on the hip. It has no primary action on the lumbar spine. The second is a respiratory muscle that sends some fibres to the lumbar vertebral column, but whose action on the lumbar spine has not been resolved.

Psoas major

Psoas major covers the lateral aspects of the lumbar vertebral bodies and the proximal quarter of the anterior aspects of the transverse processes (Fig. 3.2). Its fibres arise from the transverse processes and from the intervertebral discs and the superior and inferior margins of the vertebrae adjacent to each disc. From these sites, the fibres stream inferiorly and slightly laterally to join a tendon that passes over the brim of the pelvis to reach the lesser trochanter of the femur. The essential action of the psoas is to flex the hip, for which purpose the lumbar vertebral column constitutes a solid base. However, the psoas has no intrinsic action on the lumbar spine. Its fibres run too close to the axes of movement of the lumbar vertebrae to be able to exert any substantial moment that might bend the lumbar spine, forwards, backwards or sideways. However, although not able to execute movements of the lumbar spine, the psoas can exert very large compressive forces on the lumbar discs, when it flexes the hip, or when it is used in the action of sit-ups.

Quadratus lumborum

The quadratus lumborum covers the anterior surfaces of the transverse processes and extends laterally beyond the tips of these processes (Fig. 3.2). Most of its fibres pass directly from the ilium and iliolumbar ligament to the twelfth rib. They are joined by other fibres that stem from the lumbar transverse process and also pass to the twelfth rib. For this reason the principal function of the quadratus lumborum is held to be to brace the twelfth rib, in order to provide a steady base from which the lower thoracic fibres of the diaphragm can act.

Additional fibres pass from the ilium to the L1 to L4 transverse processes. However, these fibres are irregular in number, frequency and development. In some individuals they are large; in others they are quite feeble or absent. Only these fibres might have an action on the lumbar spine, either to bend it laterally or to control bending in the opposite direction. The strength of their action in this regard, however, is unknown.

POSTERIOR BACK MUSCLES

Interspinales

The interspinales are thin, rectangular sheets of fibres that connect the edges of apposing spinous processes (Fig. 3.1). They are too small to exert actions on the lumbar vertebra and, like the intertransversarii, are believed to contribute to proprioception from the lumbar spine.

The other posterior muscles of the lumbar spine are massive, and are the principal, if not the

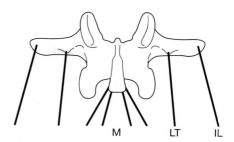

Figure 3.3 A sketch of the systematic attachments of the lumbar back muscles. Each lumbar vertebra is subtended by fibres of the iliocostalis lumborum (IL) stemming from the transverse processes, by fibres of longissimus thoracis (LT) stemming from the accessory processes, and by multiple fibres of the multifidus (M) radiating from the spinous process.

only muscles, responsible for controlling its movements. They are arranged in three columns and two layers. From medial to lateral, the three columns are formed by multifidus, longissimus thoracis, and iliocostalis lumborum, which systematically arise from the lumbar spinous processes, the accessory processes, and the transverse processes, respectively (Fig. 3.3). The longissimus thoracis and iliocostalis lumborum, however, are each formed by two parts. The deeper parts of each muscle arise from the lumbar vertebrae, and lie in the same plane as the multifidus. The superficial parts of each arise from thoracic vertebrae and ribs, and cover their respective lumbar parts. Moreover, the tendons of the thoracic parts of these muscles form the erector spinae aponeurosis, which covers the multifidus and thereby completes the superficial layer of the posterior lumbar back muscles.

Multifidus

The fibres of multifidus are centred on each of the lumbar spinous processes. From each spinous process, fibres radiate inferiorly in a systematic order to assume a variety of attachments inferiorly (Fig. 3.4). The arrangement of fibres is such as to pull downwards on each spinous process, thereby either causing the vertebra of origin to extend, or controlling its movement into flexion.

At each level, short fibres arise from the lamina and inferior edge of the spinous process and pass

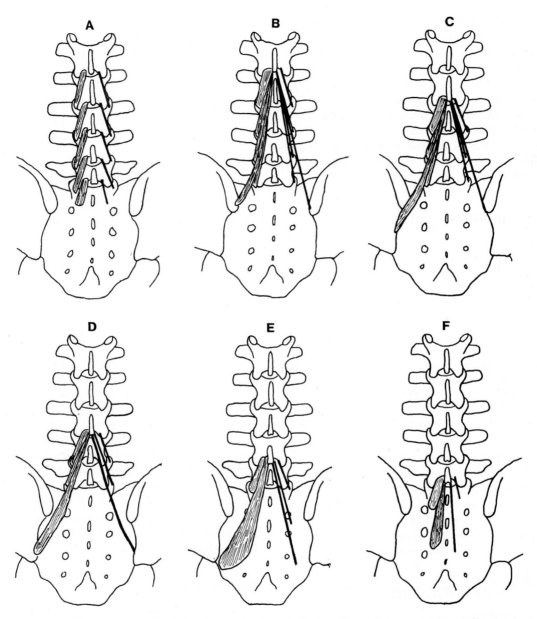

Figure 3.4 The component fascicles of multifidus. (A) The laminar fibres of multifidus. (B to F) The fascicles from the L1 to L5 spinous processes respectively. (From Bogduk N 1997 Clinical Anatomy of the Lumbar Spine and Sacrum, 3rd edn, with permission of Churchill Livingstone, Edinburgh.)

to the mamillary process of the vertebra two levels below. These are flanked by fibres from the inferior corner of the spinous process that pass to mamillary processes three, four and five levels below.

Fibres that extend below the L5 vertebra lack mamillary processes into which to insert. Instead, they find anchorage on the ilium and on the posterior surface of the sacrum.

The fibres of multifidus are arranged in laminated bands. The fibres from L1 cover those from L2 laterally and posteriorly. Those from L3 cover those from L4 and so on. This arrangement allows the multifidus to act on each spinous process individually and separately.

By some authorities in the past the multifidus has been regarded as a rotator of the lumbar spine. It has no such action. The obliquity of the fibres provides them with only a minor transverse action; the predominant action of the multifidus is to pull downwards on the spinous processes.

Longissimus thoracis pars lumborum

This is a relatively slender muscle that lies immediately lateral to multifidus. Its fibres arise from the tips of the L1 to L4 accessory processes and converge to a common tendon, flattened in the sagittal plane, and known as the lumbar intermuscular aponeurosis, that inserts into the ilium just above and medial to the posterior superior iliac spine (Fig. 3.5). These fibres are joined by a bundle of fibres from the posterior surface of the L5 transverse process that insert into the ilium just ventral to the site of insertion of the common tendon.

These fibres pull downwards and slightly backwards on the transverse processes, thereby being able to extend the lumbar vertebrae, or control their flexion. Acting unilaterally, these muscles contribute to controlling lateral bending of the lumbar spine.

Iliocostalis lumborum pars lumborum

The fibres of this muscle arise from the tips of the L1 to L4 transverse processes. Fibres are lacking from L5, having been incorporated into the posterior division of the iliolumbar ligament. In addition, at each level, fibres arise from the posterior surface of the middle layer of thoracolumbar fascia that attaches to the transverse processes (q.v.). From these origins the fibres pass inferiorly as flat sheets, in a laminated fashion, those from L1 covering those from L2 and so on,

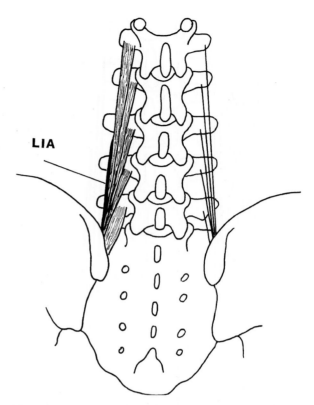

Figure 3.5   The longissimus thoracis pars lumborum. On the left, the five fascicles of the intact muscle are drawn. The formation of the lumbar intermuscular aponeurosis (LIA) by the lumbar fascicles of longissimus is depicted. On the right, the lines indicate the attachments and span of the fascicles. (From Bogduk N 1997 Clinical Anatomy of the Lumbar Spine and Sacrum, 3rd edn, with permission of Churchill Livingstone, Edinburgh.)

to insert into the crest of the ilium distal to the posterior superior iliac spine (Fig. 3.6). These fibres pull downwards and backwards on the transverse processes, thereby being able to extend the lumbar vertebra, or control their flexion. Acting unilaterally, they contribute to controlling lateral bending of the lumbar spine.

Longissimus thoracis pars thoracis

This muscle consists of a series of aggregated muscle bellies that arise at thoracic levels. Individual bellies arise from the tip of the transverse processes from T1 or T2 to T12. Additional bellies arise from the posterior surfaces of the ribs

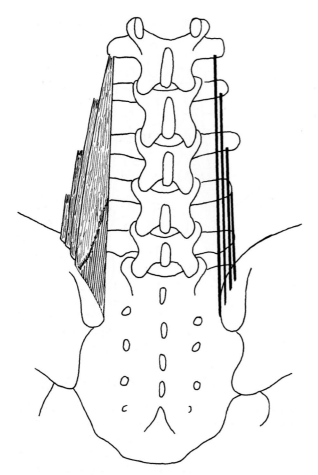

Figure 3.6 The iliocostalis lumborum pars lumborum. On the left, the four lumbar fascicles of iliocostalis are shown. On the right, their span and attachments are indicated by the lines. (From Bogduk N 1997 Clinical Anatomy of the Lumbar Spine and Sacrum, 3rd edn, with permission of Churchill Livingstone, Edinburgh.)

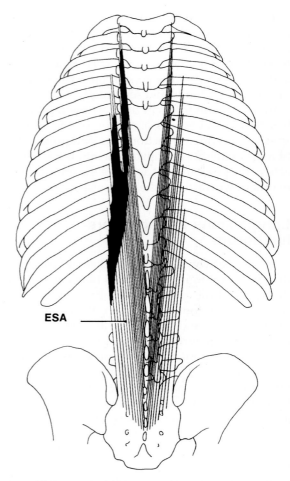

Figure 3.7 The longissimus thoracis pars thoracis. The intact fascicles are shown on the left. The darkened areas represent the short muscle bellies of each fascicle. Note the short rostral tendons of each fascicle, and the long caudal tendons, which collectively constitute most of the erector spinae aponeurosis (ESA). The span of the individual fascicles is indicated on the right. (From Bogduk N 1997 Clinical Anatomy of the Lumbar Spine and Sacrum, 3rd edn, with permission of Churchill Livingstone, Edinburgh.)

adjacent to the transverse processes from T4 to T12. Each belly is some 1–2 cm wide and 9–12 cm long, and ends in a long caudal tendon. These tendons pass into the lumbar region where they are aggregated side-to-side to form the medial half of what is known as the erector spinae aponeurosis, which covers the multifidus and the longissimus thoracis pars lumborum. The individual tendons are inserted systematically to the lumbar and sacral spinous processes, across the lower end of the sacrum, and onto the posterior

segment of the iliac crest (Fig. 3.7). The tendons from muscle bellies arising from the highest thoracic levels insert into the L1 spinous process. Tendons from lower muscle bellies insert at progressively lower levels. The tendons from T12 reach the posterior superior iliac spine.

As the tendons reach the lumbar spinous processes they form a longitudinal bundle of

The fibres of this muscle are arranged to extend the thorax in relation to the pelvis, or to control flexion of the trunk. They do not act directly on the lumbar vertebra but those that span the entire lumbar spine can exert an extension moment on it, acting like the string of a bow to bend it.

Iliocostalis lumborum pars thoracis

This muscle consists of a series of small, overlapping muscle bellies located in the thoracic region. The bellies arise from the angles of the lower eight ribs. From each belly a long caudal tendon extends into the lumbar region. These tendons are aggregated side-to-side to form the lateral part of the erector spinae aponeurosis, which covers the iliocostalis lumborum pars lumborum, and inserts into the iliac crest (Fig. 3.8).

These muscles are arranged to extend the thorax on the pelvis, or control forward or lateral flexion of the trunk. They do not act directly on the lumbar vertebrae but exert a bowstring effect on them.

ERECTOR SPINAE APONEUROSIS

Traditional anatomical textbooks describe the erector spinae aponeurosis as a large flat tendon arising from the lumbar and sacral spinous processes, the sacrum and the ilium, that gives rise to the erector spinae muscle that assumes a variety of insertions into the lumbar and thoracic vertebrae. This description disguises the true anatomy of this region.

The erector spinae aponeurosis is, indeed, a broad, flat tendon that covers the lumbar region posteriorly (Fig. 3.9). However, its fibres consist exclusively of the caudal tendons of the muscle bellies of longissimus thoracis pars thoracis and iliocostalis lumborum pars thoracis, that lie in the thoracic region. The tendons simply cover underlying muscles, and offer no attachment to them.

In sequence, from medial to lateral, lying deep to the erector spinae aponeurosis are the multifidus, longissimus thoracis pars lumborum and iliocostalis lumborum pars lumborum. These muscles arise from various elements of the lumbar vertebrae and anchor them to the sacrum and ilium.

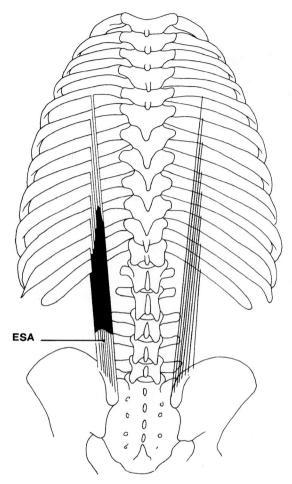

ESA

Figure 3.8 The iliocostalis lumborum pars thoracis. The intact fascicles are shown on the left, and their span is shown on the right. The caudal tendons of the fascicles collectively form the lateral parts of the erector spinae aponeurosis (ESA). (From Bogduk N 1997 Clinical Anatomy of the Lumbar Spine and Sacrum, 3rd edn, with permission of Churchill Livingstone, Edinburgh.)

fibres running dorsal to the tips of the spinous processes. This bundle constitutes the deep part of what is known as the supraspinous ligament. However, this structure lacks the features of a ligament. Its component fibres are clearly tendons. The deepest tendinous fibres curve into the interspinous space to find insertion onto the superior border of a spinous process. These fibres form the dorsal parts of the interspinous ligament.

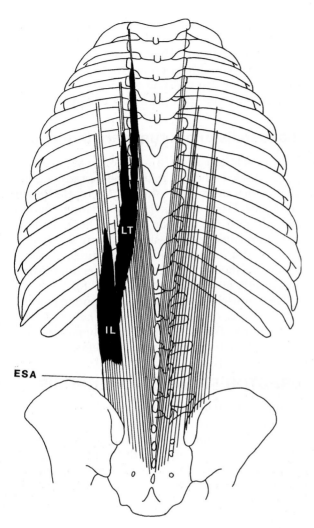

Figure 3.9 The erector spinae aponeurosis (ESA). This broad sheet is formed by the caudal tendons of the thoracis fibres of longissimus thoracis (LT) and iliocostalis lumborum (IL). (From Bogduk N 1997 Clinical Anatomy of the Lumbar Spine and Sacrum, 3rd edn, with permission of Churchill Livingstone, Edinburgh.)

FORCES AND LINE OF ACTION

No single force or line of action can be ascribed to any one of the lumbar back muscles. These muscles act on or across each of the five lumbar vertebrae, and each muscle consists of several, individual fascicles. In this regard, a fascicle is defined as a bundle of muscle fibres that share the same origin and insertion, such that they exert forces on the same bones. The forces exerted on a given lumbar vertebra will be those exerted by the fascicles that attach to it and by those fascicles that cross that vertebra but without attaching to it.

The force exerted by a given fascicle is determined by its orientation, its size, and its degree of activation. The extent to which a fascicle is activated requires information about its electromyographic activity. To date, it has not been possible to obtain electromyographic data on each and every fascicle of the back muscles. However, dissection studies have determined the size and orientation of each fascicle. These data can be used to provide estimates of the maximum possible force exerted by any fascicle, using the relationship that maximum force is the product of the physiological cross-sectional area of the fascicle and a force co-efficient. The physiological cross-sectional area is the volume of the fascicle divided by its length, and is a better estimate of the force exerted by the fascicle than an anatomical cross-section taken at an arbitrary point along the fascicle. The force co-efficient that has been found to apply to the back muscles[98] is about $0.46 \, N \, mm^{-2}$. In order to determine the force exerted by a fascicle in any given plane, the maximum force is corrected trigonometrically according to the orientation of that fascicle with respect to that plane.

Not only is the orientation of the fascicle critical with respect to the vertebra from which it arises, but also its line of action with respect to any vertebrae that it crosses. This arises because the lumbar vertebral column is not a single bone but a series of five vertebrae, each with a different orientation in the lumbar lordosis. Consequently, the force exerted on a distant vertebra will not necessarily be the same as that exerted by the same fascicle on an intervening vertebra.

The multifidus essentially consists of 11 fascicles on each side. At each segmental level a fascicle (ms) arises from the lateral aspect of the spinous process, and three arise from the tip of the spinous process (mt1–3). Those fascicles from L1 each assume a separate insertion and, therefore, need to be considered separately. The ms fascicle from

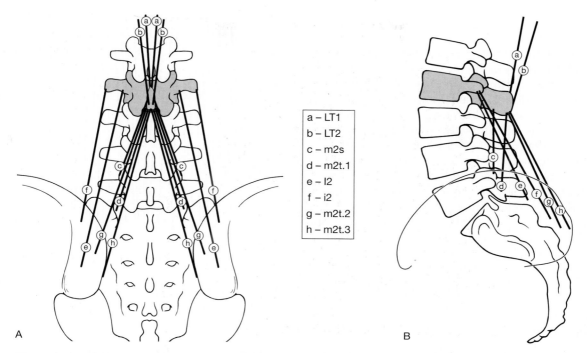

a –	LT1
b –	LT2
c –	m2s
d –	m2t.1
e –	l2
f –	i2
g –	m2t.2
h –	m2t.3

A   B

Figure 3.10   The attachments and lines of action of the individual fascicles of multifidus, iliocostalis lumborum, and longissimus thoracis that attach to the L2 vertebra. (A) posterior view. (B) lateral view. m2s: fascicles of multifidus that arise from the caudal edge of the L2 spinous process. m2t.1–m2t.3: the three fascicles of multifidus that arise from the tip of the L2 spinous process. i: fascicles of iliocostalis lumborum. l: lumbar fascicles of longissimus thoracis. LT: thoracic fascicles of longissimus thoracis.

L1 inserts into the L3 mamillary process, and the mt fascicles insert respectively into the mamillary processes of L4, L5, and S1. From the L2 spinous process, the ms and mt1 fascicles insert into the L4 and L5 mamillary processes, but the mt2 and mt3 fascicles both insert into the sacrum and can be treated together for biomechanical purposes (Fig. 3.10). The ms fascicle from L3 reaches the L5 mamillary process, but all three mt fascicles insert into the sacrum and can be treated collectively. From L4 all fascicles insert into the sacrum and can be treated collectively, as can the fascicles from L5.

There are five fascicles of the longissimus thoracis pars lumborum, each arising from a separate accessory process, and named by number according to the segment of origin. All reach the ilium. There are four fascicles of iliocostalis lumborum pars lumborum, which arise from the first four lumbar transverse processes and insert into the ilium. A fascicle from L5 is lacking.

Twelve fascicles of longissimus thoracis pars thoracis arise from thoracic levels and insert systematically into the lumbar spinous processes, across the base of the sacrum, and the posterior segment of the iliac crest. Eight fascicles of iliocostalis lumborum arise from the lower eight ribs and insert into the iliac crest.

In a posterior view, the fascicles of multifidus all exhibit a downward and lateral orientation (Fig. 3.10A). The lateral obliquity is about 15° at L1, increasing to about 20° at L2 and L3 as the multifidus widens over the sacrum, but decreasing to 16° at L4 and 6° at L5.[483] This obliquity reduces the force exerted by the fascicle in the sagittal plane in proportion to the cosine of its obliquity, but the angle is so small that virtually all of the force of each fascicle is exerted in the sagittal plane.

In a lateral view, the fascicles of multifidus exhibit a variety of orientations (Fig. 3.10B). Those from upper lumbar segments pass downwards and ventrally to their mamillary processes, whereas those from lower spinous processes pass downwards but dorsally to reach the sacrum. The orientation of fascicles varies from 11° ventral to the long axis of the vertebra of origin to 23° dorsal to this axis.[98] These differences in orientation affect the moment arm of each fascicle on each vertebra. Any accurate determination of the force and moments exerted by multifidus requires precise attention to the orientation of each fascicle.[98]

In a posterior view (Fig. 3.10A), the fascicles of longissimus thoracis pars lumborum assume an increasing obliquity from above downwards, with the fascicles from L1 and L2 being orientated at about 5° to the sagittal plane, and that of L5 at some 27° to the sagittal plane.[484] The fascicles of iliocostalis lumborum pars lumborum are uniformly orientated at only 5° to the sagittal plane,[484] except for the fascicle from L4 which assumes an angle of 15°. However, these inclinations are so small that virtually all of the force of each fascicle is exerted in the sagittal plane.

In a lateral view (Fig. 3.10B), the L2–L4 fascicles of longissimus thoracis pars lumborum are oriented at about 30° to the long axis of their vertebra of origin. The fascicle from L1 is inclined some 10° less, and that from L5 some 10° more. The fascicles of iliocostalis lumborum pars lumborum are all oriented at about 20° to the long axis of their vertebra of origin.

The thoracic fascicles of longissimus thoracis and iliocostalis lumborum run essentially along a sagittal plane, deviating not more than about 4–8° from this plane (Fig. 3.11). In lateral projection, these fascicles all run essentially parallel to the lumbar spine. Consequently, essentially all of the force exerted by any of these fascicles is directed parallel to the long axes of the lumbar vertebrae.[98]

Table 3.1 records the physiological cross-sectional areas of the fascicles of the posterior lumbar back muscles, together with the maximum

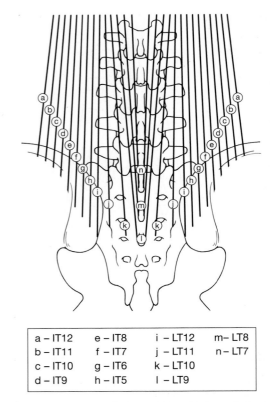

a – IT12	e – IT8	i – LT12	m– LT8
b – IT11	f – IT7	j – LT11	n – LT7
c – IT10	g – IT6	k – LT10	
d – IT9	h – IT5	l – LT9	

Figure 3.11   The lines of action and caudal attachments of the thoracic parts of longissimus thoracis and iliocostalis lumborum.

force exerted by each fascicle in the sagittal plane, the moment arms of each fascicle for each segment, as measured to the average location of the instantaneous axis of rotation of each lumbar vertebra, and the maximum moment exerted by each fascicle on each segment.[98] These data, which apply to the upright, standing position, show that half or more of the extension moment exerted on any lumbar segment is provided by the thoracic fibres of longissimus thoracis and iliocostalis lumborum. The remainder is provided by the lumbar fibres of these muscles and the multifidus, in almost equal proportions.

Upon flexion of the lumbar spine, the orientation of the fascicles of the back muscles changes, but not in a uniform manner. Some decrease their obliquity with respect to the longitudinal axis of the lumbar vertebral column; others increase

Table 3.1 The physiological cross-sectional areas (PCSA) of the fascicles of the lumbar back muscles, their maximum force in the sagittal plane (F_{sag}), their moment arms, and the maximum moments exerted on individual segments. Maximum forces and moments are expressed in terms of a force co-efficient – K, which is the maximum force that can be generated by unit cross-sectional area of muscle. An indicative value of K is 0.46 (N/mm^2). Absent values occur where the fascicle does not act on the segment in question. Negative values obtain for those fascicles of longissimus thoracis pars thoracis that insert into lumbar spinous processes and, therefore, pull upwards on those vertebrae. ms: fascicles of multifidus that arise from the caudal edge of the spinous process indicated

Muscle and fascicle	PCSA (cm^2)	F_{sag} (N)	Moment arm (cm) by segment					Maximum moment (Nm) by segment				
			L1–2	L2–3	L3–4	L4–5	L5–S1	L1–2	L2–3	L3–4	L4–5	L5–S1
Multifidus												
L1ms	0.40	39.5K	4.4	4.2	3.5	–	–	1.7K	1.7K	1.4K	–	–
L1mt1	0.42	41.6K	5.5	5.1	4.2	2.8	–	2.3K	2.1K	1.8K	1.2K	–
L1mt2	0.36	35.7K	5.5	5.6	5.2	4.0	2.5	2.0K	2.0K	1.8K	1.4K	0.9K
L1mt3	0.60	59.4K	5.3	6.4	7.0	6.8	6.0	3.1K	3.8K	4.2K	4.1K	3.6K
L2ms	0.39	38.2K	–	4.6	4.2	3.0	–	–	1.7K	1.6K	1.2K	–
L2mt1	0.39	38.4K	–	5.6	5.2	4.0	2.5	–	2.2K	2.0K	1.5K	0.9K
L2mt2–3	0.99	97.1K	–	5.3	6.3	6.5	6.0	–	5.2K	6.2K	6.4K	5.8K
L3ms	0.54	52.0K	–	–	4.5	3.9	2.8	–	–	2.4K	2.4K	1.4K
L3mt1–3	1.57	151.8K	–	–	5.2	6.0	5.9	–	–	7.9K	9.0K	8.9K
L4 all	1.86	179.2K	–	–	–	4.9	4.7	–	–	–	8.7K	8.5K
L5 all	0.90	88.5K	–	–	–	–	4.2	–	–	–	–	3.7K
TOTAL								9.1K	18.7K	29.3K	35.9K	35.9K
LTpL												
L1	0.79	78.8K	3.3	4.8	5.8	6.1	5.6	2.6K	3.8K	4.6K	4.8K	4.4K
L2	0.91	90.7K	–	3.6	4.9	5.5	5.2	–	3.2K	4.4K	4.9K	4.7K
L3	1.03	102.7K	–	–	3.5	4.6	4.8	–	–	3.6K	4.7K	4.9K
L4	1.10	108.6K	–	–	–	3.3	4.2	–	–	–	3.5K	4.5K
L5	1.16	115.7K	–	–	–	–	2.8	–	–	–	–	3.3K
TOTAL								2.6K	7.0K	12.8K	17.9K	21.8K
ILpL												
L1	1.08	107.4K	3.5	5.0	6.2	5.7	5.7	3.8K	5.6K	6.7K	6.7K	6.1K
L2	1.54	153.8K	–	3.6	4.6	4.8	4.2	–	5.6K	7.1K	7.4K	6.5K
L3	1.82	181.8K	–	–	3.5	4.1	3.8	–	–	6.4K	7.4K	7.0K
L4	1.89	188.6K	–	–	–	3.2	3.5	–	–	–	6.0K	6.6K
TOTAL								3.8K	11.2K	20.3K	27.5K	26.2K
LTpT												
T1	0.29	28.7K	5.3	–	–	–	–	2.0K	−2.1K	–	–	–
T2	0.57	56.4K	5.3	–	–	–	–	3.9K	−4.1K	–	–	–
T3	0.56	55.4K	5.3	4.7	6.2	–	–	3.8K	4.0K	−4.0K	–	–
T4	0.45	44.6K	5.3	5.7	6.2	–	–	3.1K	3.2K	3.2K	−3.0K	–
T5	0.44	43.6K	5.3	5.7	6.2	–	–	3.0K	3.1K	3.2K	−3.0K	–
T6	0.64	63.4K	5.3	5.7	6.2	5.7	–	4.4K	4.6K	4.6K	4.3K	−3.8K
T7	0.78	77.2K	5.3	5.7	6.2	5.7	4.5	5.3K	5.5K	5.6K	5.3K	4.6K
T8	1.25	123.8K	5.3	5.7	6.2	5.7	4.5	8.5K	8.9K	9.0K	8.5K	7.4K
T9	1.46	144.5K	5.3	5.7	6.2	5.7	4.5	9.9K	10.3K	10.4K	9.9K	8.6K
T10	1.60	160.0K	4.6	5.7	6.2	5.7	4.5	10.4K	11.2K	11.8K	11.7K	10.3K
T11	1.67	167.0K	3.8	4.9	6.2	5.7	4.5	10.4K	11.7K	12.5K	12.5K	11.6K
T12	1.38	138.0K	3.1	4.0	5.2	5.7	4.5	8.2K	9.6K	10.5K	10.4K	9.9K
TOTAL								72.9K	65.9K	66.8K	56.6K	48.6K
ILpT												
T5	0.23	22.8K	5.3	5.7	6.2	5.7	6.8	1.5K	1.6K	1.7K	1.6K	1.6K
T6	0.31	30.7K	5.3	5.7	6.2	5.7	5.7	2.1K	2.2K	2.3K	2.2K	2.1K
T7	0.39	38.6K	5.3	5.7	6.2	5.7	4.5	2.5K	2.7K	2.8K	2.8K	2.6K
T8	0.34	33.7K	5.3	5.7	6.2	4.6	3.6	2.2K	2.4K	2.5K	2.4K	2.3K
T9	0.50	49.5K	5.3	5.7	5.2	4.6	2.6	2.9K	3.1K	3.3K	3.2K	2.8K
T10	100	99.0K	5.3	4.9	5.2	4.6	2.6	5.8K	6.3K	6.6K	6.4K	5.6K
T11	1.23	121.8K	3.1	4.0	5.2	4.6	2.6	5.7K	6.7K	6.7K	6.4K	5.1K
T12	1.47	147.0K	3.1	3.0	4.3	3.6	2.6	4.7K	5.3K	5.6K	5.3K	3.8K
TOTAL								27.4K	30.3K	31.5K	30.3K	25.9K
TOTAL for all muscles acting on each segment (on each side)								116K	133K	161K	168K	158K

mt1–mt3: the first to third fascicles of multifidus that arise from the tip of the spinous process indicated. LTpL: longissimus thoracis pars lumborum. ILpL: iliocostalis lumborum pars lumborum. LTpT: longissimus thoracis pars thoracis. ILpT: iliocostalis lumborum pars thoracis. (After Bogduk et al.[98])

their obliquity. Some increase their moment arm; others decrease their moment arm. The net effect is that there is only a small reduction in the total moments exerted on each lumbar segment.[487] Nor is there any appreciable change in the compression load exerted by the back muscles on any lumbar segment. However, there are major changes in the posterior shear forces exerted by the multifidus and lumbar parts of longissimus and iliocostalis.

In the upright position, these muscles exert a posterior force on L1 to L4 but paradoxically an anterior force on L5. This arises because of the shape of the lumbar lordosis and the lumbosacral angle. Essentially, maximum contraction of the back muscles draws the upper lumbar vertebrae backwards but also drives them downwards under compression. As a result of this compression, the L5 vertebra is forced forwards across the sloping upper surface of the sacrum. Upon flexion, the lumbar spine is straightened, and the posterior shear force on the upper lumbar vertebrae is reduced; but at L5, the force is reversed to become a posterior shear force.[487]

With respect to axial rotation, the back muscles contribute little action. They are oriented far too longitudinally to produce rotatory moments. At best, they can exert about 2 Nm, which is only 5% of the maximum torque exerted during rotation of the trunk.[486]

THORACOLUMBAR FASCIA

The muscles of the lumbar spine are enveloped by three layers of fascia known as the thoracolumbar fascia. The anterior layer covers the quadratus lumborum and is formed by the deep fascia of that muscle. The other two layers are misnamed because they are not fascial in nature. A fascia consists of collagen fibres oriented in a variety of directions, with no particular orientation predominating. In contrast, an aponeurosis consists of collagen fibres derived from the tendon of a muscle, that assume a conspicuous predominant orientation.

The middle layer of thoracolumbar fascia intervenes between the quadratus lumborum and the iliocostalis lumborum, and is continuous with the intertransverse membranes. It consists of tendinous fibres of the transversus abdominis. Whereas the upper fibres of transversus abdominis arise from the costal margin, and whereas its lower fibres arise from the ilium and inguinal ligament, its middle fibres spring from the tips of the middle lumbar transverse processes. Between the transverse processes these tendons interlace to form the middle layer of thoracolumbar fascia.

The posterior layer of thoracolumbar fascia is formed by the aponeurosis of latissimus dorsi. The caudal tendons of the latissimus dorsi cover the erector spinae aponeurosis as they descend obliquely towards the lumbar spinous processes. In the midline they interlace with the tendons from the opposite side, to form the superficial layer of the so-called supraspinous ligament. From the midline the tendons can be traced into the opposite side. As a result of this arrangement the posterior layer of thoracolumbar fascia obtains a bilaminar structure (Fig. 3.12). The superficial layer is formed by the tendons of the ipsilateral latissimus dorsi, passing caudally and medially. The deep layer is formed by the tendons of the contralateral latissimus dorsi, passing downwards and laterally. Lateral to the iliocostalis lumborum, the two laminae are fused with the middle layer of thoracolumbar fascia along a seam known as the lateral raphe. From the lower end of this raphe, some of the most posterior fibres of external oblique take origin, in some individuals.

The latissimus dorsi exerts no direct action on the lumbar vertebral column. Rather, it uses the lumbar spine and pelvis as a wide base from which to exert its actions on the upper limb. When the upper limb is braced, however, as in climbing, the latissimus dorsi uses its attachments to the lumbar spine and ilium to lift the trunk as a whole. But it does not bend or move the lumbar spine.

Nevertheless, the posterior layer of thoracolumbar fascia acts as a retinaculum around the posterior back muscles, ostensibly helping to keep them applied to the lumbar vertebral column. The criss-cross arrangement of fibres in the posterior layer allows them to exert an extension moment on the lumbar spine, if the lateral raphe is tensed laterally by the transversus abdominis. However,

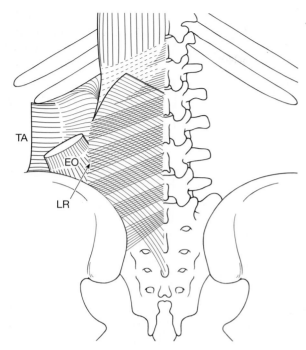

Figure 3.12 The structure of the posterior layer of thoracolumbar fascia. Fibres of the superficial lamina pass downwards and medially to the midline. Fibres of the deep lamina pass downwards and laterally from the spinous processes. Both laminae fuse in the lateral raphe (LR) lateral to the iliocostalis. To the lateral raphe are attached the middle fibres of transversus abdominis (TA) and the most posterior fibres of external oblique (EO).

this effect is trivial, amounting to no more than about 3–6 Nm,[485] compared to the 200 Nm required to sustain a moderately heavy lift.[217]

VERTEBRAL CANAL

The vertebral canal is a well-protected channel used by the nervous system to transmit nerves to and from the lower limb and pelvis. Its floor is formed by the posterior surfaces of the lumbar vertebral bodies and the intervertebral discs. Along the floor, like a carpet, lies the posterior longitudinal ligament. The roof is formed by the laminae of the lumbar vertebrae, and the ligamenta flava. The lateral walls are formed by the pedicles of the lumbar vertebrae. Between

the pedicles, the intervertebral foramina constitute windows through which nerves may enter or leave the vertebral canal.

The spinal cord reaches into the lumbar vertebral canal, terminating opposite the L1–2 intervertebral disc. Anchored to the spinal cord are the ventral and dorsal roots of the lumbar, sacral and coccygial spinal nerves. Systematically, these descend from the spinal cord to their respective intervertebral foramina (Fig. 3.13A). Nerve roots of a given segmental number are directed to the intervertebral foramen below the vertebra of the same segmental number. Because the several nerve roots resemble the fibres of a horse's tail, they are known collectively as the cauda equina.

The spinal cord and cauda equina are enclosed in a sac of meningeal tissue – the dural sac, which contains cerebrospinal fluid that bathes and nourishes the nerve roots (Fig. 3.13B). By this sac and fluid, the delicate nerves are protected from the hazards of movements of the lumbar vertebrae. Where pairs of nerve roots leave the dural sac to enter their intervertebral foramen they take a sleeve of dura mater with them, that constitutes the dural sleeve of the nerve roots. Typically, the nerve roots and their dural sleeve curve around the medial aspect of the pedicle above the intervertebral foramen to which they are destined (Fig. 3.14).

While so long as the vertebrae, their joints and their ligaments, remain normal in shape, the nerve roots in the vertebral canal remain immune to injury. However, alterations in the smooth internal surface of the vertebral canal threaten the nerves. Common alterations in this regard include osteophytes from the edges of the vertebral bodies or zygapophysial joints, herniations of disc material, bulges of the ligamentum flavum, and cysts of the zygapophysial joints.

SPINAL NERVES

The lumbar spinal nerves are short nerves lying in the intervertebral foramina. They are little longer than the intervertebral foramen is wide

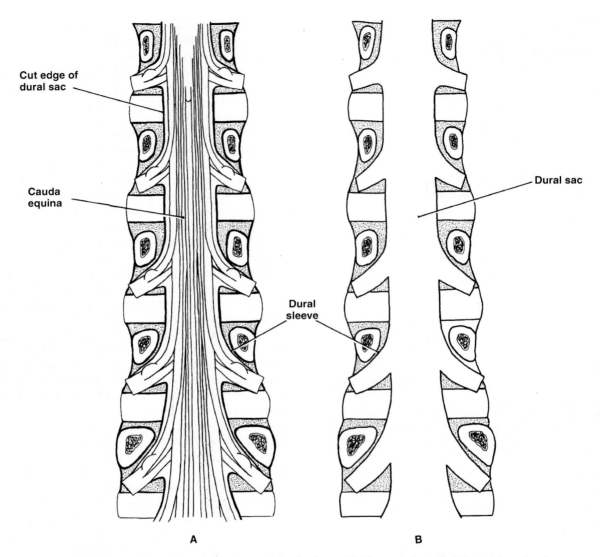

Figure 3.13 A sketch of the lumbar nerve roots and the dural sac. (A) The posterior half of the dural sac has been removed to reveal the lumbar nerve roots as they lie within the dural sac, forming the cauda equina. (B) The intact dural sac is depicted, as it lies on the floor of the vertebral canal (From Bogduk N 1997 Clinical Anatomy of the Lumbar Spine and Sacrum, 3rd edn, with permission of Churchill Livingstone, Edinburgh.)

(Fig. 3.14). Each is a mixed nerve, containing sensory and motor fibres. Those at L1 and L2 also contain preganglionic sympathetic axons. Each spinal nerve is connected to the spinal cord by a dorsal root and a ventral root. Each is enclosed by the tapering apex of the dural sleeve of the nerve roots.

The spinal nerves lie obliquely in their intervertebral foramina. Each passes downwards and laterally across the back of the lower corner of the vertebral body below the pedicle, skirting across the upper edge of the lateral end of the posterior surface of the intervertebral disc, just as it leaves the intervertebral foramen. At this

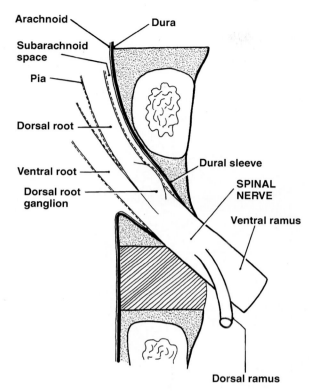

Figure 3.14 A sketch of a lumbar spinal nerve, its roots and meningeal coverings. The nerve roots are invested by pia mater, and covered by arachnoid and dura as far as the spinal nerve. The dura of the dural sac is prolonged around the roots as their dural sleeve, which blends with the epineurium of the spinal nerve. (From Bogduk N 1997 Clinical Anatomy of the Lumbar Spine and Sacrum, 3rd edn, with permission of Churchill Livingstone, Edinburgh.)

point the spinal nerve divides into ventral and dorsal rami.

VENTRAL RAMI

The ventral rami of the lumbar spinal nerves are destined to supply structures in the ventral compartment of the lumbar region, and the lower limb. Upon leaving the intervertebral foramina they enter the substance of the psoas major muscle (Fig. 3.15), in which they communicate with one another, forming the lumbar plexus of nerves. Deep branches of this plexus innervate the psoas and quadratus lumborum. Peripheral branches emerge from the lateral, ventral and medial surface of the psoas major.

The iliohypogastric and ilioinguinal nerves, and the lateral cutaneous nerve of the thigh emerge from the lateral surface of psoas. The former two supply the muscles and skin of the lower abdominal wall and groin. The latter supplies the skin over the lateral thigh.

The genitofemoral nerve emerges from the ventral surface of the psoas, and supplies the cremaster muscle in the groin, and the skin over the femoral triangle of the thigh.

The femoral nerve emerges from the lateral surface of psoas, and the obturator nerve emerges from its medial surface. Also emerging from the medial surface is the lumbosacral trunk, which provides fibres of the L4 and L5 spinal nerves to the sacral plexus, which innervates the lower limb.

The intimate relationship between these nerves and the psoas major means that the nerves can be secondarily involved in pathological processes that affect the psoas, such as infections and spread of spinal tumours. Back pain associated with neurological abnormalities in the lower abdominal wall or proximal thigh strongly imply some such process.

DORSAL RAMI

The dorsal rami of the lumbar spinal nerves are tiny branches that leave the spinal nerves at the intervertebral foramina and pass dorsally over the transverse processes to enter the posterior compartment of the spine, which is all those structures that lie behind the plane of the transverse processes (Fig. 3.15). Here they divide into lateral, intermediate, and medial branches. The lateral branches innervate the iliocostalis lumborum. Those from L1, L2 and L3 also furnish cutaneous branches that emerge from the iliocostalis, penetrate the erector spinae aponeurosis and thoracolumbar fascia, and cross the iliac crest to supply the skin over the upper and lateral regions of the buttock. Collectively these nerves are known as the superior clunial nerves. The intermediate branches of the lumbar dorsal rami end in the longissimus lumborum pars lumborum, which they supply.

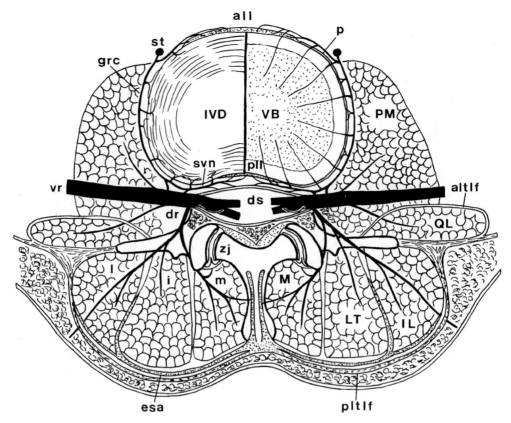

Figure 3.15 Innervation of the lumbar spine. A cross-sectional view incorporating the level of the vertebral body (VB) and its periosteum (p) on the right and the intervertebral disc (IVD) on the left. PM: psoas major; QL: quadratus lumborum; IL: iliocostalis lumborum; LT: longissimus thoracis; M: multifidus; altlf: anterior layer of thoracolumbar fascia; pltlf: posterior layer of thoracolumbar fascia; esa: erector spinae aponeurosis; ds: dural sac; zj: zygapophysial joint; pll: posterior longitudinal ligament; all: anterior longitudinal ligament; vr: ventral ramus; dr: dorsal ramus; m: medial branch; i: intermediate branch; l: lateral branch; svn: sinuvertebral nerve; grc: grey ramus communicans; st: sympathetic trunk. (From Bogduk N 1997 Clinical Anatomy of the Lumbar Spine and Sacrum, 3rd edn, with permission of Churchill Livingstone, Edinburgh.)

The medial branches of the lumbar dorsal rami cross the root of the transverse process and hook medially around the base of the superior articular process, at each level. They send articular branches to the zygapophysial joints above and below their course, and finally ramify in the multifidus and interspinalis muscles. Their distribution is segmental. Each medial branch supplies only those muscle fibres that arise from the spinous process of the vertebra below which emerges the spinal nerve that gives rise to the medial branch. In this way, the nerve of a particular lumbar vertebra innervates only the muscles that act directly on that same vertebra.

INNERVATION OF THE DISC

Each lumbar intervertebral disc receives an innervation from multiple sources (Fig. 3.15). Anteriorly and laterally the anulus fibrosus receives nerves from a plexus of fine nerves that covers the vertebral column, and is derived from branches

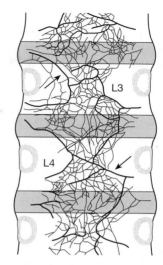

Figure 3.17 A sketch of the nerve plexus accompanying the posterior longitudinal ligament at the levels of the L3 and lower vertebrae, as seen in whole mounts of human foetuses. (After Groen et al.[316]) The large fibres arrowed represent the sinuvertebral nerves. (From Bogduk N 1997 Clinical Anatomy of the Lumbar Spine and Sacrum, 3rd edn, with permission of Churchill Livingstone, Edinburgh.)

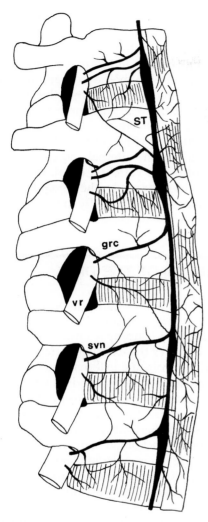

Figure 3.16 A sketch of the lateral plexus of the lumbar spine and its sources. The plexus innervates the lateral aspects of the vertebral bodies and discs. The plexus is formed by branches of the grey rami communicantes (grc) and branches of the ventral rami (vr). Posteriorly the lateral plexus is continued as the sinuvertebral nerves (svn) entering the intervertebral foramina. Anteriorly the plexus blends with the anterior plexus and sympathetic trunks (ST). (From Bogduk N 1997 Clinical Anatomy of the Lumbar Spine and Sacrum, 3rd edn, with permission of Churchill Livingstone, Edinburgh.)

of the sympathetic trunks and its grey rami communicantes (Fig. 3.16). Posteriorly the anulus receives branches from a plexus that covers the floor of the vertebral canal, and which is derived from the sinuvertebral nerves (Fig. 3.17).

The sinuvertebral nerves are the recurrent meningeal branches of the lumbar ventral rami. Each is formed by a somatic root from the ventral ramus and an autonomic root from the grey ramus communicans. Often the sinuvertebral nerve is represented by a single trunk that enters the intervertebral foramen just below the pedicle. Such a trunk may be accompanied by smaller filaments, or be replaced by multiple small filaments that enter the intervertebral foramen. Upon entering the vertebral canal the nerve divides into branches that ramify over the back of the disc at that level and branches that pass cranially towards the disc above (Fig. 3.17). In addition to innervating the anulus fibrosus, the sinuvertebral nerves innervate the posterior longitudinal ligament, the dural sac, and blood vessels in the vertebral canal.

Within the anulus fibrosus, nerve fibres are abundant in the outer third, notably in the ligamentous portion of the anulus[174,498,673,885] (Fig. 3.15). They are fewer in the middle third and absent from the inner third and from the nucleus pulposus. Some of these nerves accompany blood vessels but others end freely amongst the collagen fibres of the anulus. Most of the nerve endings in the anulus fibrosus are free nerve endings, but encapsulated and complex unencapsulated endings occur, particularly in the superficial layers of the lateral anulus. The complex receptors are believed to subserve a proprioceptive function as do similar endings in other joints of the body. The free nerve endings are believed to subserve a nociceptive function on the grounds that they contain the same neuropeptides as do nociceptive fibres elsewhere in the body. However, the cardinal evidence for a nociceptive function of at least some of the nerves in the anulus fibrosus is that needling the anulus, during the performance of discography, evokes pain (see Ch. 5).

Recent studies have also demonstrated nerve endings in the subchondral bone of the vertebral endplates of lumbar discs.[124] These fibres are probably derived from nerves that accompany blood vessels into the vertebral bodies. Their function is not known, but they could well be nociceptive.

BLOOD VESSELS

Vertebral bodies and muscles of the lumbar spine receive a rich blood supply. Lumbar arteries arise from the back of the aorta and pass dorsally around the waists of the lumbar vertebral bodies towards the intervertebral foramina. En route they furnish penetrating branches that enter the vertebral bodies from their anterior and lateral surfaces. Outside the intervertebral foramina they divide into external and spinal branches. The external branches basically follow the branches of the spinal nerves to supply the muscles of the ventral and dorsal compartments of the lumbar spine. The branches of the ventral compartment also contribute to the supply of the posterior abdominal wall. The spinal branches enter the vertebral canal in company with the sinuvertebral nerves. They supply the nerve roots, and enter the vertebral bodies from behind. Nerves derived from the anterior, lateral, and posterior sympathetic plexuses surrounding the lumbar vertebral column accompany penetrating blood vessels deep into the vertebral bodies.

The veins of the lumbar spine emanate from the vertebral bodies and form extensive plexuses around the vertebral bodies. An anterior internal vertebral venous plexus covers the floor of the vertebral canal, and an anterior external vertebral venous plexus covers the anterolateral aspects of the lumbar vertebral column. A similar pair of plexuses covers the internal and external aspects of the roof of the vertebral canal. Ultimately all these plexuses drain to the ascending lumbar veins that pass longitudinally in front of the roots of the transverse processes.

NUTRITION OF THE DISC

The lumbar intervertebral discs receive a relatively poor blood supply. No arteries enter the disc. Their blood supply is limited to tiny vessels that ramify over the external surface of the anulus, derived from the external arteries that supply the adjacent vertebral bodies. Otherwise, the nearest other arteries lie inside the vertebral bodies, separated from the disc by the vertebral endplates and their subchondral bone.

Lacking a direct blood supply, the discs rely on diffusion for their nutrition. Some 50% of this supply stems from the vessels around the periphery of the anulus. The remainder comes through the vertebral endplates from within the vertebral bodies. Nutrients such as glucose and oxygen pass into the disc down concentration gradients, and waste products such as lactic acid and carbon leave the disc in a reciprocal manner, but passage is slow and limited because of the density of proteoglycans in the disc. Nutrition is improved and aided by movement, for movement causes bulk flow of water into and out of the disc, and this bulk flow carries nutrients with it (p. 166).

FURTHER READING

Bogduk N 1997 Clinical Anatomy of the Lumbar Spine and Sacrum, 3rd edn. Churchill Livingstone, Edinburgh.

4

Biology of spinal tissues

INTRODUCTION

One of the purposes of this book is to describe the mechanisms by which spinal tissues can be injured by excessive mechanical loading. The concepts used to describe these mechanisms, such as 'fatigue failure' and 'elastic limit', are derived from mechanical studies of engineering materials, and this terminology might lead the unwary into thinking of biological structures as inert and passive. This would be unfortunate, because the same mechanical loading which deforms and damages spinal tissues also stimulates their cells to repair any damage, and perhaps even to strengthen the extracellular matrix as a precaution against future damage. The outcome of repetitive loading applied to living tissues can therefore vary from fatigue failure, on the one hand, to hypertrophy and strengthening, on the other. Furthermore, the metabolic rates of different spinal tissues varies greatly: at one extreme is muscle, which has a rich blood supply and a remarkable ability to increase or decrease its strength in a matter of weeks; and at the other extreme are the intervertebral discs, the largest avascular structures in the body, which are able to respond only slowly, and perhaps incompletely, to changes in their mechanical environment. Large imbalances in the ability of spinal tissues to respond to applied loading means that different tissues could be at risk of damage depending on how quickly the applied loading changes.[17] Therefore the risk of fatigue damage to the spine, and the location of that damage, depend on factors such as the number and severity of loading cycles, the time scale over which they are applied, and the age and health of the individual whose tissues are being loaded. Clearly, it is essential to consider the biological activity of spinal tissues when attempting to understand mechanical failure of the spine.

The following sections review the biology of musculoskeletal tissues. The description of each tissue starts with the structure and composition of the extracellular matrix, then considers cellular metabolism, including adaptive remodelling in response to external loading and healing in response to injury, and finally compares the effects of aging and degeneration. Muscle is considered first, because it applies most of the mechanical loading to the other tissues. Bone comes next, because its responses to changes in applied loading have been studied most, and are best understood. Less is known about the biology of articular cartilage, tendons, ligaments and intervertebral discs, and in these sections it will be necessary to interpret preliminary data by drawing analogies with bone. From a histological perspective, regions of the intervertebral disc resemble several other tissues, so discs are considered last. The final section compares the biological activity of spinal tissues, and considers some likely consequences of their differences.

MUSCLE

Skeletal or 'striated voluntary' muscle is a tissue specialised for forceful contraction, which enables it to produce movement and maintain posture. It has a rich blood supply, and contains a variety of nerve endings capable of monitoring tissue stress and strain. Nociceptive nerve endings capable of signalling pain are mostly located in the collagenous sheaths within and surrounding muscle.

STRUCTURE AND COMPOSITION

A human skeletal muscle is composed of bundles of contractile muscle fibres, separated by sheaths of collagenous connective tissue which coalesce

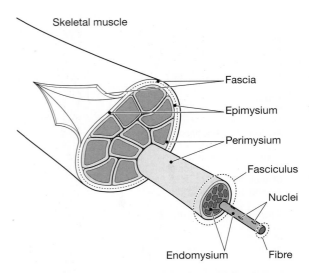

Figure 4.1 Gross structure of a skeletal muscle, showing the collagenous sheaths which surround muscle fibres, fibre bundles (fasciculi), and the whole muscle.

at each end into tendons or aponeuroses for attachment to bone (Fig. 4.1). Each individual muscle fibre is a multinucleated cell with its own cell membrane, the sarcolemma. Invaginations along the length of the sarcolemma form a transverse series of tubules, the t-tubules, which are continuous with the exterior of the muscle fibre and are filled with extracellular fluid. Running longitudinally along the muscle fibre is another series of channels, the sarcoplasmic reticulum, which stores calcium ions in high concentrations. A delicate layer of reticular fibres, the basal lamina, lies outside the sarcolemma, and this is surrounded by a thin connective tissue sheath, the endomysium. The endomysial tissue around each cell is continuous with that of adjacent cells, forming an array of endomysial tubes (Fig. 4.2) in which the muscle fibres are housed.[799] Groups of muscle fibres are bound into bundles or fascicles by the perimysium. This is the most abundant connective tissue within muscle and is composed of a cross-ply arrangement of crimped collagen I fibres which re-orientate as the muscle lengthens.[668] Tension in the perimysium contributes to muscle tension during eccentric contractions, and it protects the muscle fibres from overstretching. Surrounding the whole muscle is a third connective

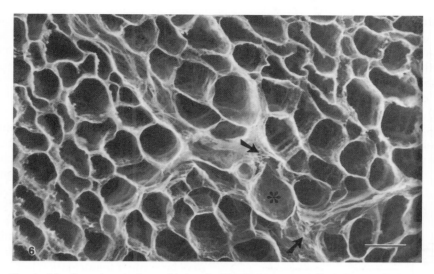

Figure 4.2 Scanning electron micrograph of bovine sternomandibularis muscle showing the collagenous sheaths (endomysium) which surround each individual muscle cell, and the coarser connective tissue (perimysium, indicated by arrows) which surrounds the muscle bundles or fasciculi. Contractile proteins have been removed as described in Trotter and Purslow.[800] (From Trotter,[799] with permission of S. Karger AG, Basel.) Bar = 50 μm.

tissue sheath, the epimysium, and lying superficial to this is the fascia which binds and compartmentalises individual muscles into functional groups. Capillaries penetrate the various connective tissue sheaths to provide muscle fibres with nutrients and remove waste products. Additional small quiescent cells, termed 'satellite' cells, lie outside the muscle fibres just below the basal lamina. These cells are thought to be stem cells that are capable of proliferation and regeneration in the event of muscle damage (see below). Healthy muscles contain very little extracellular matrix, apart from the collagenous sheaths.

Each muscle cell or fibre is packed with numerous myofibrils which are composed of a series of repeating sarcomeres. The sarcomere is the functional unit of muscle, and is composed of parallel arrays of fibrous proteins, actin and myosin (Fig. 4.3). When an action potential travels along the muscle fibre, calcium ions released from the sarcoplasmic reticulum initiate cross-bridge formation between actin and myosin, which are then able to move relative to each other and thus cause the muscle to contract.

Individual muscle fibres can be orientated parallel, or at an angle, to the long axis of the muscle, and this architectural arrangement confers different mechanical properties upon the muscle. Parallel-fibred muscles, which tend to be long and thin with fibres extending the full length of the muscle, are able to contract the greatest distance. Greater forces (but smaller contractions) can be generated by pennate muscles which consist of bundles of relatively short muscle fibres orientated at an angle to the line of pull (Fig. 4.4). This arrangement ensures a larger physiological cross-sectional area and hence a greater capacity for force production. Individual muscle fibres are tapered at their ends, where microscopic interdigitations serve to strengthen the interface between each muscle fibre and its tendon.

The mechanism by which muscles generate force has been defined by the 'sliding-filament hypothesis'[375,376] (Fig. 4.3). Several details are relevant to this book. Firstly, the maximum 'active' tension that a muscle can generate increases with muscle length up to an optimum length (L_o), and then decreases (see Fig. 10.13). This can be explained in terms of the optimum interactions between actin and myosin. On the other hand, 'passive' tension in a stretched but relaxed muscle increases greatly with muscle length, because stretching generates tension in the connective tissue sheaths described above, and within the muscle fibres themselves. During eccentric muscle contractions, active and passive processes can combine to generate peak forces considerably larger than the maximum active tension. Forces

are particularly high if the muscle is stretched rapidly. This explains why rapid forward bending movements can generate such high forces within the lumbar erector spinae (page 101).

METABOLISM

Skeletal muscle contains three main types of fibre which have different mechanical and metabolic properties (Table 4.1). Type I muscle fibres, which rely heavily on oxidative metabolism, are supplied by a more extensive capillary network than type IIB fibres, which rely mostly on anaerobic metabolism. It is generally accepted that the relative proportions of type I and II fibres in human muscle are genetically determined, although there may be some transformation between IIA and IIB fibres with training. Each muscle cell normally lives for the entire life of the individual, with new cells being produced only following acute traumatic disruption of muscle cell membranes. At puberty, muscle mass in males increases under the influence of male sex hormones, but this increase in muscle mass is achieved by an increase in the size of individual muscle fibres (hypertrophy) rather than an increase in fibre number (hyperplasia). In adult muscle tissue, the rate of protein turnover is so rapid that the half-life of contractile proteins is probably between 7 and 15 days.[293] This enables muscle to adapt to altered mechanical requirements much more rapidly than other tissues.

Muscle adaptation is influenced greatly by the type of exercise. Repeated contractions at low force

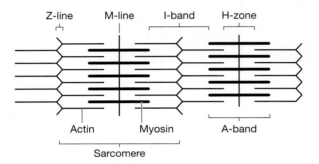

Figure 4.3 Diagram showing the arrangement of actin and myosin within sarcomeres which comprise the contractile machinery of skeletal muscle cells. Contraction is achieved by the actin molecules sliding between the myosin molecules propelled by cross-bridges which repeatedly form, change orientation, and break. The various lines and bands can be visualised by electron microscopy. Compare with Figure 4.5.

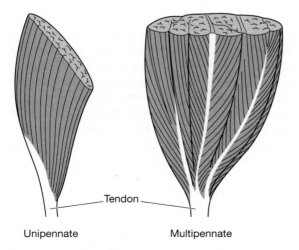

Figure 4.4 Typical arrangement of muscle fibres in unipennate and multipennate muscles.

Table 4.1 Characteristics of the main fibre types found in human skeletal muscle. A fourth type (IIC) can be distinguished in regenerating muscle. Fibre types are defined on the basis of their histochemical staining properties. (After Lane,[451] with permission of Marcel Dekker, New York.)

	Type I	Type IIA	Type IIB
Aerobic capacity	High	Intermediate	Low
Mitochondrial density	High	Intermediate	Low
Capillary density	High	High	Low
Anaerobic capacity	Low	Intermediate	High
Speed of contraction	Slow	Fast	Fast
Force of contraction	Low	Intermediate	High
Fatigue resistance	High	Intermediate	Low

levels (endurance training) produce the greatest changes in the slow twitch (type I) fibres which are preferentially recruited at low loads. In response to endurance training, type I fibres show increased vascularisation,[363] increased size and number of mitochondria, and consequently an increased concentration of oxidative enzymes.[294] Depending upon the intensity and duration of endurance training, similar changes may also occur in other fibre types. These changes enable the muscle to contract for longer before it becomes fatigued. An experiment on dogs has suggested that vigorous aerobic training can transform fibres from one type to another.[671] In human muscle, any transformation of fibre types resulting from endurance training probably occurs within the type II fibre population and not between types I and II.

Strength or power training, in which high forces are generated for short periods of time, produces the greatest changes in the fast twitch (type II) fibres. This type of exercise does not normally create more muscle fibres,[295] but appears to cause some transformation between type II fibres[311] as well as an increase in their diameter.[166,295,311] Such mechanically-induced hypertrophy is caused by changes in gene expression that result in increased synthesis of specific proteins, including actin and myosin, particularly in the type II fibres. Increased activity of myokinase, which helps maintain a high ATP/ADP ratio, has also been reported in response to strength training.[793] Muscle cells can grow in length as well as girth if they are stretched.[177,346] This occurs primarily by the addition of new sarcomeres to the fibre near the musculo-tendinous junction, so that each muscle fibre becomes longer.[865,866] Transient muscle lengthening can be achieved by creep stretching of the collagenous tissues, but this is reversed once the load is removed.

Physical inactivity reduces muscle mass (muscle atrophy) with protein synthesis falling within hours. If muscle is immobilised in a shortened position then its length is reduced along with its girth, and the proportion of collagen to contractile protein in the muscle increases.[867] The muscle becomes stiffer and less extensible.[296] This may explain the reductions in joint mobility which are often reported following injury and/or disuse.

Changes in muscle size and performance have been quantified in many studies. Typically, complete immobilisation of the leg reduces the cross-sectional area of the quadriceps by 15–20% in 6 weeks, with most of this loss being due to type I fibre atrophy resulting from a reduction in protein synthesis rather than an increase in protein catabolism.[285,287] Similarly, the capacity of muscle to respond to increased levels of loading is also marked: it is a common experience that the maximum weight that can be lifted repeatedly during weight-training exercises can increase by 100% in 12 months. Some of this is attributable to increased endurance, and some to improvements in neuromuscular activation increasing the proportion of muscle fibres that can fire at the same time, but a considerable proportion is attributable to hypertrophy. Animal experiments indicate that muscles overloaded in the stretched position can increase their muscle mass by as much as 30% in just 4 days.[293] This value will include increases in muscle fibre length as well as girth, but it serves as a useful yardstick by which to judge the adaptive ability of the skeletal tissues which must withstand the increased muscle forces.

The precise mechanical stimulus for muscle hypertrophy is controversial, although high stress, high strain and high strain rate have all been implicated. Excessive or unusual muscle activity, especially when eccentric contractions are involved, is effective in producing exertion-induced damage and subsequent repair and hypertrophy.[465] The damage initiated by this type of activity is characterised by changes in the sarcoplasmic reticulum,[57] disruption of the cell membrane,[548] and a disturbance of normal sarcomere structure),[148,284,393,596] as shown in Figure 4.5. Damage to the sarcoplasmic reticulum can affect calcium homeostasis resulting in decreased excitation of muscle cells and hence a reduction in force generating capacity that persists for several days.[595,700] Disruption of the muscle cell membrane allows proteins such as creatine kinase and histamine to leak out gradually into the extracellular environment, where they can stimulate nociceptors and cause delayed-onset muscle soreness and swelling 24–72 hours after exercise.[393,700] Muscle damage can be detected in biopsies taken

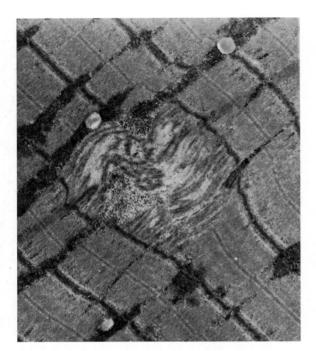

Figure 4.5 Electron micrograph showing focal disruption of sarcomeres in skeletal muscle, resulting from eccentric contractions. The myofilaments are disorganised in this region and the Z-lines are displaced. (From Newham[596] with permission of Elsevier, Amsterdam.) Magnification × 19 000.

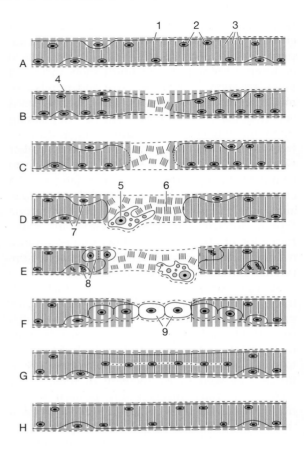

Key	1. Sarcolemma (N.B. solid line on diagram)
	2. Nuclei
	3. Sarcomere structure
	4. Basement membrane (dashed line)
	5. Macrophage
	6. Necrotic debris
	7. Satellite cells
	8. Myoblasts
	9. Myotubes

Figure 4.6 Diagram showing the stages of repair to a damaged skeletal muscle fibre. (A) Healthy intact fibre. (B) Fibre becomes locally disrupted, basement membrane intact. (C) Sarcolemmal membrane proliferates to compartmentalise damaged areas. (D) Macrophages infiltrate and phagocytose cell debris. (E) Quiescent satellite cells are activated and migrate to damaged areas where they proliferate to form myoblasts. (F) Myoblasts fuse to form myotubes. (G) New myofilaments are synthesised to form myofibrils; nuclei remain centrally located. (H) Completely repaired fibre with peripherally displaced nuclei. (From Hodgson and Rose,[358] with permission of Springer Verlag, New York.)

within an hour of completing the exercise, but the damage then worsens over the following few days. Type II fibres are probably more susceptible to this type of damage than type I fibres[262,393] although this is not certain.[57]

The damage that occurs during or immediately after exercise has been attributed to protein degradation initiated by non-lysosomal proteases, such as calpain.[80] Together with other pro-inflammatory mediators, calpain is thought to initiate an inflammatory response that begins 2–6 hours after injury. This results in an infiltration of macrophages and other phagocytic cells into the damaged muscle tissue, where they remove cell debris and release proteases that rapidly break down the damaged myofibrils. These cells also produce cytokines that stimulate cellular repair and initiate the proliferation and migration of satellite cells.[80,147] Once at the site of injury, satellite cells differentiate into myoblasts which fuse to form myotubes that repair damaged cells or develop into new multinucleated muscle cells if the original fibres are completely necrosed. The processes involved in regeneration of a skeletal muscle fibre are depicted in Figure 4.6. Collagenous tissue also regenerates, and if the damage is severe, it can proliferate to such an extent that it interferes with normal muscle function. These repair processes generally take place over a matter of days or weeks[199] and result in muscle hypertrophy. If damage is severe then recovery times are longer, being dependent on the extent of damage to nerves and blood vessels. In a rabbit model involving complete muscle division by laceration, the wound healed by extensive scar formation; after a healing period of 12 weeks, 50% of muscle strength was regained, at which time the muscle's ability to shorten was 80% of normal.[278] Some residual weakness may persist at the musculo-tendinous junction where overuse injury often involves the rupture of attachments between the perimysium and tendon. In such cases, healing is slow, and resembles that of tendon (see below).

AGEING AND DEGENERATION

Muscle mass and strength both decrease with age,[172,315] a process known as sarcopenia. The extent of these age-related changes varies between different muscles[370,560,561] and with limb dominance[370] and can be accelerated by chronic disease. It is greater in men than women[274] and in people who are less physically active.[370] Other possible influences include: reduced levels of growth hormone and sex steroids, increased production of catabolic cytokines, insufficient dietary intake of calories and protein, and reduced rates of protein turnover in the elderly. Sarcopenia can be reversed by high-intensity progressive resistance exercise, although ageing human muscle is less responsive to exercise training than younger muscle,[454] and animal studies suggest that aging muscle takes longer to regenerate following injury.[199]

As well as becoming weaker, old muscles have a reduced oxidative capacity which cannot be explained simply by the reduction in muscle mass.[171,172] This may be due to an age-related increase in the number of fibres that are deficient in cytochrome c oxidase (COX), a mitochondrial enzyme involved in aerobic energy metabolism.[436] Muscle collagen content increases with age, especially in the endomysium and perimysium[293] and this will contribute to an increase in passive muscle stiffness. Proprioceptive ability is impaired in the elderly, contributing to slower reactions and poorer motor control. The end result of these changes is to make old muscles slower, weaker and more fatiguable, so that they become a major cause of disability and frailty in the elderly.

Apart from ageing, and apart from specific muscle diseases which lie outside the scope of this book, there are no degenerative conditions of muscle comparable to those which affect the underlying skeletal tissues. This interesting fact suggests that degeneration of skeletal tissues may be attributable, at least in part, to their poor blood supply, and the relative inability of a small cell population to turnover and repair an extensive extracellular matrix.

BONE

Bone is a type of connective tissue with an abundant extracellular matrix specialised to provide a strong and rigid framework for the body. It has a rich blood supply. Nerve endings capable of signalling pain are mostly located in the collagenous sheaths which surround bone.

STRUCTURE AND COMPOSITION

Bone tissue is found in solid blocks or sheets ('cortical' bone) or arranged as a lattice-work of slender struts ('trabecular' bone). In both cases, the adult tissue is composed of mature cells, osteocytes, trapped in small cavities ('lacunae') within a rigid extra-cellular matrix. The extracellular matrix is approximately 5–8% water, and 60–70% micro-crystalline solid, composed predominantly of hydroxyapatite. These plate-like crystals are 10–40 nm long, and 2–5 nm thick. Their chemical composition is variable, but is similar to hydroxyapatite, $Ca_{10}(PO_4)_6OH_2$, where Ca is calcium, and PO_4 is phosphate. Individual crystals are very small, irregularly shaped, and contain impurities such as carbonate, sodium and magnesium. The remainder of the bone matrix is termed 'organic', and consists mostly of collagen type I (90%), other proteins such as osteocalcin and bone sialoprotein, and the small proteoglycans biglycan and decorin. Collagen I fibres are bundles of fibrils, each made up of many collagen molecules lined up in a parallel array and held together by several types of cross-links (Fig. 4.7). Each molecule is a triple helix, with short non-helical regions on either end. After secretion from a cell, part of these terminal regions are removed by matrix enzymes, and this allows the remaining part of the molecule to self-assemble (polymerise) into a long fibril. Systematic gaps between collagen molecules (Fig. 4.7) are sites for the initiation and growth of bone mineral.

The presence of crystals gives bone its rigidity and compressive strength, whereas collagen fibres confer tensile strength and toughness. The water-binding properties of proteoglycans enable them to 'capture space' in developing tissue, and then to regulate the diameter of collagen fibrils. Non-collagenous proteins appear to play a role in the mineralisation process.

The matrix is mostly arranged in concentric cylindrical lamellae with a central channel for blood vessels and nerve fibres, and with numerous bone-maintenance cells (osteocytes) lying between adjacent lamellae (Fig. 4.8). The whole cylindrical

A   Collagen molecule: triple helix

Non-helical terminal region

B   Microfibril   Collagen molecule

'Quarter stagger'   Cross-links

C   Fibril (in electronmicrograph)

300 nm

Figure 4.7   Each molecule of collagen type I or II consists of three polypeptide chains, twisted into a long triple helix, with a short non-helical region on each end (A). After the molecules are secreted from a cell, part of each non-helical region is removed by enzymes, and this permits the molecules to 'self-assemble' into a microfibril (B). The 'quarter stagger' structure is stabilised by various cross-links between parallel molecules. Microfibrils aggregate to form fibrils (C) and fibrils make up collagen fibres. Fibrils can be identified on electron micrographs from their distinctive striations (periodicity of 67 nm) which are due to the overlap and gap regions of the quarter-stagger structure.

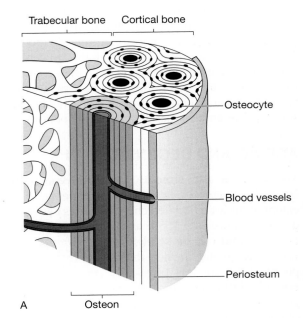

Trabecular bone   Cortical bone

Osteocyte

Blood vessels

Periosteum

A   Osteon

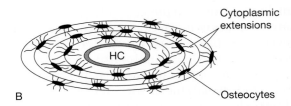

Cytoplasmic extensions

HC

B   Osteocytes

Figure 4.8   (A) Mature cortical bone is made up of cylindrical 'osteons', comprising a series of concentric layers of bone surrounding a central blood vessel. (B) The bone maintenance cells, osteocytes, become trapped in small lacunae between the lamellae, but they can communicate with each other via long cytoplasmic extensions which extend radially outwards along small cannaliculi (channels) in the solid matrix. (HC: Haversian canal.) Compare with Plate 4 (C).

structure is termed an osteon, or 'Haversian system'. Irregular spaces between osteons (which comprise a considerable proportion of the slender struts of trabeculae) are filled with less-organised lamellae of similar composition. The outer surface of a bone is covered with a fibrous membrane, the periosteum, and a similar membrane, the endosteum, lines the central medullary cavity of long bones. Each membrane consists of two layers, an outer protective layer containing many strong collagen fibres, which in the case of the periosteum blend in with the fibres from tendons, and an inner layer which contains two other types of bone cell, osteoblasts and osteoclasts.

METABOLISM

Long bones, and vertebrae, develop from a 'model' of hyaline cartilage, which gradually turns into a bone as it grows and ossifies. Internal bone growth continues into adolescence at two growth plates by a process known as endochondral ossification, which involves an intermediate stage of calcium carbonate deposition and resorption. Growth plates enable a bone to increase in length while preserving the articular cartilage covering at each end. In addition, the width of a growing bone is increased by direct deposition of bone from the inner layer of the periosteum. Active bone-forming cells, osteoblasts, secrete osteoid, which mineralises into bone during the following few hours. Initially, the mineral structure and collagen alignment are disorganised, and the tissue is referred to as woven bone. This is then 'remodelled' by two types of bone cell working in concert as a bone-forming unit to create Haversian systems of mature bone: osteoclasts dissolve the old matrix, and osteoblasts then secrete new matrix in precisely orientated lamellae (Fig. 4.8). The mineralising process traps each bone-forming osteoblast in a rigid cell or lacuna, turning it into a less active osteocyte. These bone maintenance cells communicate with each other by means of long cell processes which lie in narrow channels (canaliculi) in the matrix. Remodelling occurs throughout adult life, so that bone matrix is turned over on a regular basis, and minor cracks

are repaired before they can accumulate to cause major defects. The presence of small cracks may actually induce bone remodelling.

Bone cells can increase or decrease bone mass, or alter its shape and micro-architecture, in response to changes in external mechanical loading. This process is correctly termed 'modelling' to distinguish it from 'remodelling' in which bone mass stays the same. However, the mechanically-adaptive response is often referred to loosely as 'adaptive remodelling' (Fig. 4.9), and the underlying principle that governs the bone's response to altered mechanical demands is known as 'Wolf's Law'. In simple terms, Wolf's Law states that bone architecture and mass adapts to best resist the forces applied to it, and there is plenty of experimental evidence to back it up.[297,452] Adaptation requires concerted action from many distant and apparently isolated cells, but in fact, osteocytes are able to communicate with each other by means of long extensions of their cell membranes, and the activities of osteoclasts and

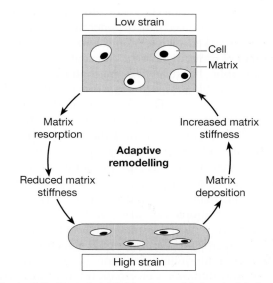

Figure 4.9 Most skeletal tissues are able to adapt their mechanical properties to match the mechanical environment. If mechanical loading increases so that tissue deformation (strain) is high, then more matrix is deposited until the matrix stiffness increases sufficiently for strain to return to the normal range. Similarly, low loading will produce low strain, and encourage matrix resorption until strain rises to acceptable levels again.

osteoblasts are 'coupled' by chemical messengers, called cytokines. Some cytokines, such as growth factors, stimulate a hypertrophic response, while others, including the interleukins, are associated with reductions in bone mass. Cytokines can be produced by bone cells responding to local circumstances. They can also be produced centrally, for example, in response to changes in hormone levels, and then distributed through the blood to many bones.

The maximum speed at which whole bones can strengthen or weaken is not well characterised. Experiments on turkeys have shown that the mineral content of a frequently loaded bone increases by approximately 40% in just 6 weeks,[692] whereas 8 weeks of continuous unloading causes a 10–15% loss of bone. A frequently quoted indicator of metabolic response is that the racquet arm of professional male tennis players contains 35% more cortical bone than the other arm.[394] Bone adaptation can be quite extreme, as evidenced by the exceptionally high bone mineral content of vertebrae in elite weightlifters.[309] Bone mineral density is closely related to strength.[310]

Bone adaptations may not always be beneficial. Scalpel-induced disc degeneration in sheep[617] leads to marked increases in sclerosis, and in the number of trabeculae, in the adjacent vertebrae,[568] presumably because the mechanically-altered disc is less able to distribute stress evenly on the bone (pp. 136–137). Denser bone could then hinder the transport of metabolites into the adjacent disc.[579] Osteophytes around the margins of the vertebral body, and in the zygapophysial joints, may represent an attempt by bones to spread high loading over a greater area, and so to reduce stress and strain within the bone. Unfortunately, these adaptations can also lead to nerve root entrapment within the intervertebral foramen.[381]

The precise mechanical signal which controls adaptive remodelling in bone is probably the maximum dynamic deformation (strain) experienced locally by the tissue. Static loading has little effect[452] whereas bone mass increases with increasing maximum strain.[693] Only 36 cycles of dynamic loading per day are capable of producing a maximal response.[692] According to the 'mechanostat theory',[267] bones strengthen when strains exceed a certain threshold value (approximately 2000 microstrains, or 0.2% change in length) and weaken when they fall below another threshold (approximately 200 microstrains). Threshold levels can be altered by disease and by circulating hormones. Bone deformation may possibly be communicated to cells by the flow of fluid, or small electrical currents, within the canaliculi, or by piezo-electric currents generated by the deformation of the crystalline matrix.

Bones can be injured by gross fracture, or by the accumulation of microdamage leading eventually to a 'stress fracture'. Bone consists predominantly of the rigid crystalline matrix, so injury mechanisms probably resemble those found in engineering materials more closely than in any other bodily tissue. Fractures heal by the migration of cells from the periosteum and endosteum to the fracture site, where they link the broken bone ends with a deformable fibrous material ('fracture callus') which subsequently mineralises to form new bone. Once the new bone has been turned over by the continuous remodelling process, it is often difficult to detect the original break, and the healed bone can regain full strength. This remarkable ability of bone to repair itself makes it highly unlikely that an injured vertebra could be a direct source of chronic back pain (unless the bone became infected).

AGEING AND DEGENERATION

Unlike muscle, bone tissue deteriorates markedly with age. Reduced levels of physical activity no doubt play a part, but so do changes in the levels of sex hormones which reduce bone mass and strength, especially in women after the menopause.[573] Hormone-related weakening of bones is termed 'osteopaenia', and when this reaches the level at which fractures are sustained during the activities of normal living[573] it is termed 'osteoporosis'. These processes do not reduce bone mass uniformly: trabecular bone is affected more than the cortical shell, and vertical trabeculae more than horizontal. If trabeculae are thinned so much that they break, then they are not replaced, at least in adults. In this way, vertebral strength depends not only on bone mass, but also on aspects of bone architecture such as the orientation and connectivity of trabeculae. Vertebral bodies are often severely affected by osteoporosis because they contain so much trabecular bone. Fracture of the vertically-orientated trabeculae which support the vertebral body endplate are so common[824] that they probably explain why endplates generally bulge into the vertebral body in old age.[811]

Thinning of trabeculae, and osteoporotic fractures, are more common in the anterior part of the vertebral body.[607] This could possibly be related to the manner in which it is loaded by the intervertebral disc, as described on pages 123–126.

Endplate fracture is often followed by the vertical herniation of nucleus pulposus tissue into the vertebral body; the displaced tissue, and the calcified shell which forms around it, are referred to as a Schmorl's node. The calcified shell can be identified using plain X-ray, but MRI is a more sensitive test because it is able to detect the displaced tissue itself. Some Schmorl's nodes are developmental in origin and often are asymptomatic. However, there is evidence linking them with disc degeneration and back pain in young sportsmen[780] and there are reasons to suspect that they are related to disc degeneration in later life (p. 137). A recent large-scale MRI study reported Schmorl's nodes in 19% of patients with lumbar symptoms, and 9% of asymptomatic controls, with only 33% of the nodes being detected by X-rays.[327]

To a certain extent, bone weakening can be countered by appropriate exercises, particularly those which involve impact loading of the bones,[68,69] and also by drug therapy (including hormone replacement therapy). However, the best solution may be to take sufficient exercise earlier in life to ensure that bone mass is sufficiently high that the normal age-related loss does not take it below the level at which the risk of fracture becomes high.

Some other causes of bone deterioration, including nutritional defects, lie outside the scope of this book.

HYALINE CARTILAGE

Hyaline cartilage is a connective tissue with an abundant extracellular matrix that combines the properties of toughness and compressive strength. It has a sparse population of cells (chondrocytes) but contains no blood vessels or nerve endings. The endplates of the intervertebral discs are composed of hyaline cartilage. Articular cartilage is a type of hyaline cartilage which covers the opposing surfaces of synovial joints, including the zygapophysial joints in the spine. It provides a low-friction and low-wear bearing surface, and is able to distribute loading evenly on to the underlying bone.

STRUCTURE AND COMPOSITION

The matrix of hyaline cartilage consists mainly of water (70%), collagen (75% of dry weight) and proteoglycans (20% of dry weight). Collagen is described on page 56. Proteoglycan molecules have a protein core, with side chains of the glycosaminoglycan (GAG) molecules chondroitin sulphate and keratin sulphate. The most common proteoglycan (90% of the total) is 'aggrecan', which combines with hyaluronan to form huge aggregates up to 10 μm in length (Fig. 4.10). GAGs attract water electrostatically, and the main role of proteoglycans is to attract and retain water within the tissue. Their tendency to absorb water and swell is resisted by tension in the network of very fine type II collagen fibrils, which holds the cartilage together and anchors it to the subchondral bone (Fig. 4.11). The structure of collagen type II fibrils is similar to that of type I (Fig. 4.7) but only the latter aggregate to form large fibres. Approximately 2% of cartilage collagen is type IX, a non-linear molecule with a projecting GAG side-chain. Type IX binds to the surface of type II fibrils, with its projecting part possibly serving to inter-connect fibrils into a three-dimensional network, or to anchor them in the proteoglycans.[748] Mechanical interactions between collagen and proteoglycans help to resist cartilage deformation,[368,709] but proteoglycan depletion does not reduce the tissue's tensile strength[123,709] possibly because at very high strains, the collagen fibrils interact directly with each other, like tangled threads of cotton.[122] The high water content of articular cartilage enables it to distribute loads evenly between opposing bones, and water loss

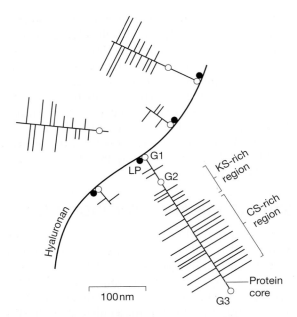

Figure 4.10 Diagram showing the structure of the proteoglycan molecule 'aggrecan'. It has a linear protein core, with three globular regions (G1, G2, G3). Linear side chains of the glycoaminoglycans chondroitin sulphate (CS) and keratin sulphate (KS) attract water into the tissue. Many individual aggrecan units aggregate together by binding on to a long molecule, hyaluronan, by means of their G1 domain. This attachment is stabilised by a link protein (LP). In mature cartilage, many aggrecan molecules are cleaved by enzyme action, leaving small fragments attached to hyaluronan, or lying free in the matrix.

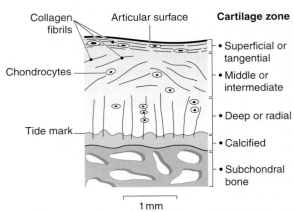

Figure 4.11 Diagrammatic interpretation of the structure of articular cartilage. Some collagen II fibrils anchor cartilage to bone, and others run parallel to the cartilage surface, but their orientation elsewhere is variable, and their length is unknown. Cartilage zones reflect differences in collagen alignment, chemical composition, and cell morphology. Below the 'tide mark', the cartilage matrix is calcified, so that its mechanical properties are intermediate between cartilage and bone.

during sustained loading allows the tissue to deform ('creep') so that the contact area increases, and the contact stress decreases.

The remainder of the cartilage matrix is composed of the small proteoglycans decorin, biglycan and fibromodulin, and non-collagenous proteins including cartilage oligomeric protein (COMP), fibronectin and anchorin. The function of these relatively small molecules is not fully understood, but they appear to regulate the formation of collagen fibrils, and help to bind the matrix components to each other, and to the cells.

Type II collagen fibrils in hyaline cartilage are so fine (10–100 nm in diameter) that they are difficult to visualise ('hyaline' means glassy). However, the gross structure of cartilage can be inferred from scanning electron micrographs of freeze-fractured tissue.[165,388] This evidence is interpreted

in Figure 4.11. The superficial ('tangential') zone has a relatively high proportion of horizontal collagen fibrils which curve over in the proteoglycan-rich middle zone, and become vertical in the radial zone, before entering a region of calcified cartilage below the 'tide mark', which forms a transition between relatively soft cartilage and stiff bone. The uppermost few microns of the tangential zone, the lamina splendens, acts like a tensile skin for the underlying cartilage, and probably plays an important role in maintaining the internal fluid pressure within the tissue.[727]

METABOLISM

Chondrocytes manufacture and turnover the matrix constituents. In adult tissue, cells cease to divide and are normally isolated from each other, each being surrounded by a 'basket' of type II collagen to form a 'chondron'.[388] Cell division, and consequent clustering, can occur when cartilage integrity is threatened, as in osteoarthritis (see below), but new cells do not appear to migrate to the location of any defect,[791] and their metabolic rate is limited by the lack of a blood supply. Nutrients must reach the chondrocytes across long distances of matrix, either by diffusion, which is important for small molecules, or by bulk fluid flow which is important for large molecules.[611]

Matrix breakdown is controlled by enzymes which include the matrix metalloproteases (MMPs) and their tissue inhibitors (TIMPS), both of which are produced by chondrocytes. Some MMPs are called collagenases because they cleave individual collagen molecules at a specific site, causing the triple helix to unwind or 'denature'. Other MMPs (gelatinases) further break down the denatured collagen. A third group of MMPs, the stromelysins, break down other matrix proteins, and also the proteoglycan molecules by cleaving their protein core. A recently discovered enzyme 'aggrecanase', which is chemically distinct from the MMPs, is primarily responsible for the cleavage of aggrecan between the globular domains G1 and G2 (Fig. 4.10) and for the subsequent loss of proteoglycans from cartilage in osteoarthritis.[453,470]

Chondrocyte activity is controlled and coordinated by cytokines, which can be produced locally by the chondrocytes themselves, or by more distant cells such as those in the joint synovium. Cell activity is also influenced by mechanical loading applied to the tissue. The synthesis of matrix constituents is maximal at an applied pressure of 5–15 MPa, and decreases when the loading is greater or less than this.[326] Generally, cyclic loading at moderate load levels tends to stimulate synthesis, whereas prolonged static loading slows it down.[817] The precise nature of the stimulus is unknown: it may be deformation of the cell membrane or cytoskeleton,[317] or changes in the fluid pressurisation within cartilage. Matrix turnover in articular cartilage is much slower than in bone, with the half-life of proteoglycans being weeks or months, depending on distance to the nearest cell. The half life of collagen could exceed 100 years.[826]

Animal experiments have confirmed that physical activity leads to thicker and stiffer cartilage, whereas inactivity or static loading has the opposite effect.[58] Results, however, depend on the size of the animal and the intensity of loading.

For example, voluntary exercise protects cartilage from degenerative changes in hamsters,[622] whereas imposed high-intensity exercise can cause cartilage deterioration in the horse.[572] The difference may be attributable to the 'cube-square law' which explains why heavy animals load their joints more severely than light ones (p. 8). Age may also play a part, because cells from old cartilage are less responsive to mechanical stimuli than cells from young tissue.[515] It is difficult to estimate from these experiments just how much exercise is good for human cartilage, or how quickly, and to what extent, human cartilage can strengthen in response to exercise. It might be expected that strengthening would be slower in cartilage than in bone, because cartilage has no blood supply. Enzymatic breakdown of cartilage, however, could conceivably be rapid. Some degree of articular cartilage adaptation must occur in humans, because variations in its thickness and stiffness across a joint surface correspond to the varying mechanical demands placed upon it.[879]

Cuts to the cartilage surface created by a sharp object do not heal, possibly because many of the cells near the wound edge die.[791] If an injury penetrates the cartilage to reach the subchondral bone, then fibrous tissue can grow from the bone to fill the defect, but this does not integrate well with surrounding articular cartilage: eventually it fails, and the joint becomes degenerated.[731]

AGEING AND DEGENERATION

With increasing age, the number of live cells in cartilage falls, and the matrix shows a range of progressive biochemical changes. Enzyme-mediated cross-linking between adjacent collagen molecules proceeds steadily, with the links becoming increasingly mature (stable). Also, non-enzymatic cross-linking occurs between collagen molecules and reducing sugars such as glucose. These latter reactions are not directly controlled by cells, and are encouraged by low oxygen concentrations in the tissue. They result in advanced glycation end products (AGEs) which discolour the tissue, make it stiffer[62] and inhibit proteoglycan synthesis by chondrocytes.[195]

It is presumed that increased stiffness makes the tissue more brittle, and therefore more vulnerable to injury.[826] This line of research provides a biochemical explanation of why articular cartilage (and other collagenous tissues) weaken with age. Previously, it had been supposed that the reduced strength of old cartilage[420,851] was attributable to fatigue damage accumulating over many years, even though this explanation was never entirely compatible with the known ability of cartilage to strengthen biologically in response to mechanical loading.

The most common degenerative disease to affect articular cartilage is osteoarthritis, which is characterised by cartilage thinning and fibrillation (surface fissuring), and hypertrophy of the subchondral bone, sometimes in the form of osteophytes (bony spurs) around the margins of the joint and sometimes as a more generalised sclerosis (thickening). Within the cartilage, large cell clusters can appear, proteoglycan turnover increases, and degradation of the collagen network allows localised tissue swelling.[63] The causes of osteoarthritis are hotly debated, and many factors appear to be important. 'Bad' inheritance can weaken cartilage and leave it vulnerable to degenerative changes, as typified by the high incidence of osteoarthritis in families with a single gene defect of collagen type II[89,667] and in mice with a defective gene for collagen type IX.[423] Age-related non-enzymatic glycation of cartilage (see above) makes the tissue stiffer and facilitates the onset of osteoarthritis in animal models of the disease.[196] Occupations which involve high loading of certain joints increase the risk of osteoarthritis in those joints.[173] It has been suggested that osteoarthritis is initiated in subchondral bone, and affects cartilage only secondarily.[674] Certainly, it is reasonable to suppose that degenerative changes in either tissue will adversely affect the other,[853] but the evidence from various animal models in support of the 'bone-first' hypothesis merely shows that degenerative changes progress more rapidly in bone, which is the more metabolically active tissue.

Osteoarthritic changes affect the zygapophysial joints of 90% of individuals aged over 40 years.[464,787,886] Early degenerative changes may explain why adult zygapophysial joint cartilage is thinner and softer than knee or hip cartilage, especially around the joint periphery.[777] Degeneration of zygapophysial joints and intervertebral discs is closely related[143,778] with changes in the disc probably coming first.

TENDON AND LIGAMENT

These connective tissues contain a few cells embedded in a fibrous extracellular matrix which is specialised for tensile strength and energy absorption. They have a blood supply, and contain a variety of nerve endings capable of monitoring tissue stress, strain and pain. The essential functional difference between tendons and ligaments is that tendons generally transmit tensile force in one direction only, from muscle to bone, whereas some ligaments must resist the separation of bones in more than one direction. This difference is reflected in the orientation of their collagen fibres, which tend to be longer and more unidirectional in tendons. The chemical and biological properties of the two tissues are similar, although ligaments generally contain slightly less collagen.

STRUCTURE AND COMPOSITION

These tissues consist mostly of a fibrous extracellular matrix containing a few elongated cells, called fibroblasts (in growing tissue) or fibrocytes (in mature, less active tissue). The matrix is 60% water, with the solid component being composed mainly of collagen type I (80%), proteoglycans and elastin. Elastin is a fibrous protein rather like collagen, but it can be stretched much further, and is abundant only in structures such as the ligamentum flavum which require great extensibility (p. 119). Small quantities of proteoglycans help to keep the tissues hydrated, and their presence may partly explain why injured tendons and ligaments can swell slightly. One of the small proteoglycans, decorin, probably acts to regulate the diameter of collagen fibres. Large proteoglycans are present in regions of tendon which are

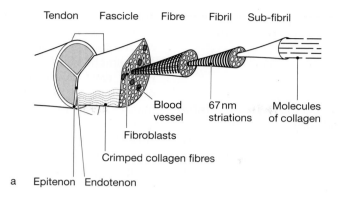

Tendon   Fascicle   Fibre   Fibril   Sub-fibril

Blood vessel   67 nm striations   Molecules of collagen

Fibroblasts

Crimped collagen fibres

a   Epitenon   Endotenon

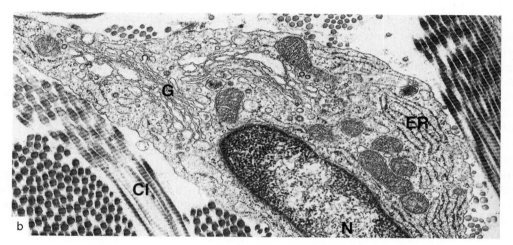

Figure 4.12 (a) Structural hierarchy of collagen in a tendon. Individual fibrils of type I collagen (Fig. 4.7) are grouped to form fibres that have a planer zig-zag shape called 'crimp'. Many fibres are bundled together, along with fibroblasts and blood vessels, to form a fascicle. Each fascicle is surrounded by a sheath of more randomly arranged collagen, the endotenon, and the entire tendon is surrounded by the epitenon. (b) Electron micrograph of tendon fibroblast secreting collagen into the extracellular matrix. Collagen molecules self-assemble into fibrils which appear striped in longitudinal section (Cl) and as dark spots in transverse section (bottom left). Active fibroblasts have a pale nucleus (N), and abundant rough endoplasmic reticulum (ER) and Golgi apparatus (G). Reproduced with permission from Young B, Heath JW 2000 Wheater's Functional Histology, Churchill Livingstone, Edinburgh.

compressed against bone, where they probably serve to maintain tissue hydration, as in articular cartilage (see above).

Most of the collagen is organised in hierarchical fashion[406] from the basic collagen molecule right up to large collagen fibre bundles which can be seen with the naked eye (Fig. 4.12). In both tissues, the gross collagen fibres exhibit a zig-zag planar waveform called 'crimp', which gradually straightens out when the tissue is subjected to high tensile forces.[701] This enables tendons and ligaments to be stretched by approximately 15% (with a stress of 100 MPa) before failure occurs.[705] The main benefit of crimping is that considerable energy is required to straighten out crimps against the elastic resistance of other matrix constituents, and this enables tendons, in particular, to function as giant elastic shock-absorbers during locomotion.[37] With reference to Figure 1.5, the great strength *and* deformability of crimped collagen fibres ensure that the area under the force–deformation curve (the strain energy) is extremely large for a stretched tendon.

METABOLISM

A sparse population of fibroblasts is responsible for the manufacture and turnover of the collagenous matrix. Their metabolic rate is low because tendons and ligaments are poorly vascularised, especially in their central regions, but there is evidence that these tissues can strengthen or weaken in response to changes in applied mechanical load. For example, the strength of spinal longitudinal ligaments is related to the bone mineral content of the vertebrae to which they are attached,[594] suggesting that they have adapted to the same mechanical demands. Spinal fixation, on the other hand, leads to softer and weaker spinal ligaments, presumably as a result of chronic underloading.[438] A tendon must surely adapt in line with any changes in strength of the muscle to which it is attached (p. 53) but it may not be capable of adapting as quickly, and this may explain why 'over-training' injuries so often affect tendons or the musculo-tendinous junction. The nature of mechanical loading, as well as its magnitude, influences the tendon matrix: compressive stresses arising from a tendon passing over a bone may cause the matrix to become more cartilaginous.[289]

Tendon damage can occur as a result of injury or repetitive loading. Achilles tendon ruptures are especially common in young to middle-aged men involved in sporting activities.[463] Fatigue injuries often occur because tendon strength (in-vitro) can fall by up to 90% if one million loading cycles are applied.[705] Injury usually occurs at the musculo-tendinous junction, although collagen fibres can rupture at mid-length, or near their attachment to bone. Damaged fibres are degraded enzymatically as fibroblasts migrate to the injury site to lay down new collagen, and this process is usually a chronic degenerative condition rather than an acute inflammatory one.[422,789] New fibres are thinner than old, and have a disorganised crimp structure, so their original mechanical properties are probably not regained even after 14 months.[298,863] Restoration of collagen fibril diameter is probably essential to restoration of ligament strength,[587] but it is not known if either can recover completely.

Ligament injuries may affect only those fibres which were orientated to resist the damaging movement. In the spine, interspinous ligament injuries are common,[681] and are characterised by apparently non-functional fibres adjacent to a smooth hole filled with fatty deposits.[269,681]

A different type of injury can affect large tendons during vigorous activity. So much heat is produced by the shock-absorbing mechanism (see Fig. 1.5) that the temperature in the poorly-vascularised centre of the tendon rises by more than 5 °C.[868] This is sufficient to denature collagen molecules by unwinding the triple-helix (Fig. 4.7) and to interfere with fibroblast metabolism.[86] However, tendon fibroblasts contain 'heat-shock' proteins which makes them more heat-resistant than fibroblasts in other tissues such as skin.[86]

AGEING AND DEGENERATION

Tendons and ligaments become stronger and stiffer up until skeletal maturity, but then tend to become weaker with increasing age.[78] This may be related to microdamage, and to gradual increases in cross-linking between collagen fibres which makes the fibres fatter and may possibly interfere with the crimping mechanism. Collagen cross-linking is a gradual chemical process which occurs in the test tube as well as in living tissue,[820] and it probably contributes to the deterioration in mechanical properties of many connective tissues in the body, including skin,[679] as discussed on page 61. With increasing age and degeneration, the ligamentum flavum becomes more calcified, and its elastin content falls.[713]

INTERVERTEBRAL DISCS

From an histological perspective, discs are classified as fibrocartilage, but they are really complex structures composed of several different tissues. Their gross structure, innervation and blood supply are considered in Chapters 2 and 3. Many details of intervertebral disc biochemistry and metabolism are assumed to be similar to those of articular cartilage, which has been investigated more thoroughly (see above).

STRUCTURE AND COMPOSITION

Disk tissue varies from a highly-hydrated gel in the centre of the nucleus, to a tough ligamentous fibrocartilage in the outer anulus, while the cartilage component of the endplates resembles amorphous hyaline cartilage. The nucleus is composed of water (70–85%), proteoglycans (50% dry weight) and collagen (less than 20% dry weight). These proportions change gradually towards the outer anulus, which is approximately 50% water, proteoglycans (10% dry weight) and collagen (up to 70% dry weight). The proportion of collagen type I (which is usually found in tensile structures such as ligaments) is highest in the outer anulus, and very low in the inner anulus and nucleus; conversely, collagen type II (which is normal in compressed tissues such as articular cartilage) is abundant in the nucleus, less common in the inner anulus, and absent in the outer anulus.[241,711] There is some evidence from work on tendons that the predominant collagen type can change from type I to type II if the habitual loading of the tissue changes from tension to compression,[289] so the varying collagen distribution in different parts of a disc probably reflects their different mechanical functions. The particularly coarse collagen fibre bundles in the outer anulus display the same crimp pattern seen in tendon and ligaments,[154] and probably for the same reason: to enable them to stretch more, and to absorb more energy before failure (see Fig. 1.5). Approximately 10–15% of disc collagen is type VI, which forms a network of short fibrils within the pericellular matrix. Small quantities of types III, V, IX, XI and XII are also present. Endplate cartilage contains collagen type X[35] which is associated with hypertrophic chondrocytes involved in calcification.

Proteoglycan molecules in the nucleus tend to be smaller, and aggregate less, than in articular cartilage. This is presumably because they are in less danger of diffusing to the edge of the (comparatively large) disc and being lost from the tissue.

METABOLISM

Tissue mechanical function appears to determine cell type. The rounded cells in the nucleus are notochordal during development and growth, but resemble articular cartilage chondrocytes in the adult. The more elongated cells in the outer anulus resemble fibroblasts, and are more deformable.[318] Each disc cell is surrounded by a collagenous 'basket' to form a chondron, with the matrix lying between the cell and basket being rich in collagen III and VI.[684] As in the other skeletal tissues, disc cells manufacture and repair the matrix, but metabolic rates are comparatively very slow because the avascular discs are so large. As far as proteoglycan synthesis is concerned, the most active cells lie in the mid-anulus region, and synthesis rates fall when the water content of the tissue is reduced or increased substantially.[76]

Metabolites of small molecular weight are transported mostly by diffusion, but the movement of large molecules is probably dominated by bulk fluid flow[611] which accompanies variations in physical activity (p. 169). These two processes can be distinguished by imagining a quantity of coloured dye thrown into a slow-moving stream: the spreading out of the dye into a large cloud is due to the random molecular movements which underlie diffusion, and the slow drift of the dye downstream illustrates the effects of bulk fluid flow. There are also two transport routes: through the peripheral anulus, and through the perforated bone and hyaline cartilage of the central regions of the endplates (Fig. 4.13). The high negative fixed charge density of the proteoglycans in the nucleus ensures that negatively-charged ions mostly enter the disc by the anulus route, whereas neutral and positively charged molecules enter by the endplate route.[609] Difficulties in metabolite transport explain the very low cell density in the nucleus, and may underlie many of the processes of ageing and degeneration. The importance of the endplate route in disc nutrition is emphasised by the fact that experimental disc injury, which leads

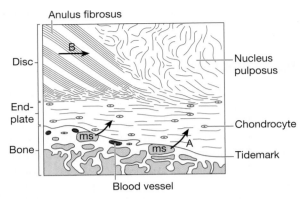

Figure 4.13 Diagram showing part of the vertebral endplate, which consists of a hyaline cartilage layer loosely bonded to a plate of perforated cortical bone. (After Roberts[683] with permission.) Note how the coarse collagen fibres of the anulus blend into the hyaline cartilage of the endplate. There are two routes for metabolite transport into the centre of the avascular disc: (A) through the marrow spaces (ms) of the endplate, and (B) through the anulus. Compare with Plates 1 and 4E.

to rapid biochemical changes in the nucleus,[551] also causes substantial increases in endplate vascularity.[567]

Cells in the nucleus and inner anulus respond to changes in their mechanical environment in a similar manner to the chondrocytes of articular cartilage: very high and very low hydrostatic pressures both decrease proteoglycan synthesis whereas moderate loading increases it.[382] Pressures in excess of 3 MPa (which would be equivalent to moderate manual labour) increase the synthesis of the matrix-degrading enzyme MMP3.[329] Proteoglycan synthesis by cells of the outer anulus is largely unaffected by hydrostatic pressure,[382] probably because they do not normally experience such pressures in life (they are embedded in a fibrous solid rather than a fluid: p. 5). Nucleus cells respond to cyclic stretching by proliferating and producing more collagen[524] suggesting that disc cells may be capable of behaving like fibroblasts or chondrocytes, depending on the prevailing mechanical environment.[328,396] During spinal flexion movements (in-vivo and in-vitro), the posterior anulus can be stretched by 50% or more,[8,312,641] and it remains to be seen what effect such large deformations have on anulus cells.

Disc metabolism is so slow that it is difficult to study in humankind or large animals. Static compressive loading of dog discs appears to stimulate collagen I synthesis and inhibit proteoglycan synthesis in the nucleus pulposus.[374] Requiring dogs to run on a treadmill for up to 40 km per day for one year showed several conflicting changes in the composition and metabolism of the discs: proteoglycan synthesis decreased at some spinal levels, but increased at others,[670] and collagen content and synthesis also were variably affected.[670] A small group of these discs were found to creep significantly more under load, suggesting that adaptive remodelling effects were being countered by the accumulation of fatigue damage during the severe exercise.[193] That discs do strengthen in response to increased mechanical loading is suggested by the finding that the disc's proteoglycan content increases in proportion to the thickness of the subchondral bone.[685] Also, a small cadaveric study showed that people who were most physically active prior to death had the strongest vertebrae and discs when spine motion segments were compressed to failure.[660] However, when specimens were loaded in a manner known to cause either vertebral failure or disc prolapse (p. 148), it was found that failure more often occurred in the disc in those spines from the most physically active people. This evidence, though far from conclusive, does suggest that discs adapt to increased mechanical demands, but more slowly than bones. Discs should therefore be vulnerable to accumulating fatigue damage when the spine is subjected to a sudden increase in the level of mechanical loading.[17] Experiments on rats and mice show that the intervertebral discs in their tails become degenerated following prolonged immobilisation, and that these changes are accelerated by static compressive loading.[378,477]

Discs show only a limited ability to heal following injury, presumably because of the difficulty in remodelling the large collagen fibre bundles of the anulus. In sheep, scalpel-induced peripheral anular tears lead to collagenous scar formation and granulation tissue in the outer anulus, and vascular ingrowth into the middle anulus.[328,396,617] However, few inflammatory cells are found in the disc[400] and the inner regions of the tear do not heal: in fact they continue to progress inwards.[617] Peripheral anular tears lead to reduced proteoglycan and collagen content within the nucleus, both in the affected and adjacent discs, but the anulus itself shows minimal biochemical changes.[551] Experimental enzymatic destruction of the nucleus leads to reduced proteoglycan synthesis,[774] but this later recovers to a certain extent. Proteoglycan–collagen interactions within the anulus[15] may partly explain why old radial fissures can 'heal' in the sense that they do not readily allow nucleus pulposus material to escape, even under severe loading.[11] In contrast, herniated tissue which escapes from the pressurised confines of the disc can undergo extensive biochemical changes, starting with rapid swelling, and leaching of proteoglycans.[213]

INTERVERTEBRAL DISC AGEING

Ageing begins at birth and involves biochemical and functional changes which resemble those found in many collagenous tissues of the body. Discontinuous lamellar 'bundles' have been observed in the posterior anulus of foetal discs,[802] but this is probably normal, and most of the evidence shows that the first age-related changes occur within the nucleus. Old cells appear to slow down and produce less of the proteoglycan molecules that serve to maintain tissue hydration.[490] As a result, proteoglycans become smaller and less aggregated, their overall concentration decreases[126,818] and the water content of the nucleus falls.[9] Brown pigmentation becomes apparent, and is probably indicative of the non-enzymatic glycation reactions[225] which render collagenous tissue more brittle and vulnerable to injury (p. 61). In the centre of large avascular discs, these reactions may well be accelerated by 'oxidative stress' arising from nutritional compromise.[590] Similar changes occur in the cartilage endplates,[88] and accompanying calcification of the endplate may compromise the nutrient supply to the adjacent nucleus (evidence reviewed by Moore[566]). Age-related biochemical changes are less pronounced in the anulus, which has a smaller concentration of proteoglycan and water

to start with. The collagen content of the disc increases with age, and the collagen molecules aggregate into increasingly thick fibrils as more and more non-reducible cross-links are formed between adjacent collagen molecules.[590,650,661] The lamellae themselves become thicker[513] and gross defects in the lamellar structure of the anulus become more frequent after the age of 40.[82]

The functional consequences of ageing are that the nucleus pulposus becomes dry, fibrous and physically stiff,[816] its volume decreases, and the region of inner anulus which exhibits hydrostatic pressure is reduced (pp. 125–126). Consequently, more of the disc's compressive load-bearing is taken by the anulus, especially the posterior anulus.[23] If disc cells are as adaptable as tendon cells, then this profound age-related change in their mechanical environment may influence greatly their appearance and function.[289] The anulus becomes weaker with age,[273] even though increased collagen cross-linking would make it stiffer.[62] This apparent contradiction may be explained by the age-related accumulation of anular defects which would weaken gross tissue samples. Disc height does not generally decrease with age;[433,811] in fact a slight increase in the height of male L4–5 discs was measured in one large study.[265]

INTERVERTEBRAL DISC DEGENERATION

'Degeneration' implies specific and deleterious changes in disc composition, structure and function. Although degeneration can occur at any age, it is much more common in older discs, so much so that many scientists speak of ageing and degeneration as if they were indistinguishable. This is unfortunate, because distinctions can be drawn between them, and a great deal of current research is aimed at making the distinctions clearer still.

Degeneration can involve all of the age-related changes in composition described above, so is difficult to distinguish from accelerated and/or exaggerated ageing. Crucially, however, degeneration also involves gross structural changes which are most evident in the anulus and endplate.[23,126,349,355,823] In the opinion of the authors, the presence of these structural changes should be a defining feature of disc degeneration, because they are not an inevitable consequence of ageing. Structural disruption tends to appear after age 20, and reaches a maximum in middle age rather than old age.[355] The fact that disc degeneration is more prevalent at lower lumbar levels, and in men[555] suggests a strong mechanical influence (see p. 87).

Typical structural changes include circumferential and radial tears in the anulus, inwards buckling of the inner anulus, increased radial bulging of the outer anulus, reduced disc height, endplate defects, and vertical bulging of the endplates into the adjacent vertebral bodies. One particular form of disc disruption (disc prolapse) is considered separately below. Anular tears can be separated into three types (Fig. 4.14), all of which appear to evolve independently of age and of each other, and all of which are common by middle-age.[825] Concentric (circumferential) clefts between adjacent lamellae are very

common, and represent delamination of the anulus. 'Rim lesions' consist of focal circumferential avulsions of the peripheral anulus, sometimes with sclerosis and osteophytosis of the adjacent bone. They are twice as common in the anterior anulus compared to the posterior, and typically affect the upper antero-lateral margin of the disc.[349] The third type of anular tear is the radial fissure, which involves radial disruption of the lamellae, starting from the inner anulus, and sometimes progressing right to the outer margins of the disc so that nucleus pulposus material can escape.[11,19] One of the most common structural defects in the anulus is inwards buckling of the inner lamellae (Plates 1C and 2C). This has been reported in the anterior and posterior anulus of 33% and 4% (respectively) of cadaveric discs of all ages[321] and in 33% of elderly cadaveric discs.[786]

Degeneration affects the cells and chemical composition of the disc. Cell clustering is common, the proportion of collagen types I and VI increases, and concentric rings rich in type III collagen can appear around some cells.[684] Blood vessels and nerves usually grow into the centre of severely degenerated discs, along the margins of clefts and radial fissures.[174,823] The simplest explanation for this is that a healthy disc has a hydrostatic nucleus (see Fig. 8.11A) which would collapse hollow blood vessels and keep them out. A severely degenerated disc, however, has a fibrous nucleus which no longer acts like a pressurised fluid (see Fig. 8.11C) and so allows blood vessels, and accompanying nerves, to grow inwards towards its centre. Matrix-degrading enzymes (including the MMPs and aggrecanase) are produced in greater quantity in degenerated discs, both by the indigenous cells and by invading cells, and enzyme levels are particularly high in herniated discs.[686] Large molecules of fibronectin, which link cartilage cells to their matrix, become more abundant in degenerated discs, and are increasingly fragmented, presumably because of increased enzyme activity.[608] Fibronectin may possibly be involved in the 'paradoxical' reaction of disc cells to structural failure (p. 200).

The various causes of disc degeneration are discussed in Chapter 6. Genetic inheritance 'explains'

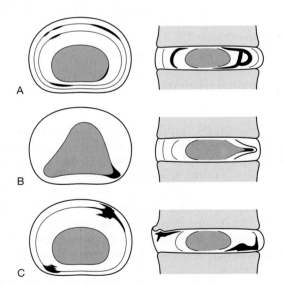

Figure 4.14 There are three common types of anular tear: concentric clefts (A), radial fissures (B), and peripheral rim lesions (C). Disrupted tissue is shown in black, and nucleus pulposus is shaded. Left: discs sectioned in the transverse plane (anterior on top). Right: discs sectioned in the sagittal plane, anterior on left. Compare with Plates 1C, 2D, 3E and 3F.

70% of it,[72,698] but environmental factors, including mechanical loading and nutrition, are also important. Some research publications appear to suggest that cytokines or matrix enzymes 'cause' disc degeneration, but the increased activity of these agents in degenerated discs probably represents an attempt by the tissue to adapt to deteriorating circumstances, rather than an initiating event. (The temptation to blame the messenger for the message should be resisted!)

Degenerative changes within the discs can affect adjacent tissues. Disc degeneration is often accompanied by arthritic changes in the zygapophysial joints, and by osteophytes (Plate 4D) around the margins of the vertebral bodies.[143,349,823]

Disc function is affected more by these degenerative structural changes than by the age-related changes in composition described earlier. Normal discs contain a soft deformable nucleus which exhibits a hydrostatic pressure even when old and pigmented.[23] Degenerated and mechanically disrupted discs, however, have either a very small hydrostatic region, or none at all, and exhibit high localised stress concentrations within the anulus (see Fig. 8.11). It appears that structural damage destroys the disc's ability to distribute compressive stresses evenly on the adjacent vertebrae, so that different parts of the disrupted tissue resist compression in a more-or-less haphazard way. When nucleus pulposus cells are deformed by non-hydrostatic loading, as they would be in a disrupted disc, then they respond by producing more collagen[524] and this could explain why degenerated discs have such a fibrous nucleus. Other mechanical changes in degenerated discs include an increased 'neutral zone' (region of minimal stiffness) in bending and torsion, combined with a reduced range of bending.[558] The range of axial rotation is increased, possibly because of loss of cartilage in the zygapophysial joints.[623]

INTERVERTEBRAL DISC PROLAPSE

Disc prolapse involves a relative displacement between nucleus and anulus which affects the disc surface. Three types of posterior disc prolapse can

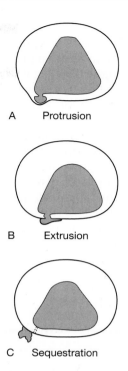

Figure 4.15 Three categories of disc prolapse (or 'herniation') are widely recognised: anulus protrusion (A), nucleus extrusion (B), and sequestration (C). Displaced nucleus tissue loses contact with the remaining nucleus in C, but not in B. Disc sections are drawn in the transverse plane, anterior on top. The site of herniation is usually posterior or postero-lateral, but can be lateral or anterior.[355,467] Distortion of the lamellae of the anulus is not always present. Compare with Plate 3.

be distinguished (Fig. 4.15): disc 'protrusion' in which the anulus bulges markedly but is not ruptured and so allows no contact between nucleus and the extra-discal space; incomplete prolapse or 'extrusion' in which the anulus is ruptured but any expelled nucleus is still attached to the rest of the disc; and complete prolapse, or 'sequestration' in which disc tissue (which may include cartilaginous endplate, especially in older patients[121,335]) is expelled from the disc and is no longer attached to it (modified from: Yasuma[880] and Moore[569]).

In adults, disc herniation shows little correlation with age or other signs of spinal degeneration[829] although it is particularly common at lower lumbar levels. In common with the evidence from epidemiological surveys (pp. 87–88) and experiments on cadaveric spines (p. 148), this suggests that disc prolapse represents a mechanical injury, or fatigue failure, rather than the end-stage in some age-related degenerative process. This is considered in more detail in Chapter 13.

There is increasing evidence that displaced nucleus pulposus can release chemicals such as nitric oxide[119] that cause morphological and functional changes in spinal nerve roots,[615] and which cause pain-related behaviour in laboratory animals.[379,409] This apparent 'pain-sensitisation' effect of displaced nucleus tissue can be modulated by inhibiting the synthesis of nitric oxide.[119] It is not yet clear if nucleus pulposus migrating down a radial fissure can similarly induce pain from the outer anulus, even when the disc is not prolapsed.

CONCLUDING REMARKS

Biological differences between spinal tissues could give rise to problems if the spine has to adapt to changing mechanical demands. The most metabolically active tissue, muscle, can change its size and force-generating capacity by a significant amount in just a few days, and it is muscle which applies most of the high forces to underlying tissues. Bone also has a rich blood supply, but it has a much higher volume of extracellular matrix per cell than does muscle, so it requires several weeks to make substantial changes to its strength and internal architecture. Tendons and ligaments are poorly vascularised, and the high proportion of large collagen type I fibres in their extracellular matrix ensures that it cannot be turned over rapidly. Adaptations in strength are possible, but they are slow, and repair following injury takes many months. The lack of a blood supply, and a low cell density, ensure that articular cartilage responds very slowly to changes in its mechanical environment. Nevertheless, significant adaptations can be measured after 1 year in young animals following exercise. The adaptive potential of mature human cartilage is largely unknown, but is almost certainly lower than that of young animals. Finally comes the lumbar intervertebral discs, the largest avascular structures in the body, with such a low cell density that they are incapable of remodelling the collagen fibre bundles of the anulus within the working lifetime of an adult. Structural damage to a disc may be patched up with scar-like tissue, but it is not fully repaired.

Consider now some consequences of these marked differences in tissue biology. Suppose a young man starts his first manual job, with a back that has been mechanically conditioned to attending school and watching television. In the new job, his muscles will presumably strengthen quickly, and his vertebrae will soon catch up. But what will happen to his tendons, to his zygapophysial joints, and his lumbar discs? What if the man is not so young, or healthy, when he starts this manual job? The research summarised in this chapter indicates that the man's spinal tissues will be unable to adapt as quickly as his muscles, especially if he is middle aged, and that the biggest problem will confront his intervertebral discs.

As another example, consider the future of an intervertebral disc that lies next to a damaged vertebral body endplate. (Minor damage to these endplates, or to the trabeculae which support them, is very common in life.[824]) The vertebra will heal rapidly, perhaps with a few micro-calluses to mark the site of injury.[824] However, the nucleus of the disc adjacent to the damaged endplate will be decompressed (p. 137) and this may leave it incapable of manufacturing sufficient matrix to restore its normal volume and pressure. Accordingly, more of the force on the disc would be resisted by the anulus rather than the nucleus, creating long-term problems for the disc rather than the adjacent bone.

Potential problems arising from the different adaptive potential of adjacent tissues remain to be investigated. Two longitudinal epidemiological studies have produced some evidence to suggest that strengthening muscles can pose a threat to the underlying spine during the first year of an arduous job,[24,430] but more work is required to rule out alternative explanations. In the mean time, the results of cross-sectional occupational surveys should be treated with some caution, because their study populations are likely to be self-selected to a certain extent: people with particularly weak backs are unlikely to survive long in the most arduous jobs, and those who do survive will include those whose backs have adapted successfully to the rigours of the job. This situation is aptly described by Nietzsche: 'what does not kill him makes him stronger!' Conversely, sedentary jobs will attract a proportion of those people who leave more arduous work because of back problems. In this way, cross-sectional surveys may systematically underestimate the adverse effects of mechanical loading on poorly vascularised spinal tissues.

5

Low back pain

In principle, any of the structures of the lumbar spine that receives an innervation could be a source of back pain. Accordingly, back pain could arise from any of the ligaments, muscles, fasciae, joints or discs of the lumbar spine. Moreover, it is quite easy to invent an explanation of how any of these structures could be affected by injury or disease in order to become painful. It is another matter, however, to prove that such explanations are realistic and obtain in a given patient.

EXPERIMENTAL STUDIES

Experimental studies in normal volunteers and patients have shown that noxious stimulation of the back muscles,[415] interspinous ligaments,[250,416] dura mater,[238,749] zygapophysial joints,[270,527,564] and the sacroiliac joint[258] can produce local and referred pain similar in quality and distribution to that seen in patients. These data corroborate that these structures can indeed be a source of back pain, but alone they do not prove what causes pain in a particular patient. The distribution of pain in a given patient does not imply any particular source.

It has been more difficult to demonstrate in normal volunteers that the discs can be painful. In individuals with intact, normal discs, discography is not painful, as a rule.[845] The intact laminae of the inner anulus fibrosus prevent the outer, innervated lamina from being distended by increased nuclear pressure. It is only in patients in whom the disc is internally disrupted that provocation discography is painful. However, probing the posterior anulus fibrosus in patients undergoing laminectomy under local anaesthesia, evokes back pain.[446,855] Indeed, the posterior anulus is the most potent source of back pain under these conditions.[446] Thus, the disc can be a source of pain, if it is affected by pathology that involves or compromises the sensitive, outer anulus.

RED FLAG DISORDERS

Tumours and infections can affect any of the spinal and paraspinal tissues of the back. They are, however, quite uncommon as causes of back pain in primary care. The prevalence of tumours is 0.7%[201] and that of infections less than 0.01%.[202]

Fractures can befall the lumbar vertebral bodies or any of their processes, but are also uncommon causes of back pain in individuals without a reason for a fracture. Such reasons are moderate to severe trauma, or a risk factor for osteoporosis, such as age or use of corticosteroids.

The vast majority of patients with back pain do not have any of these red flag disorders, so named because they pose a threat to the general health of the patient, and should be recognised as soon as possible. Most patients have some other disorder that is the basis of their pain. However, although many contentions abound, few have been validated.

LIGAMENT SPRAIN

Ligament sprain is an attractive explanation for acute low back pain following exertion or effort. However, the criteria prescribed for this diagnosis by the International Association for the Study of Pain (IASP)[553] require that the ligament be specified, and that the diagnosis be made by reliable and valid tests specific for that ligament. In contemporary practice these criteria cannot be satisfied. There are no reliable and valid clinical tests. Palpation for tenderness is not specific for

sprain of an underlying ligament, and no active or passive motion test has been shown to be specific for ligament sprain in the lumbar spine.

Selective injection of the suspected ligament with local anaesthetic is an attractive, target-specific test for ligament pain, but it has not been rigorously evaluated. Some studies report a 14%[759] or 10%[858] prevalence of interspinous ligament pain, diagnosed by local anaesthetic blocks, but no such studies have been controlled for false-positive responses. No other ligaments of the lumbar spine have been so investigated. If ligament sprain is a cause of back pain, it is uncommon.

MUSCLE SPRAIN

The IASP criteria for muscle sprain require that the muscle be specified and that sprain be diagnosed by reliable and valid tests.[553] Tenderness over muscles is an insufficient sign, for it is neither reliable nor valid. Such tenderness may be quite non-specific. Motion tests are not specific for muscle sprain. Virtually any cause of low back pain could impair motion in the same way.

MUSCLE SPASM

Muscle spasm is a diagnosis that is both unreliable and invalid. Inter-observer agreement on the detection of muscle spasm is extremely poor,[843] and there is no independent objective correlate of muscle spasm against which the diagnosis might be validated. Studies have failed to demonstrate electromyographic or other features that independently correlate with pain from the allegedly affected muscle.[42]

TRIGGER POINTS

Myofascial pain is an attractive explanation for back pain that is widely entertained. However, it lacks both reliability and validity. Inter-observer agreement about the presence of trigger points in the back muscles, quadratus lumborum and gluteus medius is poor,[42,843] and there are no objective correlates for this entity. Its pathophysiology is unknown.

ILIAC CREST SYNDROME

Tenderness over the superomedial aspect of the posterior superior iliac spine is a common feature in patients with back pain.[169] Moreover it is readily recognised. Inter-observer agreement is quite good for this sign.[603] However, there are no objective data as to its significance. It has variously been interpreted by different authors as a sign of muscle sprain, sprain of the iliolumbar ligament, or non-specific tenderness.

SEGMENTAL DYSFUNCTION

Although recognised by the IASP,[553] this entity is relatively ambiguous. It amounts to physical examination indicating that something is wrong at a particular spinal segment. However, the nature of the abnormality is entirely speculative or non-specific. It may amount to zygapophysial joint pain, discogenic pain, muscle tightness, or any combination of these or other conjectures. Objective evidence is lacking. Moreover, no studies have shown that two observers can consistently agree on this diagnosis.

DURAL PAIN

Although it is well-established that the dura mater can be a source of back pain and referred pain, there are no data on the pathology that might cause dural pain. Dural tethering has not been validated by any objective investigations, and no clinical test has been shown to be reliable or valid for dural pain. It is conceivable that the dura could be involved in inflammatory reactions to prolapsed disc material in the epidural space, but this model has not been explored.

SPONDYLOLYSIS

Spondylolysis is an acquired defect in the pars interarticularis, usually affecting the L5 or L4 vertebra. It arises most commonly as a result of fatigue failure of the pars following repeated extension or flexion, or in twisting movements of the lumbar spine (p. 156). However, it is present in some 7% of asymptomatic individuals.[570] Its radiographic presence, therefore, is not diagnostic of the cause of pain. The condition is more common in athletes, in whom the imperative lies in diagnosing the condition before fracture occurs, i.e. while the pars is being stressed and first becoming painful. Bone scan is the singular means of diagnosing this phase of the condition. In patients with frank fracture of the pars, painful fractures can be distinguished from painless, incidental defects, by anaesthetising the defect.

SACROILIAC JOINT PAIN

Traditional clinical tests for sacroiliac joint pain have been shown to be very reliable but quite invalid.[224] The only proven means of diagnosing this condition are intra-articular sacroiliac joint blocks. Using such blocks, controlled studies have shown that the prevalence of sacroiliac joint pain is about 20% in patients with chronic low back pain below L5–S1.[717,496] Its prevalence amongst patients with acute back pain is unknown.

Data on the pathology of sacroiliac joint pain are meagre. Inflammatory disorders are uncommon. In patients with ostensibly mechanical sacroiliac joint pain, there is a suggestion that sprain or rupture of the anterior sacroiliac ligament is the most likely pathology.[717]

ZYGAPOPHYSIAL JOINT PAIN

Despite several studies, no clinical test, or combination of tests, has been shown to be diagnostic of pain stemming from the lumbar zygapophysial joints.[718,719,720] However, these are a potent source of low back pain. Controlled studies using diagnostic blocks of these joints have shown that, in an elderly population, the prevalence of zygapophysial joint pain is about 40%.[718] In younger, injured workers, the prevalence is only about 10–15%.[719] This figure is nonetheless substantial.

There are no data that directly link zygapophysial joint pain with any demonstrable pathology. There are no features evident on CT that correlate with the joint being painful.[722] However, biomechanics studies and post-mortem studies indicate what might be the underlying pathology.

Forced extension of the lumbar spine causes injuries to the zygapophysial joints, in which the joint capsule is disrupted by posterior rotation of the inferior articular process.[878] Torsion injuries to the lumbar spine can cause impaction fractures on the contralateral side, and avulsions of the capsule on the ipsilateral side.[247] In patients with a history of lumbar trauma who undergo postmortem, capsular injuries and small fractures have been demonstrated in the zygapophysial joints.[788,814] Such lesions are absent in subjects with no history of trauma. The challenge remains, however, to demonstrate such lesions in living patients with proven painful zygapophysial joints.

DISCOGENIC PAIN

Discogenic pain cannot be diagnosed clinically with any degree of certainty. Conventional medical examination offers no signs that are specific for lumbar discogenic pain.[721] Testing for centralisation and peripheralisation of pain offers positive correlations with proven discogenic pain,[223] but the correlations fall short of being diagnostic.[99] They offer a positive likelihood ratio barely greater than 2, which means that the odds in favour of the diagnosis before the test is performed are increased by only a factor of 2 if and once the test is positive. In this instance, the pre-test prevalence of internal disc disruption is 40%,[721] which amounts to a pre-test odds of 40:60. A likelihood ratio of 2 converts the odds to 80:60, which amounts to a diagnostic confidence of only 57%.

The mainstay for diagnosing discogenic pain is disc stimulation and discography. This is achieved by injecting the nucleus pulposus of the target disc with contrast medium. The critical component of the test is whether or not injection reproduces the patient's accustomed pain. Secondarily, the contrast medium outlines the shape of the nucleus and the interior of the disc. The recommended criterion for discogenic pain is that the patient's pain is reproduced by disc stimulation provided that stimulation of adjacent discs does not reproduce their pain.[553] This form of control is necessary to avoid false-positive interpretations of single-level disc stimulation.

Internal disc disruption (IDD) appears to be the cardinal pathological basis for lumbar discogenic pain (p. 136). This condition is characterised by disruption of the internal architecture of the disc, perhaps in the form of radial fissures extending from the nucleus to the outer anulus.[92] The further the radial extent, the more likely the disc is to be painful.[821] The pathology, however, is confined to the interior of the disc. Its outer perimeter remains essentially intact. Population studies, using multivariate analysis, have shown that general age-related disc degeneration does not correlate with discogenic pain, but radial fissures do.[562] This is discussed on page 85.

Internal disc disruption can be diagnosed on the basis of a positive response to controlled disc stimulation, coupled with the demonstration of radial fissures on CT-discography. According to these criteria, the prevalence of IDD is at least 40% in patients with chronic low back pain.[721] Another means of diagnosis is the demonstration of a high-intensity zone on MRI of the posterior anulus. This zone represents circumferential extension of a radial fissure between the outer laminae of the anulus fibrosus, and is apparent on MRI when the plane of section transects the long axis of the circumferential fissure. This sign, however, is evident in only about 30% of patients, but when present it is highly predictive of the affected disc being painful.[55,94,383,706]

Although the presence of IDD can be demonstrated by CT-discography, its aetiology remains in dispute. IDD may arise as a result of degradation of the nuclear matrix following fracture of a vertebral endplate.[92] Perhaps as a result of an inflammatory reaction, or as a result of a disturbance to the pH of the nucleus, the proteoglycans of the nucleus de-aggregate, and the water-binding capacity and the load-bearing capacity of the nucleus is compromised. More stress is transferred to the anulus (p. 136). Radial fissures develop either as a result of mechanical stress in the disc (p. 149), or as a result of peripheral extension of the degradation of the nuclear matrix. The disc becomes painful as a result of a combination of inflammation about the peripheral end of the radial fissure, and increased strain in the few remaining intact laminae of the outer anulus fibrosus.[92]

Discs painful on discography exhibit abnormal stress profiles.[383,547] Loads applied to the disc are not borne uniformly. Stress concentrations in the nucleus are erratic and low, but are high in the anulus fibrosus, particularly posteriorly.[547] Similar patterns of stress distribution can be produced experimentally by subjecting the disc to compression loading which fractures the vertebral endplate (p. 137).[26,30,94] Coincident with this failure is a sudden increase in loading of the posterior anulus fibrosus. These data suggest that IDD is an acquired lesion most likely due to fatigue failure of the vertebral endplate.

DISC PROLAPSE

Discogenic pain and IDD need to be distinguished from disc prolapse. Discogenic pain means pain arising as a result of stimulation of nociceptive nerve endings in the intervertebral disc. It requires and implies a pathological process confined to the disc which is capable of stimulating its intrinsic nerve fibres. IDD is one such condition. Another is discitis. In both conditions, the external contour of the disc is essentially normal, for the pathology lies within the substance of the disc. In IDD, although the structure of the anulus fibrosus is disrupted, the outer anulus is intact, at least macroscopically. In particular, the anulus fibrosus does not bulge outwards, and no nuclear material is displaced beyond the normal perimeter of the disc.

Disc prolapse involves displacement of a mixture of nuclear and anular material beyond the normal perimeter of the disc, usually into the vertebral canal or intervertebral foramen (p. 69). The nuclear material is displaced through a radial fissure in the anulus fibrosus, where it gathers debris from the anulus. The prolapse may be contained, in that it remains covered by a layer of anulus fibrosus or by the posterior longitudinal ligament; or the prolapsed material may breach this covering layer, in which case it is sometimes described as an extrusion. If the prolapsed material loses continuity with material still within the disc, it is described as a sequestrated fragment.

Disc prolapse may be totally asymptomatic. Indeed, it occurs in some 24% of asymptomatic individuals,[90,389] and with increasing frequency with advancing age.[389] If disc prolapse does become symptomatic, it does so by compromising a spinal nerve or its roots. The classical symptom is radicular pain (sciatica). This pain is perceived as a shooting or lancinating pain in the lower limb, and is quite distinct from either back pain or somatic referred pain in the lower limb. Radicular pain is also usually, but not necessarily, associated with objective neurological signs (of weakness or numbness) in the distribution of the nerve roots affected.

Radicular pain is caused by inflammation of the affected nerve roots, by compression of the dorsal root ganglion or its blood supply, or by microscopic damage to the nerve roots. Compression of the roots is not a critical factor for the genesis of pain, for radicular pain can occur in the absence of frank compression, and pain may be relieved despite the persistence of compression.

Patients with radicular pain may complain of back pain. However, their cardinal complaint is of pain in the lower limb. Indeed, a classical feature of disc prolapse is pain in the lower limb worse than in the back. The back pain has traditionally been ascribed to the disc prolapse, but the relationship is both imperfect and specious.

There is a positive correlation between disc prolapse and back pain,[101] but the relationship is weak, for reasons discussed on page 201. Some disc prolapses are associated with back pain but the majority are not.[389] Meanwhile, most patients with back pain do not have disc prolapses.

In patients with a disc prolapse, back pain can arise in a variety of possible ways, none of which involve inflammation or compression of nerve roots. The prolapsed disc material may irritate the dura of the nerve root sleeve (p. 70), in which case the back pain arises from stimulation of nociceptive nerves in the dura mater. If the pro-lapsed material is contained, it may cause pain by stretching the overlying anulus fibrosus or posterior longitudinal ligament. Alternatively or additionally, the back pain that the patient suffers may be unrelated to the actual disc prolapse and arises from the IDD that may have preceded the prolapse.[223] The latter is most concordant with clinical experience that records that excision of prolapsed disc material is very effective for the relief of leg pain but offers no guarantee for the relief of back pain.

SYNOPSIS

Although many lesions have been implicated as the cause of low back pain, few are supported by objective evidence. Tumours, infections and fractures are rare. Ligament sprains and muscle sprains are attractive explanations for acute low back pain, but there are no clinical features by which these conditions might be reliably and validly diagnosed. Muscle spasm and trigger points are neither reliable nor valid diagnoses. Spondylolysis is most often asymptomatic, but is perhaps a cause of back pain in athletes. Data are lacking on the diagnosis and prevalence of dural pain.

The best available data implicate the sacroiliac joint, the zygapophysial joints and the inter-vertebral discs as the leading sources of chronic low back pain. Sacroiliac joint pain accounts for some 20% of patients, but its pathology remains unknown. Zygapophysial joint pain accounts for some 10–15% of patients. Small fractures or tears of the joint capsule are the most likely lesions in injured patients. Discogenic pain caused by inter-nal disc disruption accounts for some 40% of patients. This condition can be diagnosed by CT-discography. Circumstantial evidence favours fatigue failure of the vertebral endplate as the cause of this condition.

6

Epidemiology of low back trouble

INTRODUCTION

The epidemiology of low back trouble is a huge subject which could fill a book on its own. The following selective account aims to summarise the evidence which is most pertinent to the title of this book, and in particular to indicate the relative importance of mechanical, biological and psychological influences on the phenomenon of back pain.

Epidemiology has been defined as 'the study of how diseases occur in different groups of people, and why'.[167] It serves to put a problem into perspective; it provides information on a number of aspects that are necessary to understand the problem and inform possible solutions. That information may include the magnitude and consequences of the problem, its natural history, and the identification of its major risk factors.

SYMPTOMS, PATHOLOGY AND DISABILITY

The title of this chapter, with the word 'trouble' replacing the more usual 'pain', needs some explanation. It reflects some of the difficulties faced when discussing the epidemiology of low back problems which do not constitute a single identifiable disease. Before the population 'at risk' can be characterised, it is necessary to establish just what is being studied.

The term low back trouble (LBT) covers a range of symptoms and pathology which are not necessarily closely related to each other. Direct experience of LBT ranges from occasional twinges of discomfort to severe and persistent symptoms. LBT can also be used to refer to the consequences of back pain, including disability, work absence, and litigation, so epidemiology needs to consider not only the reported symptoms, but also their effects on life. The difficulty, in epidemiological terms, is compounded by the fact that there is usually no clinically identifiable diagnosis (or disease process) that can be identified reliably as the source of symptoms. There are, of course, various pathological states that occur in spinal structures but often they do not readily fit a traditional 'disease' model, which further complicates epidemiological study.

The basic epidemiology of LBT will be considered under three main headings: symptoms (pain in the lower back and/or legs), pathology (disc disorders and other degenerative changes) and disability (limitation of daily activities and/or work). Each of these may variously be associated with care-seeking. Four additional sections will then consider the influence of specific risk factors for LBT (other than age and gender), grouped under the following headings: genetic, individual, environmental and psychosocial. Social influences will not be covered in detail, and specific disease processes such as infection, tumours, osteoporosis and spondylolysis lie outside the scope of this review.

RISK FACTORS

Risk factors for LBT can be grouped in various ways (Fig. 6.1), and this 'taxonomy' is important when it comes to interpreting the epidemiological evidence. Genetic risk factors are risks associated with specific genes inherited from parents. They can be studied by comparing disease prevalence in unrelated people and in identical twins, with the confounding influence of childhood environment being controlled for by comparing identical with non-identical twins. It is relatively easy to show the overall influence of genetic inheritance on a given disease, but the techniques of molecular biology are required to identify which particular gene or genes are responsible for the increased risk. 'Individual' risk factors such as body height,

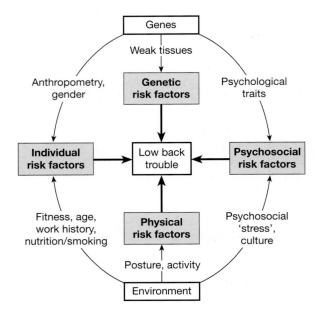

Figure 6.1 Suggested classification of risk factors for low back trouble, indicating possible relationships to each other.

weight, and spinal mobility are considered separately because they are partly genetic and partly environmental: for example, you might be born with a predisposition to obesity which nevertheless requires access to sufficient food to be fully realised. Individual risk factors are of practical importance because most are easy to quantify, and so could conceivably be employed in the workplace to identify those at risk of LBT. Environmental risk factors for LBT mostly concern the physical environment, such as occupation and sporting activities, but also include nutritional factors, smoking, and social policy. Psychosocial risk factors include clinical factors such as depressive mood and somatisation, attitudes and beliefs about the activity/pain/damage relationship, and occupational psychosocial interactions.

Biomechanical risk factors need not be environmental. The inheritance of small intervertebral discs, for example, or short spinous processes (see Fig. 7.2) could increase the compressive stress acting on the discs. Alternatively, the inheritance of defective collagen or proteoglycans could weaken spinal tissues so that they are more vulnerable to injury.

THE NATURE OF EPIDEMIOLOGICAL EVIDENCE

'Systematic reviews' assemble the evidence in a given subject area from previously published 'source' papers, which are systematically identified and graded for methodological quality according to pre-set criteria. Systematic reviews are the foundation of evidence-based medicine, and are particularly well suited to evaluate the results from clinical trials of treatments where the randomised controlled trial is the scientifically preferred methodology. However, systematic reviews are less well suited to examining other types of evidence where it is more difficult to specify acceptable investigative methodologies and exclusion criteria. Interesting studies can sometimes be excluded on the grounds of perceived methodological limitations, some of which might have limited bearing on the results presented. Systematic reviews are less likely to introduce bias than narrative reviews, but they can come to inconsistent findings that are not entirely due to the variable quality of the papers reviewed.[271] Another potential problem is that the evidence from a few innovative source papers can be swamped by that from more mundane studies. It is all too easy to fail to find a statistical relationship between two variables if they are not quantified very well, even though the study itself is well designed. For example, it would be difficult to establish a statistical association between disc degeneration and back pain if the term 'degeneration' was used to include any age-related changes visible on magnetic resonance imaging (MRI), and if 'back pain' was used to include self-reporting of even the mildest symptoms. As a result, systematic reviews have a tendency to come to somewhat nihilistic conclusions.

'Meta-analyses' pool and analyse data from multiple studies. As far as epidemiology is concerned, they can have similar limitations to systematic reviews, and consequently their results can be negative (e.g. 'no predictive value') for reasons discussed above.

The evidence presented in this chapter will be based largely on recent systematic reviews, because this is the most appropriate way of summarising a large body of evidence in an impartial manner, while at the same time giving due attention to its methodological quality. However, several well-focused and incisive source papers are also discussed, because they can give additional insights, emphasis and direction in certain areas.

EPIDEMIOLOGICAL TERMINOLOGY

Two key concepts in epidemiology are incidence and prevalence. Incidence is the percentage of individuals in a given population who develop a disease during a specified period of time. Prevalence is the percentage of individuals in a given population who have a disease during a specified period of time. Typical prevalence rates are lifetime, 1-month and 1-year prevalence, with point prevalence being the percentage with the disease at a given moment in time.

The influence of specific risk factors is sometimes expressed in terms of R^2 (where R is the correlation coefficient). An R^2 value of 0.56 means that 56% of the disease prevalence is statistically associated with the risk factor in question. This could mean that the risk factor is entirely responsible for the disease in 56% of people, or that it contributes 56% of the risk in each person, or anything in between.

'Odds ratios' usually express the increased or decreased risk of disease associated with having a particular factor. In the case of a continuous variable such as body height, it is customary to define the odds ratio (OR) in terms of two different values: for example, it could refer to the increased risk associated with having a body height equal to the mean of the population plus one standard deviation, compared to having a height equal to the mean minus one standard deviation. An OR of 4.5 means that risk is increased by a factor of 4.5, which is equivalent to saying that the risk is increased by 350%. If a risk factor is relatively rare in the population studied, then it is usual to express its influence in terms of an odds ratio (or 'relative risk', which is similar) but if the risk factor is common, then its influence is more likely to be expressed in terms of R^2. If a risk factor is rare, but decisive whenever it does occur, then it will have a high OR, but low R^2.

Statistical significance is expressed in terms of a probability 'P'. It is conventional to accept a relationship between two variables as being statistically significant if there is a less than one-in-20 (5%) probability that it is simply due to chance ('$P < 0.05$'). Note that P does not indicate how important or strong the relationship is: a large epidemiological survey may be able to detect small influences (low R^2) with high probability (low P) simply because data were collected from a large number of subjects. For example, smoking is a highly significant but relatively unimportant risk factor for intervertebral disc degeneration (see below).

SYMPTOMS

BACK PAIN AND SCIATICA IN ADULTS

It is important to appreciate that pain is a symptom which may reveal little or nothing about the nature of any underlying disorder or disease. Thus, in large part, epidemiological studies of low back pain tell us about the people who experience the symptom, and how they experience it. Of necessity, the data-collection method is restricted to questionnaires in which the precise wording of the questions influences the responses, and leads to difficulties when comparing surveys. For example, descriptions of the location of back pain differ between surveys, as does its definition. Some studies take the precaution of specifying the type of pain (e.g. 'low back pain other than the normal aches and pains after, say, gardening'), but others simply ask about 'pain in the back'. As a result, some studies record what may be considered troublesome symptoms while others will include trivial discomfort. By way of example, one recent study found that some physical risk factors were significant predictors of 'serious' low back pain (which involved medical consultation or time off work) but they did not predict

more trivial backache,[24] so the definition of pain is important.

In addition, studies use different target populations, ranging from community suveys to investigation of specialised groups. Not surprisingly, the literature reports differing incidence and prevalence rates for back pain in different populations. However, a recent review concluded that most international studies of adult back pain report a point prevalence of 15% to 30%, a 1-month prevalence of 19% to 43% and a lifetime prevalence of 60% to 70%.[585] No substantial difference in prevalence rates for back pain can be established across the developed countries and, indeed, similar prevalence rates seem to occur in native populations.[362] The fact that between 40% and 90% of people with back pain also report pain in other (perhaps unrelated) regions, suggests that back pain should not necessarily be considered a local pain problem.[577,678,840] The lifetime prevalence of back pain in adults does not seem to increase substantially with age,[678] indeed there is some evidence that the prevalence decreases modestly in older people,[577] although back pain in the elderly has not been well-investigated.[108]

The 'true' incidence rate (first ever onset) for back pain is especially difficult to determine, partly because of the high but poorly recalled prevalence in adolescence (see below). The incidence rate for new 'episodes' of back pain is more easily determined, but again estimates vary. The most recent, robust evidence in the UK comes from the South Manchester Back Pain Study, which found a 1-year incidence rate of 36%, with 40% of these being reported as the first-ever episode.[181] Reigo[678] found a somewhat lower 1-year incidence of 24% for a new episode in Sweden.

The symptom of sciatica should be considered separately, but robust epidemiological data are scarce. Whilst leg pain (as a referred symptom associated with back pain) is not uncommon – perhaps occurring in about 35% of cases – the lifetime prevalence of true sciatica as determined by strict diagnostic criteria is far lower, amounting to between 2% and 5%, with a slight preponderance in males.[585] Sciatica is strongly associated with herniated lumbar discs, peaking between the ages of 40 and 45 years. Obesity is predictive of sciatica only when patients are considerably overweight.[577]

BACK PAIN IN CHILDREN

Adolescents seem to have prevalence rates similar to those for adults, although the pain is readily forgotten, and disability is rare.[137] The lifetime prevalence in children rises from 12% at age 11 to 50% at age 15, when the point prevalence reaches 13%. There is insufficient evidence to conclude that childhood back pain, in itself, is a predictor of adult back pain, but seemingly familial factors may be important.[577] Radiological abnormalities in adolescence were not found to be predictive of adult back pain during a 25-year follow-up in one study,[337] but another study[697] found that early evolution of degenerative changes in the lower lumbar discs predicts the reporting of persistently recurrent symptoms up to age 23.

THE TIME COURSE OF BACK PAIN

Back pain is conventionally described as acute, subacute or chronic. Wood and Badley[873] proposed a simple taxonomy based on their review of the epidemiology in the late 1970s, in which there are three classes: the transient twinges experienced by most people, acute episodes of pain experienced by many, and chronic back pain and disability afflicting a minority. The authors raised the interesting (but unanswered) question: are chronic backs chronic from the beginning, or do they develop from an unfavourable response to acute pain? It is now becoming apparent that the overall picture of the complaint is that of a recurrent, intermittent and episodic phenomenon, leading to a new epidemiological concept of looking at the pattern of pain over long periods of the individual's life.[585,840] This view is well supported by the evidence. A careful prospective study showed that 75% of patients presenting to primary care had failed to recover completely in terms of pain and disability after 1 year, leading the authors to suggest that we should stop characterising low back pain as a series of acute

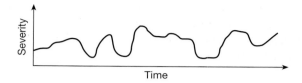

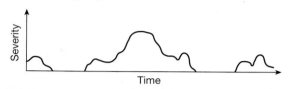

Figure 6.2 Conceptual pattern of low back pain over a period of years. Top: fluctuating severity of symptoms with no pain-free periods. Bottom: fluctuating severity of symptoms with episodic pattern. (After[179,200,840,850].)

problems, and accept it as a chronic problem.[180] Another study, in manipulative practice, found that 70% of patients reported multiple episodes during the follow-up period of 4 years.[140] It is apparent that even persistent (chronic) presentations are characterised by a fluctuating level of symptoms and disability, rather than a constant dismal state.

This conceptualization of adult back pain is illustrated diagrammatically in Figure 6.2, which shows examples of 'typical' lifetime patterns of fluctuating symptoms of varying severity. The key feature suggested by the epidemiology is one that Croft et al. described as 'a chronic problem with an untidy pattern of grumbling symptoms and periods of relative freedom from pain and disability interspersed with acute episodes, exacerbations and recurrences'[180] which is incompatible with frequently voiced claims that 80–90% of episodes of back pain end in complete recovery. Croft's description neatly accommodates the fact that the best single predictor of future back pain is a previous history of back pain; this has been consistently demonstrated and substantially outweighs any other predictor.[24,505,577,633,678,841]

Back pain, then, can be considered a common complaint affecting most people at some point in their lives, and for the majority will be a recurrent event. This depiction is somewhat generalist (for that is the nature of the evidence) and it is accepted that for some individuals the pattern may be different – this is true for any disease or disorder – but the reasons for that variation can be obscure.

CARE-SEEKING

The extent to which the experience of back pain provokes care-seeking helps to put the problem into perspective. A community survey[849] found that only about 50% of people sought treatment for their back pain during a 12-month period. Consultation for episodes lasting less than 2 weeks was associated with greater than median pain; consultation for episodes lasting more than 2 weeks was associated with increased disability; and consultation for episodes lasting more than 3 months was associated with increased depression.[849] Even for those consulting their General Practitioner, only about 10% continue to attend beyond 3 months despite the fact that they are experiencing symptoms and disability.[180] By contrast, care-seeking can be common for recurrences of back pain: most patients attending an osteopathic clinic generally returned to the same osteopath with recurrences during a 4-year follow-up period.[140] The same has been reported for patients visiting chiropractors.[150] Hadler[324] suggested that this recurrent/chronic nature of the back pain experience is an indication that what many patients are saying when they consult is not simply 'My back hurts', but 'My back hurts, but the reason I'm here is that I can't cope on my own any longer'.

PATHOLOGY

Various pathologies affecting the lumbar spine, and potential sources of pain, are considered briefly in Chapters 4 and 9. The present section considers the epidemiology of only the most common conditions, including intervertebral disc herniation and degeneration, zygapophysial joint osteoarthrosis, spinal stenosis, spondylolisthesis,

and segmental instability. It should be remembered that most patients who present to primary health care with simple backache (by far the largest proportion of complaints) have no objectively identified pathology to account for that pain.[95,256] This may indicate either a failure of current clinical methods to identify pathology, or a true absence of significant pathology.

INTERVERTEBRAL DISC HERNIATION AND DEGENERATION

Unlike symptoms, certain types of pathology constitute a 'hard' (objective) outcome measure that may be easier to link to causative risk factors. (Hence the epidemiologists' joke about the hardest of all outcome measures: 'where there's death, there's hope!') Disc herniation (or extrusion – as opposed to simple protrusion or bulge) is one such hard outcome, because it can be visualized on MRI with a fair degree of reproducibility, and it is not consistently associated with any other age-related findings on MRI scans.[387,829] Evidently it is a pathological entity in its own right, and should not be included with disc degeneration. Nevertheless, the epidemiology of back pathology remains at the mercy of the variable methodological designs of reported studies[803] and the problem of interpreting spinal images,[48] which may lead to uncertainties and inconsistencies; furthermore, a clear distinction between disc herniation and disc degeneration has not always been made.

Disc herniation, whilst being the major cause of sciatica, does not necessarily produce symptoms. MRI scans reveal disc herniations in many asymptomatic volunteers: Boden et al.[90] found at least one herniated disc in 20% of those aged 60 years or less, and in 36% of older subjects, while Boos et al.[101] reported a prevalence of 76% among 46 subjects aged 20 to 50 years. Nevertheless, the prevalence was increased to 96% in a symptomatic group matched for age, sex and work-related risk factors,[101] so the MRI finding of a disc prolapse is not clinically irrelevant. A 5-year follow-up of the asymptomatic subjects showed that disc herniations and neural compromise did not worsen, whereas disc degeneration progressed in 41.5%.[102]

The prevalence of asymptomatic disc herniation in children is unknown, but symptomatic herniation does occur and may represent between 0.8% and 3.2% of all disc protusions or herniations.[106] Arguably, the lifetime prevalence of 'true sciatica' (i.e. between 2% and 5%: see above) may be taken to represent the lifetime prevalence of symptomatic disc herniation,[585] which is similar to the prevalence of 'extrusions' (6%), largely uninfluenced by age, reported by Jarvik and Deyo.[387]

Lumbar disc degeneration (revealed by X-ray, MRI or autopsy) is even less easy to define than disc herniation (see p. 67). Usually, any age-related changes in the disc, including reduced water content of the nucleus, are included as 'degeneration'. Consequently, 'disc degeneration' as so designated is extremely common, of little clinical relevance, and difficult to relate to any risk factor other than age. Generally, disc degeneration is more severe and starts earlier at the L4 and L5 levels than at L3, and the L2 and L1 levels are less frequently affected.[48,355] A prevalence of 31% has been found in 15-year-old schoolchildren.[696] This rises linearly with age until by 50 years of age virtually 100% of lumbar spines show disc 'degeneration'.[48] Preliminary findings from a prospective MRI study indicate that physical job characteristics and psychological aspects of work are more powerful than MRI-identified disc abnormalities in predicting the need for back pain-related medical consultation and resultant work incapacity.[102]

If disc degeneration is more specifically defined by the presence of disc space narrowing, osteophytes and sclerosis, then it is associated with non-specific low back pain with odds ratios ranging from 1.2 to 3.3.[803] Associations between disc degeneration and back pain are to some extent corroborated by a cadaveric study which found that disc degeneration, anular ruptures, and vertebral osteophytosis were related to a history of back injury, and to heavy work.[828] Radiographically defined severe disc degeneration is more common in Westernised societies than in certain native populations.[244] This has been attributed to a protective effect from the increased spinal mobility[392] and habitual flexed 'squatting' postures of the latter,[243] although factors such as genes and diet could also play a role.

OTHER SPINAL PATHOLOGY

Spondylolysis, spondylolisthesis, spina bifida, transitional vertebrae, spondylosis and Scheuermann's disease do not appear to be associated with low back pain.[803] In view of perceived methodological deficiencies in many of the reported studies, it was concluded that there is no firm evidence for the presence or absence of a causal relationship between radiographic findings and low back pain.[803] The term lumbar spondylosis should be reserved to refer to vertebral osteophytes secondary to disc degeneration. Thus, the epidemiology of spondylosis follows closely that for disc degeneration: it increases markedly with age, but seems to occur somewhat later, and is uncommon below 45 years of age.[48] The prevalence of zygapophysial (facet) joint osteoarthrosis also increases with increasing age; it seems to be related to disc degeneration and the indication is that discs degenerate before zygapophysial joints.[48]

DISABILITY

Disability (loss of ability to perform activities of daily living or work) often accompanies low back pain; it varies in extent, and may be temporary or essentially permanent. Much of the available information comes from surveys in which disability is self-reported, so there is no objective evidence or pathological basis for the following figures. Approximately 7–14% of adults in the USA experience disabling back pain during the course of a year, and just over 1% will be permanently disabled.[840] In the UK, 11% of adults experience back pain-related restrictions of their daily activities during a month, and 8% resorted to bedrest during a 12-month period.[840] The lifetime prevalence of disability tends to rise with age, and the extent of disability may be slightly greater in males: a UK population survey that used clinical measures of disability revealed that the 1-year prevalence of a disability score of 50% or more was 5.4% for men and 4.5% for women, whereas the lifetime prevalence was 16% and 13% respectively.[844]

Accurate information on disability, defined as workloss, is particularly difficult to obtain, being dependent on social policy and local issues such as compensation systems and job availability. Taking the UK as an example, a 1-year prevalence of time off work due to back pain has been reported as 11% for men and 7% for women, with a lifetime prevalence of 34% and 23%.[844] Approximately 85% of people are off work for short periods (a week or so) but account for only about half the lost work time – the remainder being accounted for by the 15% who are off work for more than 1 month.[840]

What can be said about disability is that the prevalence of 'compensated' back pain disability increased exponentially in most industrialised countries through the latter part of the twentieth century (Fig. 6.3) though there are signs that this curve is leveling off, at least in the UK.[840] The social context needs to be considered, and a clear distinction made between the 'epidemiological sea' of low back symptoms and the small proportion of sufferers who receive long-term sickness benefits.[840]

An overview of the epidemiological evidence on back pain was included in the UK Occupational Health Guidelines for the Management of Low Back Pain at Work.[152] These guidelines were based on a comprehensive review[841,842] and presented a synthesis of the evidence reported in a variety of previous reviews, supplemented with individual studies where reviews were unavailable. The guidelines documentation represents the output from the Blue Circle Industries plc, Faculty of Occupational Medicine and British Occupational Health Research Foundation project on occupational health aspects of low back pain. It is convenient to reproduce here some of the relevant evidence statements presented in that review. (Full text for the guidelines and evidence review can be found at www.facoccmed.ac.uk). The star rating against each statement represents the strength of the evidence (*** = strong evidence; ** = moderate evidence; * = limited or contradictory evidence – = no scientific evidence). The following evidence statements relating to disability are taken from that review.

** There is moderate evidence that patients who are older (particularly >50 years), have more prolonged and severe symptoms, have radiating leg pain, whose symptoms impact more on activity and work, and who have responded less well to previous therapy are likely to have slower clinical progress, poorer response to treatment and rehabilitation, and more risk of long term disability.[48,61,159,325,342,380,450,613]

*** There is strong epidemiological evidence that most workers with LBP are able to continue working or to return to work within a few days or weeks, even if they still have some residual or recurrent symptoms, and that they do not need to wait until they are completely pain free.[48,132,207,323,338]

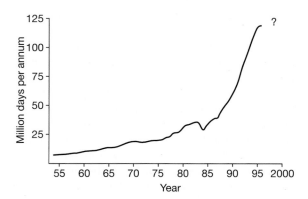

Figure 6.3 The exponential rise in the back pain problem shows recent signs of flattening out. (From Waddell[840] with permission from Churchill Livingstone, Edinburgh.)

GENETIC RISK FACTORS

Identical twins studies have shown that approximately 70% of intervertebral disc degeneration is statistically associated with genetic factors (p. 80), even after many environmental factors have been controlled for.[72,698] This applies both to lumbar and cervical discs, and when degeneration is defined in a number of different ways.[698] However, disc prolapse in the lower lumbar spine has a much weaker dependence on genes than other aspects of disc degeneration.[71] Preliminary findings suggest that 60% of back pain may be similarly attributable to genetic inheritance.[540] Only a few of the genes responsible for disc degeneration have so far been identified: they include genes for the vitamin D receptor,[831] for collagen type IX[624] and for proteoglycans.[408] Osteoarthrosis, which affects the zygapophysial joints in 90% of individuals aged over 45,[464] is strongly influenced by similar genetic risk factors, as discussed on page 62.

INDIVIDUAL RISK FACTORS

Several large prospective studies have sought to establish links between future LBT and individual factors such as height, weight, flexibility, strength, fatigability, and fitness. Generally, the results have been inconsistent, and this may be due, in part, to differing definitions of back trouble. Overall, back muscle strength and general levels of fitness appear to be of little significance,[24,73,83,145] and although easily fatigued back muscles were associated with more back pain in men, the same was not found for women.[83] There is no persuasive evidence of substantial or meaningful differences in prevalence rates for back pain dependent on gender, and leg length discrepancy.[577,578] Methodological differences between studies (as well as methodological weaknesses such as poor follow-up rates) will contribute to inconsistent findings, leading to the tendency for summary statements of systematic reviews (see below) to indicate weak links between individual characteristics and LBT.

However, a recent prospective study with 90–99% follow-up rates has shown that certain physical and psychological risk factors are significant predictors of future back pain.[24] Of particular interest is the high risk associated with having poor lumbar mobility, and a long back, in young health care workers who are newly exposed to heavy physical work: these two individual factors explained almost 12% of future back pain in this population.[24] Presumably tall people with long backs tend to lift weights at the end of greater

lever arms (see Fig. 7.2) and this may explain why tall people have a greater risk of disc prolapse as well.[344]

The UK Occupational Health Guidelines for the Management of Low Back Pain at Work review[841] offered the following evidence statements:

** There is moderate evidence that examination findings, including in particular, height, weight, lumbar flexibility and straight leg raising (SLR), have little predictive value for future lower back pain (LBP) or disability.[48,259]

** There is now moderate evidence that the level of general (cardiorespiratory) fitness has no predictive value for future LBP.[48]

* There is limited and contradictory evidence that attempting to match physical capability to job demands may reduce future LBP and work loss.[48,49,276,277]

*** There is strong evidence that X-ray and MRI findings have no predictive value for future LBP or disability.[85,102,680,704,783,803]

ENVIRONMENTAL (PHYSICAL) RISK FACTORS

The risks of a physically demanding workplace can be quantified adequately only if the risk exposure itself (the magnitude and intensity of spinal loading) is also quantified. Epidemiological studies which accurately quantify the exposure tend to show stronger associations between exposure and LBT than those which rely on vague categories or self-assessment of work intensity.[251] Bearing this in mind, there are numerous studies that show relatively high risks from work activities such as lifting heavy weights from the ground while in a twisted position (for disc prolapse[419,571]), and from activities involving a combination of rapid bending and twisting (for back pain[248,523]). In addition, sudden unexpected incidents that require sudden muscular efforts[507] have been found to lead to back pain.[495]

Turning to objective evidence of mechanical overload damage, disc height can be severely and significantly decreased in workers exposed to exceedingly heavy manual work (much more arduous than current regulations would permit), but vertebral height decrease seems rare.[118] In the same study, substantial exposure to whole body vibration on unsprung operators' seats (but not on sprung seats) was associated with a reduction in disc height. A recent twins study showed that job description and leisure time physical activity accounted for 7% and 2% respectively of lumbar disc degeneration.[72] Previous injury to a vertebral body was found to lead to disc degeneration several years later in a high proportion of subjects, although this degeneration was rarely painful.[421] The main value of this small study was that the subjects were aged between 9 and 21 years at follow-up, so there was little disc degeneration in the age-matched control group.

The UK Occupational Health Guidelines for the Management of Low Back Pain at Work review[841] offered the following evidence statements to reflect what was seen as the balance of the evidence:

*** There is strong evidence that physical demands of work (manual materials handling, lifting, bending, twisting, and whole body vibration) are a risk factor for the incidence (onset) of LBP, but overall it appears that the size of the effect is less than that of other individual, non-occupational and unidentified factors.[24,129,207,251,482,832]

*** There is strong epidemiological evidence that physical demands of work (manual materials handling, lifting, bending, twisting, and whole body vibration) can be associated with increased reports of back symptoms, aggravation of symptoms and 'injuries'.[48,105,127,251,601,832,129,207,856]

Note: the above two statements are not incompatible. Whilst the epidemiological evidence shows that low back symptoms are commonly linked to physical demands of work, that does not necessarily mean that LBP is caused by work. Although there is strong scientific evidence that physical demands of work can cause individual attacks of LBP, overall that only accounts for

a modest proportion of all LBP occurring in workers.

* There is limited and contradictory evidence that the length of exposure to physical stressors at work (cumulative risk) increases reports of back symptoms or of persistent symptoms.[127,139,251,482,523,601,606]

** There is moderate scientific evidence that physical demands of work play only a minor role in the development of disc degeneration.[72,827]

*** There is strong epidemiological and clinical evidence that care-seeking and disability due to LBP depend more on complex individual and work-related psychosocial factors than on clinical features or physical demands of work.[129,207,634,840]

Evidence on the role of sports and leisure activities as risk factors for LBT is somewhat inconsistent,[48] with sports participation variously being reported to have a protective effect, a detrimental effect, or no effect on prevalence rates. Vigorous sports such as weightlifting and gymnastics can carry an increased risk of disc degeneration[781,830] and vertebral damage,[780] some of which is symptomatic.[780,781] Running carries no increased risk of back pain or spinal degeneration.[830] Athletes in general have no more back pain than non-athletes, suggesting that vigorous physical activity can increase resistance to back pain.[830] There are, of course, substantial physiological benefits from physical fitness, and there is some evidence that physically fit individuals recover more rapidly from episodes of back pain[43] and that exercise programs are an effective prevention intervention.[469]

There is limited evidence that sports participation may represent an additional hazard for first-onset back pain when superimposed on another physical hazard,[139] whilst sports participation over and above normal school sport may be a hazard in 15-year-old schoolboys (but not in girls or younger children).[137]

It should not be assumed that the risk of LBT increases uniformly with the spine's exposure to high physical loading. On the contrary, there is evidence that reported LBT is common in sedentary workers[345,488] although this does not imply that the pain is caused by sitting. A recent systematic review, whilst accepting the generally high prevalence of back pain in the population, failed to find support for the popular notion that sitting-while-working is a risk factor for LBP.[339] Whilst it is accepted that whole body vibration is a risk factor for back pain (see evidence statements above), car driving may also carry an increased risk of disc prolapse,[417] which could be related to vibration, to reduced muscle protection of the spine following prolonged flexion[751] (p. 172) or to fatigued muscles having a reduced ability to protect the spine.[211] There is possibly a 'U-shaped' relationship between spinal loading and risk of back injury, with too little exposure being almost as detrimental as too much (Fig. 6.4). This can be explained in terms of the ability of spinal tissues to adapt to increased or decreased mechanical demands (see Ch. 4). Those who avoid vigorous activity run the risk of developing a 'weak' back which is then vulnerable to injury during slips and falls.

The different rates at which spinal tissues are able to adapt to increased mechanical demands could lead to an increased risk of injury to poorly vascularised tissues (such as intervertebral discs and ligaments) when levels of physical activity are suddenly increased, perhaps as a result of a new job or sporting activity (p. 70). In cross-sectional epidemiological studies, people who have survived in a heavy job without developing back pain will often, but not necessarily, be over-represented compared to those who have had to give up their job because of back pain. The true impact of mechanical loading on low back pain can, therefore, be higher than cross-sectional studies suggest, and will only be quantified accurately when controlled prospective studies are carried out. Already, the physical dangers of a new job are suggested by several longitudinal studies,[24,430] and the effects can occur with only short term exposure.[586] Another prospective study of nurses found that time spent in nursing without suffering an attack of LBP was negatively correlated with future episodes of LBP[505] suggesting some protective adaptation over time to the increased spinal loading.

Other environmental risk factors include cigarette smoking, which accounts for approximately 2% of disc degeneration[72,74] and slightly increases the risk of disc prolapse.[418] Presumably, smoking interferes with the precarious supply of metabolites to the centre of the disc (p. 166), yet a systematic review concluded that smoking should be considered a weak risk indicator and not a cause of LBP.[457]

PSYCHOSOCIAL INFLUENCES

The relationship between back pain and psychological and psychosocial factors has received much attention in recent years. The tendency for the terms psychological and psychosocial to be used interchangeably can lead to confusion. There is an argument that the term psychological should be reserved for those factors that embody a clear-cut psychological construct, and the term psychosocial should be used to describe factors having a 'social' element (e.g. work stress). In common with many of the papers in this field, the term psychosocial will be used here to embody both concepts.

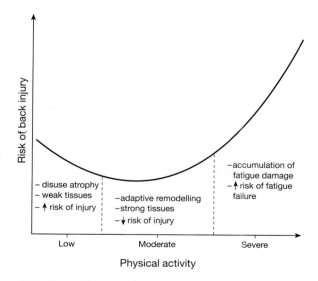

Figure 6.4 Proposed 'U-shaped' relationship between mechanical loading and low back trouble.

Psychosocial influences are related more to what people do about their back trouble than what caused it. Nevertheless, there is some evidence that psychosocial factors can predict up to 3% of reports of new onsets of LBP.[505,634] It is difficult to draw strong causal inferences, yet employees' reactions to psychosocial work characteristics such as job satisfaction and job stress are more consistently related to LBP than the psychosocial work characteristics themselves (e.g. job demands and social support).[191] In addition, it seems that there is an interaction between physical and psychosocial risk factors to increase the risk of low back disorders.[198] Psychosocial stress can increase spinal loading due to muscle tension, suggesting a mechanical explanation for some of the related back pain.[522] However, the psychosocial influences on LBP are usually considered in relation to outcomes: that is, they may predict reporting patterns, attribution of cause, care-seeking, response to treatment and the development of chronicity. Recently, psychosocial factors have been viewed in terms of them acting as 'obstacles to recovery'[133] both in occupational settings as well as clinical environments.

A recent systematic review of the role of specific psychological factors as predictors of unfavourable outcome concluded that there was good evidence to implicate psychological factors (notably distress/depressive mood and somatisation) in the development of chronicity (persisting symptoms and/or disability). Acceptable evidence generally was not found to link other psychological factors to back pain chronicity, although weak links emerged for catastrophising as a coping strategy. There was a basic lack of information on the potentially important role played by fear avoidance beliefs.[647] The influence of these variables was found to be generally consistent across environments (primary care, clinics and workplace) and have been reported by other recent reviewers.[468,801] Considering specifically non-return to work due to LBP, additional predictive factors have been found to include subjective negative appraisal of one's ability to work, and job satisfaction[801] and the importance of confounders (e.g. age and education) has been stressed.[127] Certainly, attribution of back pain to work is common. In a UK survey, nearly 80% of those with musculoskeletal symptoms identified a work task (or tasks) as leading to their complaint.[395] For LBP, the most commonly perceived causes were manual handling (66%) and posture (33%), along with workload/pace, and lack of social support.[395] Perhaps surprisingly, attribution to work remained high even for symptoms that started after ceasing work.[395]

The UK Occupational Health Guidelines review[841] considered the evidence on psychosocial influences and offered the following evidence statements:

*** For symptom-free people, there is strong evidence that individual psychosocial findings are a risk factor for the incidence (onset) of LBP, but overall the size of the effect is small.[182,505,840]

*** There is strong evidence that low job satisfaction and unsatisfactory psychosocial aspects of work are risk factors for reported LBP, health care use, and work loss, but the size of that association is modest.[100,191,601,832]

*** There is strong evidence that individual and work-related psychosocial factors play an important role in persisting symptoms and disability, and influence response to treatment and rehabilitation. Screening for 'yellow flags' can help to identify those workers with LBP who are at risk of developing chronic pain and disability. Workers' own beliefs that their LBP was caused by their work and their own expectations about inability to return to work are particularly important.[132,151,251,254,276,450,604,699,840]

CONCLUDING REMARKS

An intuitive 'injury/damage' model for the phenomenon of LBT would suggest that high exposure to physical stressors results in some form of damage to spinal tissues, and that further exposure leads to further damage and/or impeded recovery. However, it is apparent from the epidemiological evidence that such a simple model does not adequately explain what is observed.[129] An alternative injury model would suggest that there is a 'U-shaped' relationship between exposure and injury (Fig. 6.4). Whilst links between injury and pain are undoubtedly complex (p. 201), it is becoming obvious that many aspects of back pain and pain behaviour are not adequately accounted for by any mechanistic model.

The biopsychosocial model was proposed in 1987 to fill this gap,[839] and it remains supported by recent research.[801] This model accounts for all of the epidemiological evidence reviewed above, including the chronic course of much LBP (Fig. 6.2). In essence, it accepts that a proportion of back trouble results from some sort of physical insult leading to spinal pathology and pain. However, that pain should resolve within a relatively short period of time (perhaps following appropriate treatment/management) as is the case with many other musculoskeletal disorders. That the problem does not resolve for many people suggests that alternative explanations are required. To date, the most promising explanation, guided primarily by the epidemiology, appears to involve a substantial influence from psychosocial factors acting as obstacles to recovery.[133] This has significant implications for society as well as science when trying to find solutions for what is evidently a substantial current health problem. The overall view of back pain shared by the authors of this book (see Ch. 13) is compatible with the biopsychosocial model, although special emphasis is placed on the emerging role of genes and cell biology in the initiation of spinal pathology and pain.

7

Forces acting on the lumbar spine

COMPRESSION, SHEAR, BENDING AND TORSION

All of the forces acting on a given part of the spine can be added up to form a single 'resultant' force (p. 4). For convenience, the resultant is usually divided into 'components' as shown in Figure 7.1. The component which acts perpendicular to the mid-plane of the disc is defined as the compressive force acting on that part of the spine, and the other component acting parallel to the disc is the shear force. In three dimensions, there would also be a lateral shear force acting perpendicular to the plane of the paper in Figure 7.1, but lateral forces are usually small, and will not be considered further.

The resultant force may cause the spine to bend or twist about its centres of rotation, which usually lie within the intervertebral discs.[642] The torque (force × lever arm) responsible for the bending and twisting can be divided up into components in a similar manner to forces. The components which cause the spine to bend in the sagittal and frontal planes are referred to as the bending moment and lateral bending moment respectively, and the component which causes the spine to twist about its long axis (Fig. 7.1) is the axial torque on the spine. Bending moments and torque have the same units (Nm), and the words are sometimes used interchangeably. The word 'torsion' can refer to the axial torque (in Nm), or the axial rotation (in degrees) that it causes.

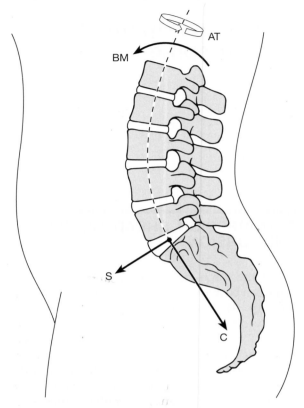

Figure 7.1 Component forces acting on the lumbar spine. C: compression; S: shear; BM: bending moment in the sagittal plane; AT: axial torque. In three dimensions, there could also be a lateral shear force and a lateral bending moment.

WHERE DO THE FORCES COME FROM?

GRAVITY, AND INERTIAL EFFECTS

Gravity exerts a vertical force on each part of the body in direct proportion to its mass (p. 5). When a person stands upright, the mass of the trunk, head and arms presses vertically on the lower lumbar spine with a force of approximately 55% of bodyweight,[694] which is 385 N for a 70 kg man. Assuming the lumbosacral disc is inclined at an angle of approximately 30° to the horizontal, the gravitational force will give rise to intervertebral compressive and shear force components of approximately 335 N and 190 N respectively.

The mass of body segments can give rise to much greater 'inertial' forces when they are rapidly accelerated or decelerated. According to Newton's second law of motion (force = mass × acceleration) the force rises in proportion to the acceleration (change of velocity divided by time). The high vertical acceleration experienced by a fighter pilot ejecting from an aeroplane generates an impulsive compressive force on the spine that may be sufficient to crush a vertebra.[356] Similarly, rapid decelerations experienced during a fall on the buttocks can be sufficient to crush the spine.[261] The maximum velocity reached by a falling body just before impact depends on the distance of fall, whereas the time taken to stop depends on the amount of cushioning at impact. Therefore the peak deceleration (and peak force) generated during a fall from upright standing depends mainly on the length of a persons legs, and the 'softness' of their landing.

MUSCLES

Muscles of the back and abdomen act to protect the spine, by stabilising it in upright postures[765] and by preventing excessive bending and axial rotation movements. However, the muscle tension required to protect and to move the spine also subjects it to high compressive forces, because many of the strongest trunk muscles lie approximately parallel to the long axis of the spine. According to circumstances, the back muscles can be the spine's best friend, or worst enemy.

Even during relaxed standing and sitting, muscle tension increases the compressive force on the lumbar discs to approximately twice the superincumbent body weight.[582,702] During activities such as bending forwards and lifting weights, the back muscles need to generate much higher forces in order to overcome the effects of gravity acting on the upper body.[40,141,142,209,220,533] These forces can be estimated by using a 'moment arm analysis' as shown in Figure 7.2. The simple analysis explained in this figure refers to a static equilibrium, where nothing is moving. In practice, manual handling activities require the upper body

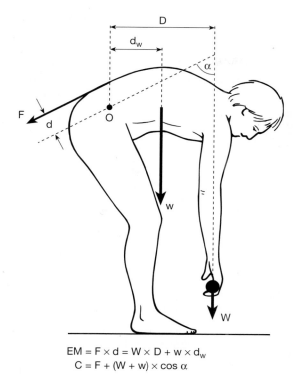

$$EM = F \times d = W \times D + w \times d_w$$
$$C = F + (W + w) \times \cos \alpha$$

Figure 7.2 During manual handling, the back muscles must generate an extensor moment (EM) to overcome the forward bending moment due to upper body weight (w) and the weight being lifted (W). The average lever arm (d) of the extensor muscles in the lower lumbar spine is approximately 7.5 cm,[534] whereas W and w act on much larger lever arms (D and d_w). For this reason, the tensile force in the back muscles (F) is much greater than w or W, and the spine is subjected to a high compressive force (C).

to be moved quickly, often from a stationary position, and so higher muscle forces are required to generate accelerations of the trunk.[217,533] Manual handling typically involves movements in several planes,[523] and these require additional lateral bending moments and axial torques which increase muscle tension further.[221,272,425,519,517,649]

FASCIA AND LIGAMENTS

Fascia and ligaments are passive (non-contractile) structures that can sustain high tensile forces when stretched. This is demonstrated by the 'flexion–relaxation' phenomenon, in which the back muscles fall electrically silent when a person

bends forwards to touch their toes.[255,322,427] The effect extends to include the hamstring muscles and much of the thoracic erector spinae.[539] Evidently, the forward bending moment generated by the upper body (Fig. 7.2) must be resisted by tension in passive tissues such as the ligaments of the neural arch, the erector spinae aponeurosis, lumbodorsal fascia and collagenous sheaths (see Fig. 4.2) in the muscle itself.

The involvement of passive tissues in lifting is an important and controversial topic, because it can be both beneficial and harmful to the spine. Stretched passive tissues store elastic energy when the spine is flexed, and then release the energy when the person straightens up again, so that the back muscles do less work.[300,445] In addition, the supraspinous ligament and the strong posterior band of the lumbodorsal fascia both lie posterior to the back muscles,[97] and so act on longer lever arms relative to the centre of rotation in the discs than do the muscles.[534] Therefore, any extensor moment generated by these passive structures has a smaller compressive 'penalty' as far as the spine is concerned. (In other words, their ratio of extensor moment to tensile force is high.) On the other hand, most of the ligaments of the neural arch act on shorter lever arms than the back muscles, so any extensor moment generated by them is at the expense of a high compressive penalty. Also, too much flexion can leave the discs vulnerable to prolapse when the compressive force is high (p. 148). These considerations suggest that, during manual handling, the spine should be flexed sufficiently to tension the lumbodorsal fascia, but not so much that high forces are generated in the intervertebral ligaments and disc.

The feasibility of doing this was investigated in a recent study on 149 healthy volunteers who lifted 10 kg weights from the ground, either with their knees flexed (squat lifts) or straight (stoop lifts).[216] On average, these volunteers flexed their lumbar spine by 83% and 96% in the squat and stoop lifts respectively, where 0% and 100% flexion refer to the erect standing and fully flexed positions (see Fig. 10.3). Complementary static experiments investigating the relationship between lumbar flexion, electrical silence in the

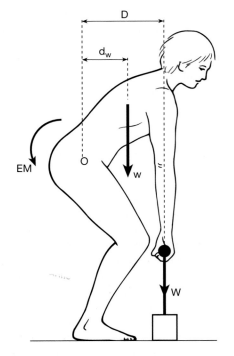

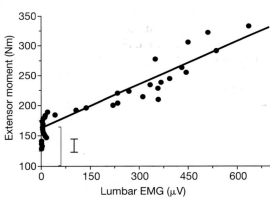

Figure 7.3 During an isometric contraction in the stooped position, the EMG activity of the erector spinae muscles is linearly related to the extensor moment generated (EM). (Upper) The subject pulled up on a load cell, reaching their maximum force in approximately 3 s. Extensor moment was calculated from D, d_w, w and W as shown in Figure 7.2. (Lower) The intercept on the y-axis (I) indicates the extensor moment generated when the erector spinae are electrically silent.

back muscles, and extensor moment generation (Fig. 7.3) showed that 'passive' structures must have contributed 22% of the extensor moment in the squat lift, and 31% in the stoop lift. Furthermore, comparisons with the bending properties

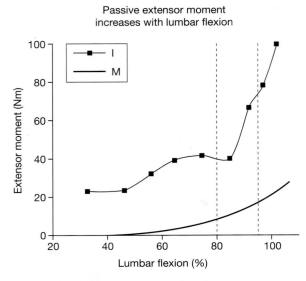

Passive extensor moment increases with lumbar flexion

Figure 7.4 Extensor moments attributable to non-contractile tissues (I) can be calculated during isometric contractions as shown in Figure 7.3. If the experiment is repeated with the subject in varying amounts of lumbar flexion, I increases markedly when flexion exceeds 80% of the in-vivo range of movement. M represents the bending-stiffness properties of cadaveric osteo-ligamentous spines (Fig. 7.8). A comparison of the two curves (I and M) suggests that, in the range 80–95% flexion, less than 25% of I is attributable to the osteo-ligamentous spine. (From Dolan and Adams.[14,216])

of cadaveric motion segments[14] showed that tension in the ligaments of the neural arch and in the posterior anulus fibrosus would have been low in both lifts, and contributed less than 25% of the total 'passive' extensor moment (Fig. 7.4). Calculations suggest that the lumbodorsal fascia, and collagenous tissue within the back muscles themselves, are indeed strong enough to generate large extensor moments during lifting activities.[216] Previous estimates of the strength of the lumbodorsal fascia were based on testing excised samples of it,[790] but the collagen fibre disruption caused by the excision of small samples can probably lead to the strength of the whole structure being underestimated.[15]

The experimental evidence therefore indicates that it is possible to make use of passive tension in the lumbodorsal fascia and stretched back muscles during lifting, without generating high tensile stresses in the intervertebral ligaments and disc. This can be achieved simply by flexing the lumbar spine by 80–95% of the range between upright standing and touching the toes. It has been suggested that the lumbodorsal fascia can be tensioned in other ways, in particular by raising the intra-abdominal pressure, and by contracting the abdominal muscles so that they pull sideways on the fascia and generate a longitudinal tension within it.[301,303] However, attempts to demonstrate these mechanisms either directly in cadavers[790] or using detailed anatomical data from cadaveric dissection,[485] showed that the effects were small.

INTRA-ABDOMINAL PRESSURE

Raising the intra-abdominal pressure (IAP) during lifting has been advocated by some as a means of transmitting load directly from the shoulders to the pelvis in order to reduce spinal compression[65] (Fig. 7.5). Pressures above 150 mmHg have been recorded during weight lifting,[236,520] which is sufficient to occlude the blood supply to the abdominal cavity and make the lifter go red in the face. However, a raised IAP is normally associated with increased abdominal muscle activity, which actually produces a flexion moment on the trunk.[77] This would act to increase spinal compression, so any benefit of the IAP mechanism is difficult to assess. A recent study (summarised in Fig. 7.4) showed that volunteers were able to generate an extensor moment of 20–25 Nm while keeping their erector spinae muscles electrically silent and without flexing forward enough to stretch the intervertebral ligaments or lumbodorsal fascia.[216] This 20–25 Nm could possibly be due to a raised intra-abdominal pressure. Holding the breath increases IAP and gives workers a subjective feeling of spinal stability.[537] Axial rotation of the trunk leads to particularly high IAP.[45]

Use of lifting belts

Wearing a wide abdominal belt helps to generate a higher IAP, and could possibly reduce the compressive force on the spine during lifting by approximately 15%.[537] However, the effectiveness of lifting belts in reducing spinal loading is debatable, and depends on the type of belt.[307] There is some evidence from experiments on

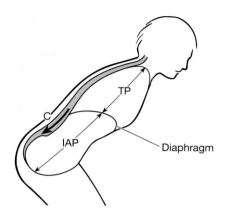

Figure 7.5 When a person lifts a heavy weight as in Figure 7.2, a raised intra-abdominal pressure (IAP) and thoracic pressure (TP) has the potential to transmit force directly from shoulders to pelvis, by-passing the lumbar spine. In this manner, it is hypothesised that a high IAP can reduce the compressive force (C) acting on the lumbar spine.

cadaveric human torsos that an increased IAP (simulating belt-wearing or breath-holding) has a greater effect on torso stiffness during lateral bending and axial rotation than in flexion and extension.[528] A raised IAP could therefore help stabilise the trunk in asymmetric manual handling tasks.[520] Some of this extra stability may be due to the belt increasing pressure within the muscles themselves.[559] It is noteworthy that abdominal belts are worn with their widest part next to the spine, rather than next to the abdominal wall they are supposed to be supporting. This raises the possibility that weight lifters like to use a belt because it helps to keep the lumbar spine flat (i.e. moderately flexed) rather than in lordosis or kyphosis. There is some evidence that a belt can reduce sudden spinal bending movements during unexpected loading events.[455] The influence of back belts (and other ergonomic interventions) on LBP is considered on page 178.

COMPRESSIVE LOADING OF THE SPINE

Until recently, spinal loading has been equated with compressive loading, which is unfortunate because mechanisms of spinal injury depend greatly on the presence of bending and torsion. Nevertheless, the spine is compressed for most of the time, day and night, and compressive loading is undoubtedly an important contributor to the fatigue failure of spinal tissues. The following sections explain briefly how the spinal compressive force is measured, and what influences it.

MEASURING SPINAL COMPRESSION

Intra-discal pressure

The 'gold standard' measurements of spinal compression were made originally by Nachemson, who inserted a pressure-sensitive needle into the L3–4 disc of conscious volunteers.[576] Measurements of pressure were later converted into compressive forces[582] using the results of cadaver experiments to calibrate the pressure readings against force.[580] Many of the results have been confirmed recently using better technology.[702,862] Intra-discal pressure techniques have limitations, however, because subjects are unlikely to move in a natural or vigorous manner with a long needle in their backs. Also, the recorded pressures in-vivo were calibrated in terms of the compressive force applied to cadaveric discs that would have been swollen by post-mortem storage, whereas the experiments on living people were performed after their discs had been dehydrated by hours of activity. In cadaveric experiments, load-induced fluid expulsion from intervertebral discs is especially marked in the nucleus pulposus, and this effectively transfers compressive loading from nucleus to anulus,[28] and from the disc to the neural arch (p. 169).[6,27] As a result, the ratio of nucleus pressure to spinal compressive force decreases by up to 36% following creep loading.[28] In-vivo estimates of spinal loading which are based on intra-discal pressure measurements may therefore underestimate true spinal loading by a similar amount.

Spinal shrinkage

An indirect approach to quantifying the compressive force on the spine is to measure the amount of disc creep that it causes over a specified time period. Procedures have been developed to detect small time-dependent changes in the length of the spine, while minimising errors due to changes in posture.[39,135,175,204,441] Inter-individual comparisons are difficult because the rate of disc creep depends on many factors, including age,[205] loading history,[28] the degree of disc degeneration,[9] disc area,[39] and posture (which influences water expulsion from the discs[9] as well as load-bearing by the zygapophysial joints: p. 162). These variable factors may help explain why spinal shrinkage has been reported to be greater in standing postures than in sitting,[39,459] less when performing overhead work compared to standing,[135] and why a stature gain has been reported following dynamic hyperextension exercises.[491] Increased spinal shrinkage following sitting on a vibrating seat[771] may be attributable to increased disc creep under oscillating loads, or increased muscle activity in the subjects being vibrated. However, another study showed that vibrations had no effect on stature over and above the effect due to sitting.[39] Despite these variable factors, spinal shrinkage does provide a simple cumulative measure of spinal loading over time which may complement measurements of peak spinal loading in ergonomic studies.[257,474] We suggest that the technique is most suitable when the spine is loaded predominantly in flexed postures (when all of the compressive load is resisted by the discs (p. 162)) and when comparisons are made between the same subjects performing different activities, so that individual variable factors such as disc area and degeneration are controlled for.

Linked-segment and EMG-assisted models

Various mathematical models essentially elaborate the 'moment arm analysis' approach (Fig. 7.2). Some are static[40,157] but most of them make allowance for the extra forces required to accelerate body segments.[141,424,533,708,798] Parts of the body such as the thigh, pelvis and lumbar spine are likened to a series of rigid segments which are linked by frictionless hinges (joints) and moved by the action of muscles which join the segments together. The position of each body segment is measured on living volunteers at frequent time intervals using a device such as a video camera. The change in position of each body segment per unit time gives the velocity of each segment, and the change in velocity per unit time yields its acceleration. Anthropometric data regarding the mass and centre of mass of each body segment can then be used to compute the net moments (force × distance) acting about each joint. Net moment is divided by the lever arm of the muscle mass responsible for the movement, yielding the muscle force acting on the joint. (Detailed anatomical data required in these calculations, including the lever arms and cross-sectional areas of individual back muscles, is presented in Table 3.1 and in previously published work.[98,487,521,534,797]) Force plate data is incorporated to account for the effects of the ground reaction force during dynamic movements. Fully dynamic linked-segment models are able to measure accurately three-dimensional forces acting on each joint of the body[424] but they do have one drawback: they are unable to detect antagonistic muscle activity which can increase joint loading without affecting the movement of adjacent body segments.

The influence of muscle activity on spinal loading has been tackled by more complicated models which acknowledge that each joint is moved by several different muscles, some of which could act antagonistically to each other. Electromyographic (EMG) measurements can be combined with data concerning muscle cross-section areas in order to determine the relative activity of each muscle, so that moments can be distributed between them.[304,518,531] Other models use optimising principles to divide up the overall moment between different muscles: for example, they may stipulate that the square of muscle power should be minimised,[302] or that spinal compression should be minimised.[716] Unfortunately, the relationship between EMG activity and muscle tension is influenced by variable factors such as muscle length and speed of contraction, and optimising principles can appear somewhat arbitrary. A direct comparison between an EMG-assisted model and a simple optimisation model suggested that the former was more sensitive and produced larger estimates of spine compression.[162]

Direct EMG estimates of spinal loading

Because most of the compressive force acting on the lumbar spine arises from tension in the back muscles (Fig. 7.2), it is tempting to try to quantify spinal compression directly from the EMG activity of these muscles.[209] This approach does not attempt to predict forces or moments generated by individual muscles. Instead, it uses the EMG activity of the erector spinae to predict the extensor moment generated by them all, and then divides the moment by an effective lever arm[534] which is representative of the whole muscle group.

Initially, the EMG activity from several sites overlying the erector spinae is calibrated against extensor moment when a volunteer pulls up with gradually-increasing force on a chain attached to a load cell (Fig. 7.3). Linear regression is used to determine the gradient and the intercept of the relationship between EMG and extensor moment during isometric contractions. By repeating these calibrations in a range of postures which require different amounts of lumbar flexion, the effect of back muscle length on the EMG-extensor moment relationship can be determined.[209] In flexed postures, the intercept indicates the moment generated when there is no EMG activity in the back muscles, so the technique can be used to determine the extensor moment resisted by passive tissues such as the lumbodorsal fascia.[216] During concentric muscle contractions, the relationship between extensor moment and EMG activity is also influenced by the rate at which the muscles shorten.[84] This effect can be accounted for by repeating the EMG-extensor moment calibrations at a range of different contraction speeds, using an isokinetic dynamometer.[209] Forces associated with an upwards thrust by the legs on the spine, and acting in the direction of the long axis of the spine, must be measured separately using a force plate, but these 'hidden' forces are generally only 2–4% of the maximum spinal compressive force.[220]

The main advantage of this EMG approach is that it requires no minimising principles, and it accounts directly for the variable effects of muscle length and contraction velocity on the EMG/moment relationship. It also measures antagonistic muscle activity, because any contractions of the abdominal muscles cause a compensatory increase in erector spinae activity which is detected by the electrodes.[220,507] The technique is portable and particularly well suited for measuring spinal compression in the workplace, especially when there are rapid movements of the trunk. It has been developed to include bilateral EMG recordings which makes it suitable for investigating asymmetric lifting tasks.[221,665] The technique's main drawback is the inherent variability of EMG signals, which may be attributable to varying recruitment strategies for individual motor units within a large muscle.[426]

Comparison between direct EMG and linked-segment model techniques

In an attempt to validate the main approaches for measuring spinal compression during dynamic lifting activities, a 3-D linked segment model and the direct EMG technique were applied simultaneously to a group of volunteers.[220,221,426] Both techniques demonstrated similar increases in spinal loading in response to changes in either the load lifted, the speed of lifting, or the technique of lifting. However, the EMG model consistently predicted higher extensor moments than the linked-segment model. In the less arduous lifts (6.7 kg lifted slowly and without any trunk rotation) the EMG predictions were approximately 8% greater,[426] and this could be due to differences in the anthropometric assumptions of the two models.[221] However, in the most arduous lifts (15.7 kg lifted rapidly with 90° of trunk rotation), the EMG predictions were up to 40% higher. Some of this large difference may be due to varying amounts of electrical filtering applied in the two techniques, and some would have been due to antagonistic muscle activity.

COMPRESSIVE LOADING IN-VIVO

Nachemson's revised measurements of intradiscal pressure,[582] and subsequent experiments in Japan[702] indicate that the compressive force on the lumbar spine rises from about 150–250 N when lying, to 500–800 N when standing erect, 700–1000 N when sitting erect, and 1900 N when stooping to lift a 10 kg weight. The higher compressive force during sitting (when the normal lumbar lordosis is flattened) can be explained in two ways: some back muscles are more highly activated in upright unsupported sitting postures than in standing,[214] and tension is increased in the stretched posterior ligaments of the spine whenever the spine is flexed.[27] A recent study (on a single volunteer) reported similar intradiscal pressures in standing and sitting, and suggested that the higher levels in sitting recorded by Nachemson may be an artefact caused by bending of the pressure-sensitive needle.[862]

Results from EMG-assisted linked segment models suggest that spinal compression at L4–5 rises to approximately 4 kN and 5.5 kN when healthy young men lifts weights of 14 kg and 29 kg respectively[663] and that about 20% of this is due to inertial forces.[533] These values are similar to those obtained using the direct EMG approach[217] but lower than those calculated by early moment-arm models which assumed that the 'lever arm' of the back muscles was only 5 cm[157] rather than the 6–8 cm currently accepted.[534] Antagonistic contraction of the abdominal muscles (sometimes called 'co-contraction') increases the stability of the trunk[275,306] but at the cost of increasing spinal compression by up to 45% during simulated lifting movements.[305] This high figure is applicable to semi-upright postures which require considerable stabilising muscle activity. When the spine is flexed and stabilised by a tensioned lumbodorsal fascia, antagonistic muscle activity probably has less effect on spinal compression (p. 171).

During forward bending and lifting tasks, compressive forces due to muscle tension are influenced by factors such as the mass and position of the load lifted, the amount of asymmetry, and the technique and speed of lifting.[141,142,209,217,249,272,305,724] The direct EMG approach was used to compare the effects of all these factors on a group of 21 young men who lifted various objects from the ground.[217] The peak compressive force on the lumbosacral disc increased from approximately 2.5 kN when lifting 10 kg, to 5.0 kN when lifting 30 kg. Lifting with the knees bent increased the compressive force by approximately 5% compared to straight-leg ('stoop') lifts. Increasing the distance of a 10 kg weight from the feet, from 0 cm to 60 cm, increased the peak compressive force from 2.8 kN to 5.2 kN, and lifting 10 kg quickly (in 1 second), increased the peak compressive force to 5.3 kN compared to 3.2 kN when the lift was performed more slowly (Fig. 7.6). In the workplace, manual handling tasks often combine several of the factors considered above, so that compressive loading would be particularly high when bulky objects are lifted rapidly from an awkward position relative to the lifter's feet.

Peak forces are not directly proportional to the weight lifted, because much of the muscle tension is generated to lift the weight of the upper body, which is usually much heavier than the weight being lifted. Similar trends were observed in 18 female subjects, but the overall forces were reduced by an amount which reflected their smaller upper body mass and shorter limbs.[217] Lifting with a rotated trunk (bending forwards and to one side) has been reported to have little effect on the peak spinal compressive force as inferred from the 'total moment' generated by the back muscles.[425] However, this experimental approach neglects antagonistic activity from the abdominal muscles, and there is other evidence that lifting in a plane rotated by 45° or more increases antagonistic muscle forces[305,456] and therefore increases spinal compression.

Values of peak compressive forces measured in these studies are approximately 50–70% of the ultimate compressive strength of cadaveric lumbar spines of similar age and gender (p. 134) so they would not be expected to cause injury. However, repetitive loading can damage cadaveric specimens at 40–50% of their ultimate compressive strength[113,334] (see Table 9.2) so compressive fatigue damage might be expected to accumulate at forces above 4 kN in a typical young man. It appears, therefore, that a change in just one variable factor (weight, distance or speed) can be enough to raise the estimated peak compressive force above the 4 kN threshold for fatigue damage during manual handling. Evidently, the risk of compressive back injury in the workplace depends on more factors than just the weight of the object lifted.

Many reported low back symptoms are associated with sudden and alarming events[495] such as stumbling while carrying a heavy weight, or misjudging the weight of an object to be lifted. Under these circumstances, muscles can over-react and apply unnecessarily high forces to the spine. A laboratory experiment showed that peak spinal compression during manual handling was increased by 30–70% when the subjects were alarmed.[507] It made little difference whether or not they were blind-folded, suggesting that the increased spinal loading was largely due to

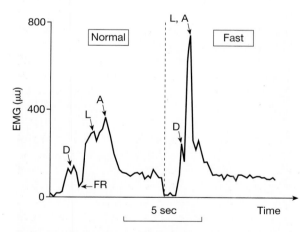

Figure 7.6 A subject bent forwards to lift a 10 kg weight from the ground at normal speed, and then as quickly as possible. EMG activity was averaged from electrodes overlying the erector spinae at T10 and L3. At normal speed, the first EMG peak (D), which represents deceleration of the upper body, is followed by a brief spell of 'flexion–relaxation' (FR). The following peaks represent lifting the weight off the ground (L), and accelerating the body and weight upwards (A). During the fast lift, L and A coincide, and the EMG peak is doubled. After EMG corrections for the effect of contraction velocity, this still indicates a 60% increase in spinal compression. (Data from Dolan et al.[217])

compensatory, reflex contractions of the trunk muscles caused by stimulation of muscle spindles and Golgi tendon organs. Similar increases in back muscle activity in response to sudden and/or unexpected loading have been reported previously.[206,493,857] Even if an unknown load proves to be lighter than expected, it can lead to increased anticipatory muscle activity prior to lifting, and a faster less-controlled movement during the lift.[206]

SHEAR

The shear force resisted by the osteoligamentous spine has never been measured in-vivo. It is probably higher at the lowest lumbar levels where the discs are inclined at a steep angle to the horizontal so that a substantial component of the gravitational forces acts to shear the joint (Fig. 7.1). If the lumbosacral disc is inclined at 30° to the horizontal, the weight of the upper body will give rise to an intervertebral shear force of approximately 190 N. This increases in stooped postures, and when weights are carried, and is estimated to oscillate between 380 N and 760 N when a man marches with a heavy backpack.[184] This is a 'worst-case' analysis, and other models based on detailed anatomical observations and EMG recordings suggest that shear is limited to 250 N by back muscle activity.[487,664] Co-contraction of the abdominal muscles has been reported to increase shear by up to 70%.[305]

BENDING

MEASURING SPINAL BENDING

The bending moment acting on the osteoligamentous lumbar spine plays a major role in damaging the intervertebral discs and ligaments (see Ch. 9) and yet few attempts have been made to measure it. Ligament forces have been calculated by some mathematical models, but the predictions are based on many assumptions[40,531] and

the results can be inconsistent.[663] A more straightforward approach is to compare lumbar flexion movements measured in-vivo with the bending stiffness properties of the lumbar spine measured in-vitro.[14]

In this technique, the bending moment acting on the spine in-vivo is determined from dynamic measurements of lumbar flexion. These can be obtained using an electromagnetic tracking device, the 3-Space Isotrak (Polhemus, Vermont), which records lumbar curvature between L1 and S1 up to 60 times per second during dynamic activities (Fig. 7.7). Values of peak lumbar flexion are 'normalised' by expressing them as a % of the

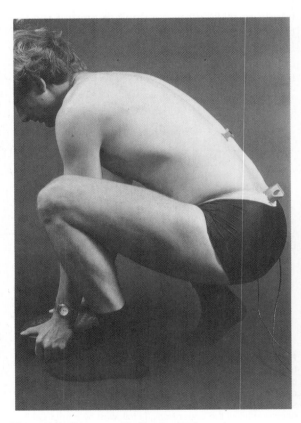

Figure 7.7 It is normal to flex the lumbar spine substantially when lifting weights from the ground, even if the knees are bent. Here, lumbar flexion is measured using the 3-Space Isotrak device mounted over the spinous processes at L1 and S1/S2. Note that the lumbar lordosis has been eliminated, so that the lower back is flat.

individual's in-vivo range of flexion between the erect standing and fully flexed (toe-touching) positions (see Fig. 10.3). Normalised flexion values are then compared with normalised bending-stiffness curves for cadaveric osteo-ligamentous lumbar spines.[14] The underlying principle is indicated in Figure 7.8. However, the normalising procedures take into account the different flexibilities and strengths of different spines, and allow the bending moment in-vivo to be predicted with an accuracy of ±8% of the bending moment required to cause the first signs of damage to a motion segment (i.e. ±5 Nm for a typical young man). The technique can be summarised by the equation:

$$M = 0.1 \times (0.093V - 2.25)^3$$

where M is the bending moment expressed as a % of that required to bend a motion segment right up to the elastic limit, and V is the flexion angle measured in-vivo, expressed as a % of the full range from erect standing to full flexion. M can be converted into absolute units by multiplying by 60 Nm, which is the approximate strength in bending of an average cadaver lumbar spine (p. 145).

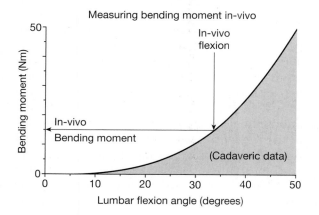

Figure 7.8 Composite bending stiffness curve for a cadaveric lumbar spine L1–S1. Values of lumbar flexion measured in-vivo can be compared to this curve in order to estimate the bending moment acting on the spine in-vivo. Note that the bending moment doubles over the last 10° of flexion. (After Adams and Dolan.[14])

SPINAL BENDING IN-VIVO

Results obtained using the above technique indicate that peak bending moments are about 10 Nm when lifting a 10 kg weight with the knees bent (Fig. 7.7), and 19 Nm when lifting with the knees straight.[217] Bending forwards and to one side increases the bending moment on the lumbar spine by up to 30% compared to lifting in the sagittal plane,[217] probably because a smaller proportion of the movement can be accommodated by the pelvis. In bent-knee 'squat' lifts, increasing the mass of the load from 0 kg (a pen) to 20 kg increased the bending moment from 7.5 Nm, to 13 Nm, whereas increasing the distance of a 10 kg load from the body increased peak bending moment up to 20 Nm (calculated from Dolan et al.[217]).

Evidently, spinal bending during lifting depends on several variable factors, but it is noteworthy that none of these factors caused the peak bending moment to exceed 25 Nm, which is 40% of its value at the elastic limit. It seems that the back muscles adequately protect the spine from excessive bending during moderate lifting tasks, at least in the group of young, healthy subjects who took part in these experiments. However, average values can conceal valuable information: several of the volunteers consistently flexed so far that the estimated peak bending moment exceeded 50% of the value at the elastic limit. These subjects actually flexed further forwards during the dynamic lifting tasks than when attempting to reach full flexion in a static posture, so that peak flexion values were up to 115% of their normal range. It would be expected that these individuals, who possibly had impaired proprioceptive or motor function (p. 173), would be more likely to sustain fatigue damage to spinal tissues during repetitive bending and lifting tasks. A recent prospective epidemiological study showed that people who applied most bending to their spine during arduous laboratory lifting tasks were indeed more likely to develop back pain in the follow-up period.[506]

Peak bending moments acting on the lumbar spine rise to higher levels in people with poor spinal mobility, and are lower than normal in those who are particularly supple.[210] This could explain why limited lumbar mobility predicted future back pain in a recent prospective study.[24] The peak bending moment can also increase when particularly heavy or large objects are lifted, or when the bending movement is forwards and to one side.[210,217] Rapid flexion movements are resisted more strongly by the spine so that peak bending moments in-vitro increase by 10–15%.[16] Sudden and alarming incidents can increase spinal bending, especially when the trunk muscles are not pre-activated.[442,507]

During repetitive lifting, fatigue of the quadriceps muscles and/or back muscles is associated with increased lumbar flexion[211,662,798] and increased bending moments on the lumbar spine.[211] Prolonged sitting or standing in flexed postures causes creep in spinal ligaments and fascia,[535] and just 5 minutes of this (simulated in-vitro) is enough to reduce by 40% the ability of intervertebral ligaments to protect the discs in bending.[16]

Muscle protection of the spine can also be compromised by sustained and repetitive flexion. The back muscles normally contract automatically in response to signals from stretch receptors in ligaments, tendons and muscles (see Fig. 10.19), but experiments on anaesthetised cats have shown that repeated stretching of the supraspinous ligament over a period of 10 minutes almost eliminates this protective reflex.[751] A similar effect was noted after just 3 minutes of simulated sustained flexion.[864] Full recovery of the protective muscle reflex can take several hours[281] and full creep recovery takes even longer.[752]

In the first few hours of each day, the increased water content of the intervertebral discs increases the bending stiffness of the spine (p. 169). Much of the effect is lost after 1 hour,[215,441] but during this first hour, the peak bending moment acting on the spine during bending and lifting activities is increased by approximately 100%.[212,215]

High lumbar flexion during lifting means that non-contractile tissues contribute to the total extensor moment. When a 10 kg weight is lifted from the floor using the stoop (straight leg) and squat (bent leg) techniques, the 'passive' contribution is approximately 20% and 30% respectively (pp. 95–96). This can be reduced if the weight is lifted from a convenient height off the ground.[161] Only a small proportion of the 'passive' extensor moment can be attributed to the intervertebral discs and ligaments[216] so most of it must be due to tension in the lumbo-dorsal fascia,[790] the supraspinous ligament,[574] and non-contractile tissue in the muscles themselves.[407]

TORSION

The lumbar spine is subjected to torsion during activities such as golf and discus throwing, and small coupled axial rotation movements generally accompany lateral bending movements.[640] However, very little is known about the torsional stresses acting on the spine in-vivo. Trunk muscles can exert torsional moments of 50–80 Nm about the long axis of the spine[532] with the back muscles contributing approximately 5 Nm.[486] These same muscles would be expected to protect the underlying spine from any externally applied torque (perhaps applied to an outstretched arm) but the extent to which they do this is difficult to quantify.

In theory, it should be possible to measure torsional stresses in-vivo by measuring axial rotation movements and comparing them with the torque-rotation properties of cadaveric spines. In practice, however, this approach has considerable difficulties. The full range of axial rotation in-vivo is only about 1° to each side for each lumbar level (Fig. 8.2), and in this range, torsional stresses acting on the posterior anulus of the disc are minimal (p. 140). However, contact stresses in the zygapophysial joints, and hence the axial torque on the spine, rise rapidly with increasing angle of rotation[7] so a small experimental error in the measurement of angular rotation would lead to a large error in the prediction of torque. Because skin movements lead to gross overestimates of axial rotation when measured by skin-surface techniques[639] this makes any attempt to predict torque from skin-surface measurements unfeasible. More accurate measurements of axial rotation can be obtained by inserting pins into the spinous processes,[314,320,480,758] but this invasive procedure could inhibit normal movement patterns.

In cadaveric specimens, torsional damage is first detectable at a torque of 15–30 Nm[7] so this is probably the upper bound of torque acting in-vivo. The normal in-vivo range of bending moment appears to be approximately 40% of the bending moment required to cause damage (p. 103); if a similar safety margin is applicable to torsion, that would suggest maximal torques of approximately 6–12 Nm acting on the lumbar spine in life.

Evidently, the precise torque acting on the osteo-ligamentous spine during vigorous activities remains elusive, and is likely to remain so. Nevertheless, non-invasive measurements of axial rotation[252,639] do give some comparative measure of torque on the spine, which may be sufficient for occupational studies attempting to assess the risk for low back pain.[523]

8

Mechanical function of the lumbosacral spine

INTRODUCTION

This chapter describes how the spine 'works' during normal daily life, and explains the mechanical function of each component part. Mechanical damage is considered separately in Chapter 9, and a discussion of how posture affects spine mechanical function is included in Chapter 10.

To a certain extent, spinal function can be inferred from a careful consideration of anatomy, and this is why form and function were described together in Chapters 2 and 3. However, this is not always good enough, because some 'common-sense' inferences regarding mechanical function can be misleading, and often it is difficult to decide between two equally plausible explanations of how something works (or fails to work) without detailed quantitative information. For example, to appreciate the relative role of the lumbar discs and ligaments in resisting torsional stresses, it is necessary to compare the amplitude of axial rotation movements measured in-vivo, with torsional stiffness data obtained from cadaveric spines in-vitro. Only then is it possible to infer the relative loading of certain structures, or to specify at what angle of rotation a given structure begins to resist strongly.

WHY IS THE SPINE CURVED?

The purpose of the 'S-shaped' curvature of the spine in the sagittal plane (Fig. 8.1) is not straightforward. The cervical lordosis develops when an infant first lifts its head to move around, and the lumbar lordosis follows when the child starts to walk upright. A lumbar lordosis can be induced artificially in growing monkeys and rats by forcing them to walk on their hind legs.[153,666] It appears therefore that spinal curves have 'something to do' with locomotion in upright posture. But what?

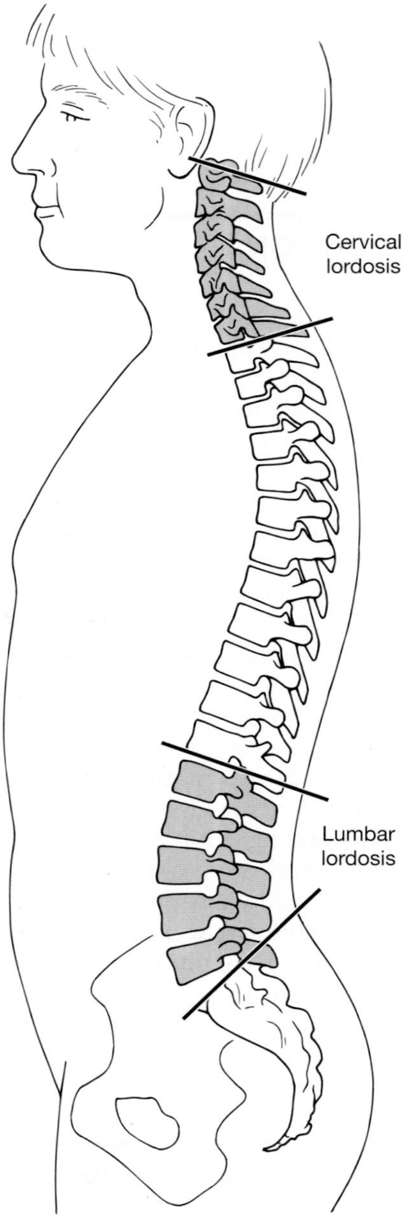

Figure 8.1 The 'S-shaped' curves of the spine assist in shock absorption during locomotion. See text for details.

Spinal curves are not required to give a level line of sight during upright walking, because a straight spine would do that just as well. To a certain extent, the curves provide rotational stability in the sagittal plane by distributing body mass away from the straight line between skull and pelvis. This mechanism can be likened to a 'tight-rope walker' extending his arms out sideways to reduce side-to-side wobble. In both cases, distributing body mass away from a central axis of rotation increases the moment of inertia about that axis, and therefore makes it easier to maintain balance. In addition, a lumbar lordosis increases motion 'coupling' in the lumbar spine (for example, linking lateral bending with axial rotation[163]) and this has been proposed as a fundamental mechanism to facilitate pelvic movements during locomotion.[300] However, the soldier's habit of swinging the arms backwards and forwards when marching can achieve pelvic rotation just as well.

The most important function of the spinal curves is revealed by the manner in which they vary during the walking cycle. Sagittal-plane curves increase and decrease during every stride, with an amplitude of approximately 1–2° per lumbar level.[782] This suggests that the curved spine can absorb and release energy during each stride, somewhat in the manner of a bed-spring. Generally, a curved shape allows a compressed structure to be deformed in bending, rather than pure compression, and this in turn enables it to act as a shock absorber.

But this is still not the whole story, because flexion-extension movements of only 1–2° per lumbar level are resisted very little by the spine (see p. 144), so spinal tissues themselves are unable to absorb much strain energy.[38] This is perhaps just as well, because a proportion of absorbed strain energy is always lost as heat (this is 'hysteresis' energy: p. 7), and the avascular discs would find it difficult to dissipate much heat during vigorous exercise. Very large and poorly vascularised tendons in the legs of race-horses have a similar problem, so that exercise-induced temperature rises may cause degenerative changes within them.[868] The usefulness of the spinal curvature during locomotion becomes apparent when it is realised that large muscles of the back and abdomen must be working vigorously to oppose gross changes in spinal curvature, in much the same way that the quadriceps and calf muscles oppose knee and ankle flexion.[37] Substantial antagonistic activity of the trunk muscles in supporting the upright spine has been measured using electromyography[305] and can be inferred from measurements of intra-discal pressure.[582] The stretched tendons of these trunk muscles are the real spinal shock absorbers. The importance of musculo-tendinous shock-absorption can be appreciated by jumping off a chair and landing with straight legs and back: the elasticity of discs, bones and articular cartilage could do little to protect from a damaging impact unless the body's joints were allowed to flex, against the resistance of their muscles. (The experiment is better imagined than performed!)

Spinal curves, therefore, allow some of the energy associated with up-and-down movements of locomotion to be absorbed by the tendons of trunk muscles and, to a lesser extent, by the ligaments and discs of the spine itself. In this way, they reduce the vertical accelerations which would otherwise be transmitted from the pelvis to the skull. These mechanisms could also operate when a person sits on a vibrating surface such as a tractor seat, although most sitting postures involve some reduction of the spinal curves (see Ch. 10) so the shock-absorption would be less. During static postures, either sitting or standing, there is no obvious benefit to be gained from the spinal curvature. It has been suggested that a lumbar lordosis strengthens the spine by allowing it to behave as an arch,[59] but the conclusions of this paper have been questioned.[2]

MOVEMENTS OF THE LUMBAR SPINE

RANGE OF MOVEMENT: RADIOGRAPHS AND IMPLANTED PINS

The range of spinal movements can be measured in-vivo most accurately using stereo radiographs[637,764] and average values for young men are given in Figure 8.2. The overall range of sagittal-plane movement is approximately 14° at most lumbar levels, although the changing proportions of flexion and extension indicate that the reference position (erect standing) involves more extension at L3–4 and L4–5 than at other lumbar levels. Figure 8.3 also shows values obtained from cadaveric spines which have been flexed and extended right up to the elastic limit of their ligaments. The similarity between in-vivo and in-vitro ranges of movement suggest that healthy people can flex and extend their lumbar spine close to their ligamentous limits, although the back muscles normally provide a small margin of safety in full flexion.[13,14]

Lateral bending movements are slightly less than in the sagittal plane, especially at L5–S1 (Fig. 8.2). Axial rotation movements of the lumbar spine are barely larger than the errors in the radiographic technique used to measure them,[640] but their small size (approximately 1°) has been confirmed by measuring the movements of metal pins inserted into the spinous processes of healthy

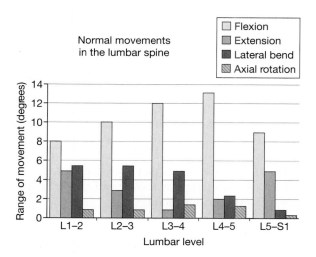

Figure 8.2 Ranges of movement in the lumbar spine in healthy young men: data from bi-lateral X-rays.[637,640] Values for lateral bending and axial rotation are averaged for movements to the left and right from the neutral position (relaxed standing).

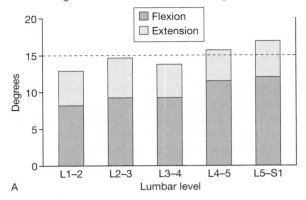

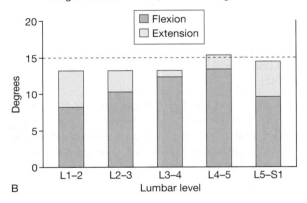

Figure 8.3 (A) Ranges of movement for cadaveric motion segments. Overall mobility is similar to that in (B), but there is rather more extension in the cadaveric spines, presumably because their reference position (unloaded) involves some flexion compared to the reference position for living people (erect standing). (B) Ranges of sagittal plane movement in young men as measured by bi-lateral X-rays.[637] The reduced range of extension at L3–4 and L4–5 suggests that these levels were already extended in the reference position, which was erect standing.

volunteers.[314,480,758] Lateral bending has also been measured in-vivo using implanted pins.[75]

RANGE OF MOVEMENT: SKIN-SURFACE TECHNIQUES

Assessment of techniques

Invasive techniques can be used on small groups of subjects, but other methods must be devised to characterise the effects of age, gender, pathology and physical training on spinal range of movement. Most of these methods use devices attached to the surface of the back. Devices such as inclinometers and flexicurves which measure spinal curvature directly agree well with radiographic measurements of vertebral rotations, with small systematic errors, and correlation coefficients greater than 0.9.[25,703] Accuracy is better for flexion than for extension.[703] Reported disagreements between skin-surface measurements and radiographs in one study can be attributed to the measurements being taken at different times in different postures.[763] It is important to realise that it is difficult for a supple person to fully flex their lumbar spine while sitting in a chair with the knees flexed.[669] Skin-stretching as measured by the Schober test does not correlate well with radiographic measurements of mobility[218,657] although an apparent correlation was obtained by Macrae and Wright[489] who (incorrectly) pooled data from normal subjects and patients suffering from ankylosing spondylitis. Schober measurements are unreliable[557,657] and are affected by body weight, lumbar lordosis and trunk length.[24,550] The electromagnetic '3-Space Isotrak' device can give accurate values of lumbar flexion if it is mounted on the back with its electrical cables running horizontally,[210,218] but if the cables run over the shoulders then flexion movements tend to be exaggerated[353] possibly because the cable tilts the sensor. Isotrak measurements of lateral bending appear reasonable, but measurements of axial rotation must include large movements of the skin and thorax because they greatly overestimate the movements measured by radiographs.[639] Optical movement-analysis devices can track the position of skin-mounted markers with considerable accuracy, but the computed values of spine angular movement do not agree closely with radiographs.[644]

Variations in lumbar mobility with age and gender

Skin-surface measurements have been used to show that sagittal mobility decreases with age,[230,773] especially in the upper lumbar spine.[128]

Mobility in the frontal plane also decreases with age, but axial rotation appears to be unaffected.[538] Gender differences in the full range of sagittal movement are generally small[230] although women extend more from the standing position, whereas men flex more.[128,231,773]

Other influences on lumbar mobility

Mobility measurements must be taken according to a strict time protocol, because during sustained or repeated flexion, the restraining ligaments 'creep', allowing flexion angles to increase by 5–10% in just a few minutes.[211,535] Attention must also be paid to the time of day, because fluid expulsion from the discs (p. 169) increases the range of lumbar flexion during the day by 5–6.5° in healthy subjects[20,230] and 11° in back pain patients.[239] The range of lateral bending also tends to increase,[230] but the range of extension is unaffected.[239]

The range of axial rotation is decreased in stooped postures because the increased forward shear force presses the zygapophysial joint surfaces firmly together.[320] It has been suggested that flexion could increase the range of axial rotation by allowing more 'free play' to the tapered inferior articular processes[639] but the Isotrak measurements in support of this theory contain large artefacts.

Appropriate physical training can increase the range of lumbar flexion and lateral bending in adults by 5% and 9% respectively[872] but it seems unlikely that the range of lumbar extension can be increased much.[444] The evident suppleness of certain athletes and dancers is mostly attributable to increased flexibility of their hamstring muscles.[444]

PATTERNS OF MOVEMENT
Intersegmental movements

The time course of lumbar flexion or extension movements during simple bending and lifting tasks has been measured using a variety of techniques. The best is videofluoroscopy, which is effectively a continuous X-ray image recorded by a video camera. It is invasive, and the image enhancement techniques required to obtain sharp pictures reduce sampling frequency to 2.5–5 Hz.[397,612] This technique has shown that when healthy subjects bend forwards slowly from the upright position, the initial and final movement must take place in the hips, and that lumbar flexion usually either starts in the upper lumbar spine and spreads smoothly to the lower levels,[397] or else all levels flex at the same time. No particular pattern predominates in the lumbar spine when subjects straighten up again,[612] and no contrary or 'paradoxical' movements at individual lumbar levels were observed.[397] Translational (gliding) movements between adjacent vertebrae were 1.1–3.3° in flexion, and 0.3–1.3° in extension.[397] Videofluoroscopy has also shown that expert weightlifters flex their lumbar spine when lifting a barbel from the ground, sometimes by a considerable amount.[161]

Patterns of intersegmental movement have also been studied using skin-mounted devices or markers, but errors arising from skin movement artefact may explain why movements of individual vertebrae appear inconsistent.[279] Oscillating intervertebral movements during treadmill walking have an amplitude of 1–2° per lumbar level in both the sagittal and frontal planes, and a similar movement appears to occur at the hips.[782]

Coupled movements

Any primary movement of the spine deforms the intervertebral discs and ligaments, and may cause the neural arches to make contact with each other. Because the material properties of spinal structures vary from place to place, and because the geometry of the neural arch is so irregular, the primary movement usually creates small 'coupled' movements in other planes, as the spine bends and twists in order to minimise resistance to the primary movement. For example, a primary movement in lateral bending may cause the bony surfaces in one of the zygapophysial joints to meet at an oblique angle, and this would cause one vertebra to move in the direction of this contact force. Generally speaking, coupled movements measured in-vitro are small, inconsistent, and depend on posture.[163,625] In living people they are small and probably modified by muscle action.[640] However, consistent motion coupling has been measured in living people by inserting steel pins into the L3 and L4 spinous processes of healthy volunteers: primary movements in lateral bending were consistently coupled with small twisting movements to the opposite side, and with some flexion.[758]

MOVEMENTS OF THE WHOLE LUMBAR SPINE

Skin-surface measurements of overall movement between L2–S1 made with the Isotrak show that when people lift weights from the floor, they flex their lumbar spine by 85–105% of the range between upright standing and full flexion.[14,216,217] Subjects with poor spinal mobility often exceed 100% of their static range of flexion[210] and this is not a contradiction in terms, because static limits can be exceeded during dynamic 'lunging' movements. Even if they bend their knees, normal subjects find it impossible to lift a 10 kg weight without flexing the lumbar spine by more than 50%[216] (Fig. 7.7). When bending forwards from a standing position, with legs straight, the initial angular movement probably starts in the hips,[397] but this is soon followed by a phase of motion dominated by lumbar flexion. The contribution from hip flexion then increases and dominates the final phase of movement.[240] Straightening up again with a weight in the hands involves hip extension at first, and then the lumbar spine extends.[589] When asked to lift a heavy weight while keeping their knees bent, young men tend to raise their hips and straighten their legs first, and then extend the lumbar spine only when the main effort of lifting is over.[192] The thoracic spine does not move much during such activities.[192]

SPINAL MOVEMENTS AND SPINAL DISORDERS

Attempts have been made to distinguish between 'normal' and 'back pain' populations on the basis of spinal movements. In general, patients with back pain move more slowly[541] and through a smaller range of movement[134,525,638,658]

presumably because full-range movements exacerbate their pain. Patients sometimes show abnormal 'coupling' of movements[764] or show 'steps' in an otherwise smooth movement.[541] Patients with degenerative spondylolysthesis tend to move the slipped level first when bending forwards, sometimes in a 'disordered' way, and when returning to the upright position again the affected level can be slow to extend.[612] Differences can be demonstrated between different groups of patients as regards their spinal movement patterns[643,785] or torque-generating capacity[598,599] and those with back pain can be identified.[87] However, the variability in mobility and movement patterns found in normal people and patients makes it difficult to assign an individual patient to a specific diagnostic group on the basis of these measurements.[541]

Movement analysis techniques can also be used to monitor patient progress during rehabilitation.[492,525] Again, the natural variability of spinal movements hinders the identification of significant progress in specific individuals or patient groups. The use of large 'isoinertial' machines to monitor the mobility and strength of patients' backs has been extensively and critically reviewed.[598]

A restricted range of sagittal-plane movement causes the lumbar spine to be subjected to increased bending stresses,[210] and reduced lumbar mobility increases the risk of future low back pain.[24] A similar increase in risk is associated with a tendency to bend the lumbar spine more than average when performing standardised lifting tasks in the laboratory.[506] This association could be interpreted in terms of impaired coordination or motor control, and is analogous to the increased risk of knee pain in those people ('microklutzes') who walk heavily.[675]

TECHNIQUES USED TO INVESTIGATE SPINAL FUNCTION

Our knowledge of spine mechanics is derived mainly from experiments on animals and cadaveric spines, and from mathematical models, so it is appropriate to consider the limitations of these techniques before dealing with the information they produce. The following account is based on a previously published methodological review.[4]

MECHANICAL TESTING OF CADAVERIC TISSUES

Load and loading rate

Most biological tissues are stiffer when high forces are applied to them (i.e. they are 'non-linear'), and they are also stiffer when forces are applied rapidly (i.e. they are 'visco-elastic'). It follows that the spine's response to loading depends on the magnitude and rate of loading, so both of these should be as realistic as possible. As described in Chapter 7, the spine is subjected to 3–6 kN of compression and 10 Nm of bending during routine manual handling tasks, and these forces are applied rapidly, typically between 0.2 and 5 s. Cadaveric specimens should be loaded with similar severity. Also, the spine's resistance to one form of loading depends on other forces which are applied at the same time (for example, a compressive preload increases resistance to bending[386]) so cadaveric experiments should aim to reproduce the combined 'complex' loading encountered in life. It is not normally necessary to apply separate forces to simulate the action of each individual muscle, because any number of forces acting in the same plane can be represented by a single 'resultant force' (Fig. 8.4), provided that the vertebrae can be assumed to be rigid, which is usually the case. Finally, cadaveric tissues must be protected from dehydration during prolonged testing, but on the other hand, intervertebral disc tissue must not be allowed to come into contact with water unless the disc is under load, because unloaded disc tissue can absorb water and swell to an unphysiological extent.

Effect of death on the spine's mechanical properties

In this materialistic age, there is no reason to suppose that the moment of death changes

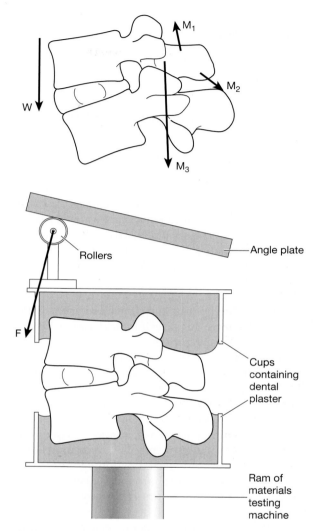

Figure 8.4   The upper diagram represents the many muscle forces (M), and body weight (W), that act on a lumbar vertebra. In cadaveric experiments, it is convenient to sum all of these forces into a single 'resultant' force (F) which has a specified magnitude, direction and point of application.

the mechanical properties of the spine. Certain changes were noted when creep tests were performed on pig spines, just before and after death,[413] but similar changes were noted in repeated tests even though the animals did not die in-between,[414] so the changes are due, at least in part, to poor reproducibility of the experimental measurements.[5] Respiration may possibly influence the spine's mechanical properties,[413] but this would constitute a very small mechanical perturbation which could be simulated on cadaveric material if considered worthwhile.

Changes in the hours following death

The loss of muscle tension after death reduces loading of the intervertebral discs, allowing them to imbibe water from surrounding tissues. The same physico-chemical process causes discs to swell up every night when a person relaxes their muscles during sleep, and it is reversed during the following day's activity. It is misleading to talk of a 'normal' or 'physiological' disc hydration because hydration depends on many factors, including loading history and age (see Ch. 10). Preliminary creep tests can be used to bring cadaveric discs into the physiological range before other tests are performed on them.[20,542,646] The water content of cadaveric discs differs slightly from that of discs removed during anterior fusion operations,[391] but it is not clear just how much of the difference is due to post-mortem changes, and how much to degenerative changes in the surgically-removed discs.[542] Apparent post-mortem changes in disc hydration and swelling pressure suggested by Johnstone et al.[391] may be an experimental artefact caused by storing discs for several hours after they have been cut away from the vertebral body: this would cause the nucleus to lose its intrinsic prestressing by the anulus and ligamentum flavum, and allow a re-distribution of water and swelling pressure throughout the disc.[542]

The cooling down of cadaveric tissues after death influences their mechanical properties. Spinal ligaments shrink slightly at 21°C so that they are less extensible,[340] and laboratory temperatures reduce the rate of creep in intervertebral discs and tendons by approximately 10–15%.[168,433] Bones are 6% less extensible at 21°C[723] and the fatigue life of vertebrae is probably higher at laboratory temperature.[113] Currently we do not know if differential thermal contraction in different spinal tissues leads to a measurable change in load-sharing between them.

Effect of frozen storage on mechanical properties

Frozen storage has a variable effect, being greater when freezing is at −20°C than at −80°C, and affecting time-dependent creep properties more than elastic. Freeze-thawing at −80°C has a negligible effect on tensile properties of the anulus,[273] ligaments[794] or bone.[723] Freeze-thawing at −20°C does not change the compressive stiffness of motion segments[745] or affect intra-discal pressure,[580] and only minor changes in the gross elastic mechanical properties of motion segments occur during subsequent prolonged laboratory testing.[629] Freeze-thaw cycles at −20°C lead to faster creep in the highly-hydrated discs of young pigs, possibly as a result of minor cracking of the vertebral body endplate[67] but this does not happen with mature human discs.[203] Freeze-thawing has been reported to increase the compressive strength of young pig spines by 24%,[146] but this result is difficult to explain, and may not be applicable to human discs. When cadaveric human motion segments are subjected to creep loading at 1 kN and 21°C, they approach an equilibrium height loss of approximately 20%[542] which is similar to the diurnal loss in height and volume of living discs, as measured from magnetic resonance imaging (MRI) scans taken in the early morning and evening.[104]

It appears that the combined effects of death, cooling, and post-mortem storage can change certain mechanical properties of cadaveric spines, but these changes are small compared to the differences in mechanical properties between individual spines. Their effects can be minimised in cadaveric experiments by appropriate experimental design: for example, by comparing mechanical properties in the same specimens before and after some planned intervention.

'Motion segment' experiments

Additional problems arise when spines are dissected into 'motion segments' consisting of two vertebrae and the intervening disc and ligaments. The longitudinal and supraspinous ligaments are weakened during dissection because they contain fibres which span several vertebrae. Also, the inferior and superior surfaces of the vertebral bodies of a motion segment must be loaded by rigid plaster or metal plates, rather than by an intervertebral disc. However, this is unlikely to have much effect because compressive failure always occurs in the inner endplates, which are loaded naturally.[115] Testing whole lumbar spine specimens, from L1–S1, avoids these problems, but it creates others, because a curved lumbar spine buckles when compressed in-vitro without any support from living muscles. Buckling can be avoided by using steel cables to simulate the action of individual muscles[860,861] or by using cables to follow the line of action of the resultant force from numerous muscles[636] but neither of these techniques is suitable for applying high forces in a rapid manner.

MATHEMATICAL MODELS

Mathematical models of the spine depend on materials properties obtained from cadaver experiments, and so incorporate the same post-mortem artefacts. In addition, they are obliged to make simplifying assumptions regarding the mechanical behaviour of complex fibre-reinforced composite materials such as the anulus fibrosus. Analytical models must simplify spine anatomy, often to an unrealistic degree. This can be overlooked if the purpose of the model is merely to demonstrate some mechanism in a qualitative manner (for example, to show that any reduction in nucleus volume will lead to increased radial bulging of intervertebral discs[111]) but simplifications become a problem if the model is used for quantitative predictions (for example, the angle at which anulus fibres become damaged in torsion[367]). Finite element models are able to represent the anatomy correctly, but for some reason, many of them concentrate on upper lumbar levels[290,734] so their conclusions may not be applicable to the wedge-shaped L4–5 and L5–S1 discs which are of most clinical interest. The precise shapes and spacing of the opposing zygapophysial joint surfaces have a critical effect on the predicted contact stresses, and even finite-element models must approximate these shapes and spacing from limited cadaveric material.[735,738] Evidently, the mathematical modellar can choose between a wide variety of assumptions, material properties, and shapes, until the output of the model appears 'reasonable', so the models have little true predictive power. However, they are able to explore internal mechanisms that would be difficult to verify experimentally[448,736,737] and they can examine how intervertebral disc function depends on variable factors such as height and water content.[478,479] Another problem with most finite-element models is that they are constructed using averaged geometrical and materials properties, so that they are unable to predict the diversity of mechanical behaviour encountered in different spines, and which may be of clinical interest.[29] Some modellers have taken diversity in geometrical and materials properties into account in order to reduce this problem.[687,775]

ANIMAL MODELS

Some mechanical properties of spinal structures can be assessed in living animals[413,414] but these experiments present severe technical problems, including poor reproducibility.[5] Experiments on small animals can be used to demonstrate underlying biological principles within living spinal tissues,[378,477] provided that allowance is made for the fact that metabolites can diffuse much more rapidly into small animal discs than large human ones (pp. 166–167). Problems of scale mean that structural failure can occur quite differently in human and animal discs. According to the 'cube-square law' (p. 8) engineering structures can not simply be scaled-up unless the materials used to make them also increase in strength: for example, a small bridge can be made of wood, but a very large one requires steel (or a different design). Similarly, it might be anticipated that the materials properties, and failure mechanisms, of spinal tissues will differ in the human and the mouse. Small inter-species differences in the shape of spinal structures may also be important, because shape affects the magnitude and location of maximum stresses within the disc[479] and it affects the ease with which cadaveric discs can be induced to prolapse.[8] The age of experimental animals must also be taken into account, because age greatly affects the distribution of compressive stress within the intervertebral discs (p. 125), and the ability of cartilage cells to respond to mechanical stimuli falls with age.[515]

The above discussion highlights one of the underlying problems of spinal research: only very limited interventions can be contemplated with the spines of living people, so it is often necessary to turn to some cadaveric, mathematical or animal model in order to make progress, and each of these types of models has its strengths, weaknesses and areas of applicability.

VERTEBRAE

VERTEBRAL BODY

Lumbar vertebral bodies (and the intervening discs) resist most of the compressive force acting down the long axis of the spine, with the exact proportion decreasing with age (p. 117), and depending on posture and loading history (see Ch. 10). Most of this load must be resisted by the dense network of trabeculae, because removal of the outer shell of cortical bone weakens the structure by between 10%[526] and 35–44%.[882] One finite-element model supports the lower of these figures[741] and another indicates that relative loading of the cortex increases from 34% near the endplates to 63% at mid-height in the vertebral body.[149]

The endplates which mark the boundary with the intervertebral discs are of thin cortical bone, perforated by many small holes which allow the passage of metabolites from bone to the central regions of the avascular discs.[682,683] These holes doubtless weaken the endplate, and may explain why it is the most easily damaged structure in the lumbar spine (p. 133).

Vertebral bodies lose strength with age to such an extent that fracture can occur during the normal activities of daily living, such as opening a window.[573] Weakening is more pronounced in women, and is associated with hormonal changes following the menopause (p. 58). Trabecular bone is affected more than cortical, and when trabeculae are lost, they probably are never regained. Vertically-orientated trabeculae which lie just behind the endplate frequently show signs of damage in elderly cadaveric spines,[824] and there is an overall reduction in the amount of trabecular bone in the centre of an old vertebral body which appears to be related to degenerative changes in the adjacent discs.[742] As a result, load-bearing by the vertebral body cortex increases with age [688,882] and the endplates bulge more and more into the vertebral body.[350,811] Vertebral bodies may possibly be hydraulically strengthened during rapid loading by the blood trapped inside them, but this theory has not been supported by experimental evidence.[373]

NEURAL ARCH

The neural arch is mostly cortical bone, with only a small volume of trabecular bone inside, so it is unlikely to weaken as much with age as the vertebral body. Numerous processes serve as attachment points for muscles and for ligaments. If muscle and ligament forces become unbalanced, then the entire neural arch can bend upwards or downwards relative to the body. For example, touching the toes generates high forces in the erector spinae, which pull down on the neural arches of lumbar vertebrae and bend them downwards (in-vivo) by 2–3° on average.[313] When full flexion is simulated on cadaveric motion segments, tension in the intervertebral ligaments causes the inferior articular processes to bend forwards and downwards by 1–6° relative to the vertebral body, pivoting about the pars interarticularis.[313] Similarly, in full extension, bony contact between the neural arches bends the inferior articular processes backwards and upwards. The relevance of this to spondylolysis is considered on page 156. The spinous processes can make firm contact in full extension, or following pathological disc narrowing, so that a proportion of the compressive force acting on the spine can be resisted by these 'kissing spines'.[21]

ZYGAPOPHYSIAL JOINTS

ARTICULAR SURFACES

These small synovial joints have gently-curved articulating surfaces with an average area of 1.6 cm^2.[779] They stabilise the lumbar spine in compression, and prevent excessive bending and translation (gliding movements) between adjacent vertebrae. Articular cartilage removed from these joints will swell up if it is immersed in saline, suggesting that the joint surfaces are permanently pre-stressed in the body,[795] presumably by the ligamentum flavum. In this manner, they are able to protect the intervertebral discs. The articular surfaces are approximately vertical in the upper lumbar spine, but are more oblique at L4–5 and L5–S1 (Fig. 8.5). This explains why the lower lumbar zygapophysial joints resist approximately 20% of the compressive force acting perpendicular to the mid-plane of the discs, while at the upper levels they resist only half as much.[6] Most of the resistance to axial compression comes from the lower margins of the articular surfaces,[229,735] but the presence of an extension moment greater than 4 Nm, causes direct extra-articular contact with the inferior lamina.[229,707] Pathological disc narrowing can lead to small hollows of eburnated bone in the laminae, and corresponding osteophytic spurs around the margins of the inferior articular processes.[6,229] In exceptional cases, the zygapophysial joints can transmit up to 70% of the spinal compressive force from one vertebra to the next.[6] Even in healthy spines, extremely lordotic postures and backwards bending movements can cause substantial compressive forces to be transmitted through the zygapophysial joints (p. 162). Flexion movements probably cause contact to occur in the superior antero-medial regions of the joint surfaces.[735]

Lumbar zygapophysial joints are best able to resist forces acting perpendicular to their broad articular surfaces, approximately in the plane of the disc. They severely limit the range of axial rotation in the lumbar spine[7,34,228] with the greatest contact stresses probably occurring in the superior–posterior margins of the joint surfaces[735] and they are capable of resisting forward shearing

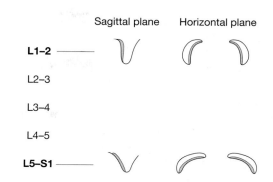

Figure 8.5 The orientation of the zygapophysial joints varies with lumbar level, in both the sagittal and horizontal planes. Changes are gradual between L1–L2 and L5–S1. Cartilage-covered articular surfaces are shown hatched.

forces of 1 kN each.[189] If the zygapophysial joints are asymmetrical in the horizontal plane (Fig. 8.5) then shear induces a small axial rotation.[186] Muscle forces pulling down on the spinous processes may serve to increase the intervertebral shear force resisted by the zygapophysial joints according to a 'door knocker' mechanism.[372] This would help to 'lock' the zygapophysial joints and enhance their stabilising action in flexed postures.[320]

JOINT CAPSULE

The joint capsule consists of a strong outer layer of collagen fibres, 13–20 mm long, and an extensible inner layer containing elastic fibres which are 6–16 mm long.[877] It is thickest in the inferior margins of the joint, where the fibres are longer and run in a superior–medial to inferior–lateral direction. Thickenings of the capsule are often referred to as the 'capsular ligaments' (see below). Full extension can stretch the joint capsule as it resists the backwards rotation of the inferior articular processes about the pars interarticularis[313,878] and there is some evidence that this can cause back pain.[156]

SPINAL LIGAMENTS

Most of the intervertebral ligaments lie posterior to the centre of sagittal plane rotation, which lies within the intervertebral discs (see Fig. 9.9).[642] Therefore their primary action is to protect the spine by preventing excessive lumbar flexion. This protective action is not entirely beneficial, because ligament tension acts to compress the intervertebral discs, so that intra-discal pressure increases by 100% or more in full flexion, even for the same externally applied compressive force.[27]

For ease of reference, typical physical and mechanical properties of the intervertebral ligaments are compared in Figure 8.6. Average lengths and cross-sectional areas of ligaments from eight cadavers with an average age of 63 years have been published.[648] Strength values are from various studies described below. Data of this sort should be viewed with caution, because some ligaments vary markedly with lumbar level, and some are orientated at an angle to the horizontal and sagittal planes. Other ligaments consist of several bundles of fibres with slightly different lines of action, so their overall strength is underestimated by simply pulling the vertebrae apart in a given direction and noting the force at which the first fibres fail. Experimental details given

below characterise the mechanical function of individual ligaments when tested to simulate specific functions in life, such as resisting flexion. The large comparative study of spinal ligament strength by Mycklebust et al.[574] was performed on old cadaveric material (average age 67 years) and so its results are supplemented by those of smaller studies performed on younger specimens.

INTERSPINOUS AND SUPRASPINOUS LIGAMENTS

The fibres of these two ligaments merge in with each other, so that a scalpel cut along their common boundary reduces their combined tensile stiffness by 40%.[226] Mechanically, therefore, they should be treated as a single unit. Together they have a tensile strength of 160 N and fail at a nominal 39% strain when resisting flexion.[18] This very high value of strain for a ligament reflects their position far behind the centre of rotation. Collagen fibres cannot be stretched much more than 10%, so it appears that these two ligaments must either be slack in the neutral position (when the motion segment is neither flexed nor extended) or else their fibres must re-orientate during flexion movements. The anatomy of the interspinous ligament (Fig. 8.6) suggests that its fibres do re-orientate in the initial stages of flexion.[347] This probably explains why the interspinous and supraspinous ligaments provide minimal resistance at small angles of flexion, but resist 19% of the applied bending moment in full flexion, and are the first structures to be damaged beyond the normal range of movement.[18,20]

When considered in isolation, the supraspinous ligament is weak or absent in the lower lumbar spine[366,681] and its tensile strength has been reported as 77 N at L1–L3, falling to 49 N at L3–L5.[226] In the upper lumbar spine, its fibres are difficult to distinguish from those of overlying structures (p. 21), which may explain why some studies accord it a much greater tensile strength.[574] The isolated interspinous ligament has been reported to have a tensile strength of 100 N.[226,574] Another study suggested that it could resist 100 N without damage.[352]

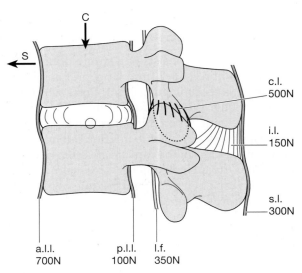

Figure 8.6   Lumbar motion segment, showing typical values (in Newtons) for the strengths of intervertebral ligaments. (9.81 N = 1 kg). Data compiled from various sources. (a.l.l. = anterior longitudinal ligament; p.l.l. = posterior longitudinal ligament; l.f. = ligamentum flavum; c.l. = capsular ligaments of the zygapophysial joints; i.l. = interspinous ligament; s.l. = supraspinous ligament.)

INTERTRANSVERSE LIGAMENT

This is stretched by up to 20% during lateral bending movements, which is more than any other ligament, and it may play a major role in resisting lateral bending.[627] However, its strength has not been assessed, and it could possibly be weak, and slack in the neutral position. In the thoracic spine, it was not considered to be a true ligament by Jiang et al.[390] who found it to be inseparable from interweaving muscle tendons in the region between the transverse processes.

LIGAMENTUM FLAVUM

This unusual ligament contains a network of un-crimped collagen fibres loosely arranged about its long axis[366] together with a high proportion of elastin, a fibrous protein which is more extensible than collagen. Elastin gives the ligament its yellow colour, and enables it to be stretched by 80% without failure.[584] At 100% strain (which would be difficult to achieve in life) the ligament fails by pulling away from the bone.[366] In an unloaded motion segment, the ligamentum flavum is pre-stretched by 11–17%, and therefore pre-stresses the disc in the normal upright posture[366,584]). It also provides much of the spine's resistance to small flexion movements.[18] Its primary mechanical function may be to provide a smooth posterior lining to the vertebral foramen, a lining which does not become slack or buckle when the spine is bent backwards.[712] This would be a considerable advantage, because anterior buckling of a ligament in this critical position could compromise the spinal cord. The ligamentum flavum provides 13% of the spine's resistance to full flexion[18] and its tensile strength is approximately 250–350 N.[574,584]

ZYGAPOPHYSIAL JOINT CAPSULAR LIGAMENTS

These localised thickenings of the joint capsule are sometimes considered as distinct ligaments. They are short but very strong, and appear to be deployed to provide maximum resistance to spinal flexion. Fibres at the antero-lateral margins of the joint capsule are shorter than those at the posterior margin, but because they lie closer to the centre of rotation, they become taut at the same angle of flexion.[3] However, if the vertebrae are simply pulled apart in the vertical direction, the two fibre bundles fail separately, the shorter ones first,[188] and the peak recorded tensile force (for left and right joints combined) is then typically 350–1100 N.[188,574] In full flexion, these ligaments provide 39% of a motion segment's resistance to bending, and transmit an average tensile force of 591 N.[18] The capsular ligaments lie lateral to the mid-sagittal plane, so are able to resist lateral bending as well as forward bending, and they could possibly be the first spinal structures to suffer injury during an excessive movement in antero-lateral bending. They also resist hyperextension[21,343,878] but offer little resistance to axial rotation, at least in the lumbar spine.[7,627]

POSTERIOR LONGITUDINAL LIGAMENT

This thin band adheres to the posterior surface of the discs, but is only weakly attached to the vertebral bodies in between. It contains crimped collagen fibres which straighten out when the ligament is stretched by 7–8%,[366] and it applies a small pre-tension to the disc of approximately 3 N.[794] Its tensile strength has been variably reported as 100 N[574] and 180 N[794] which may reflect some difficulty in determining the precise boundary between disc and ligament. It lies close to the centre of rotation, so can play only a negligible role in protecting the disc from excessive flexion. On the other hand, it is capable of protecting the spinal cord from herniated disc material: when cadaveric discs are induced to prolapse in the laboratory, the displaced fragment of nucleus pulposus can be contained, or even deflected upwards, by this ligament (Plate 3F). Because it is so much weaker than the posterior anulus, the ligament could perform this function only by yielding to the posteriorly displaced disc material until it is sufficiently far from the nucleus that it is de-pressurised. The posterior longitudinal ligament is innervated by a plexus of nerves from the sinuvertebral nerve (p. 47), with capsulated and un-encapsulated nerve endings,[357,437] so it may possibly function as a 'nerve net' to detect abnormal posterior deformations of the underlying disc.

ANTERIOR LONGITUDINAL LIGAMENT

This is thicker and stronger than its posterior counterpart, and adheres to the anterior margins of the vertebrae rather than to the discs. Its crimped collagen fibres straighten out at a stretch of 8–10%.[366] Its strength increases with the speed at which it is stretched[592] and is typically 600 N when tested in-situ[574] and 330 N when stripped from the underlying bones.[794] Interestingly, its strength has been shown to correspond to the mineral content, and presumably strength, of the underlying vertebral body, suggesting that the ligament is capable of mechanically-adaptive remodelling in a manner similar to bone.[594] The anterior longitudinal ligament helps to resist spinal extension movements, but its proximity to the centre of rotation, and to the much stronger anterior anulus, suggest that this is not an important function. Excessive extension would be resisted more effectively (but perhaps, more painfully) by impaction of the neural arches. The anterior longitudinal ligament is very broad, so it could conceivably protect the inferior vena cava and dorsal aorta from rubbing against antero-lateral vertebral body osteophytes.

ILIOLUMBAR LIGAMENTS

Like the intervertebral ligaments, they resist bending and axial rotation of the L5 vertebra relative to the pelvis.[164,462,876] Lateral bending is particularly restricted.[876] The extra stability conferred by the iliolumbar ligaments may explain why L5–S1 is less mobile than L4–L5 in living people, but not in cadaveric motion segments in which this ligament is cut through (Figs 8.2 and 8.3).

INTERVERTEBRAL DISCS

These complex structures lie between the vertebral bodies, and their primary function is to transfer

compressive forces evenly from one vertebral body to the next, while allowing small intervertebral movements. They are too stiff to be good shock absorbers, and are not well suited to resist high bending, shearing or twisting forces acting on the spine. The soft nucleus pulposus ensures that an even distribution of compressive stress acts on the vertebral bodies, with the hyaline cartilage endplates acting as a buffer between nucleus and bone, and the encircling lamellae of the anulus holding the nucleus in place. Hydrostatic pressure within the nucleus generates a tensile 'hoop stress' in the surrounding anulus as indicated in Figure 8.7.

The tendency of the proteoglycan-rich nucleus to swell up in tissue fluid is resisted by tension in the collagen fibres of the anulus and longitudinal ligaments, so that the nucleus exhibits

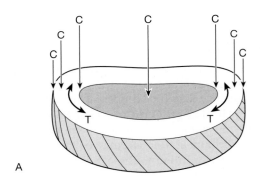

A

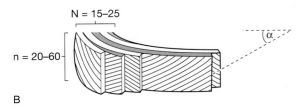

B

Figure 8.7   (A) When an intervertebral disc is loaded in compression (C), a hydrostatic pressure is generated in the nucleus (shaded), and this creates a restraining tensile stress (T) within the anulus. (B) Detail showing individual lamellae of the anulus: note the discontinuities in lamellar structure. The alternating fibre angle (α) is approximately 30°, but varies locally. N = number of lamellae in a typical region of anulus. n = number of collagen fibre bundles visible in a vertical section of a typical lamella. (From[513].)

a pressure of approximately 0.05 MPa in a cadaveric vertebral body-disc vertebral body unit, even when it is unloaded. Pre-tension in the ligamentum flavum[584] raises the intrinsic nucleus pressure in an intact, but unloaded, cadaver motion segment to 0.05–0.12 MPa, with degenerated discs being at the low end of this range.[28,626] Low level muscle activity in living subjects lying prone raises the nucleus pressure to 0.10–0.15 MPa.[672,862] However, small tensile forces in the anulus, ligaments and muscles are not sufficient to prevent the disc from swelling, and this is why people grow 2 cm in stature overnight (p. 169), and why astronauts exposed to zero gravity for long periods of time are reputed to return to Earth up to two inches taller. Under normal gravity, everyday loading of the spine is sufficient to expel water from the intervertebral discs, leading to a diurnal cycle of nocturnal swelling and daytime height loss (p. 169).

ANULUS FIBROSUS

The anulus consists of approximately 15–25 concentric lamellae[154,513] which contain a high proportion of large collagen fibre bundles arranged in alternate directions as shown in Figure 8.7. The structure shown in the Figure is an idealisation, because individual fibre bundles often take a curved course from bone to bone, and irregularities in the lamellar structure are common, especially in the postero-lateral anulus.[513] Note that the alternating dark and light banded appearance of the anulus is due to the way incident light is reflected by collagen fibres reaching the surface at different angles in successive lamellae; it is not due to bands of collagen alternating with bands of softer matrix.

Different regions of the anulus have different functions. The outer lamellae have a high proportion of thick type I collagen fibres, and they function as a strong ligament which resists excessive bending and twisting of adjacent vertebrae.[22,27,111] The middle lamellae are sufficiently deformable that they can behave like a fluid in young non-degenerated disc, although after the age of 35 years they usually behave like a fibrous solid and

directly resist high compressive loading, even when unsupported by the nucleus.[111,514] The vertical compressive stiffness of anulus tissue is greatest anteriorly, and decreases with age and degeneration.[816] The innermost lamellae are sufficiently deformable that they normally behave like a pressurised fluid, even though their collagen fibres are distinct and form a 'capsule' around the nucleus (see Fig. 2.7).

Tensile properties of the anulus

Tensile tests performed on small samples of anulus show that adjacent lamellae are only weakly bound together and can be pulled apart with a tensile stress of 0.2–0.3 MPa at a strain of 100–250%.[268,512] This stress probably represents an upper bound on the strength of the proteoglycan matrix, though it may include the strength of small collagen fibres binding the lamellae together. The anulus is much stronger in the plane of individual lamellae, especially when stretched in the horizontal direction or parallel to one of the two predominant fibre directions.[273] If small horizontal samples of outer anulus are stretched very slowly (0.01% per s) then failure occurs at a stress of 1–3 MPa and a strain of 10–25%, with the anterior anulus being stronger than the postero-lateral, and the outer anulus stronger than the inner.[1,233] These variations may be due to structural differences within the collagen network,[513] because they cannot be explained by differences in chemical composition.[743] At faster strain rates, the stress at failure rises to approximately 3.5 MPa in the horizontal direction[273,874] and 10 MPa in the direction of the collagen fibres.[273,512] When large samples of outer anulus are stretched in the vertical direction, in order to simulate spinal bending, then failure occurs at a stress of 2–4 MPa, and a strain of 30–70%.[312] The anterior anulus is softer and weaker in tension than the posterior anulus, and the inner anulus is much weaker again.[312] Comparisons between studies are difficult, because small specimens appear to be disproportionately weak, especially when stretched vertically, on account of the extra disruption to their collagen fibres (see below). Because of this effect, the vertical tensile strength of the outer anulus in-situ may be 4–9 MPa.[312]

These results suggest that the disc's primary role is to resist compressive force (which generates approximately horizontal tensile stresses in the anulus) rather than bending (which stretches the anulus vertically) and that stretching of the posterior anulus needs to be resisted more vigorously (or more often) than stretching of the anterior anulus. The reduced strength of the inner anulus might be expected from its collagen composition, and from the fact that tensile stresses in the walls of thick pressure vessels are lowest near their inner surface.

As with most skeletal tissues, the tensile strength and stiffness of the anulus falls with age and degeneration.[1,268,273] It also falls during cyclic loading, presumably because microdamage accumulates within the tissue. If 10 000 loading cycles are applied, then anulus tissue fails at approximately 40% of the tensile stress required to damage it in a single loading cycle.[312]

Fibre-composite behaviour of the anulus

The marked effect that specimen size has on anulus stiffness and strength[15] is typical of chopped-fibre composite materials,[365] and indicates that the tensile properties of the anulus depend on collagen-proteoglycan interactions rather than the strength of intact fibres passing from bone to bone. In effect, the collagen fibres provide tensile reinforcement of the anulus in the manner of a material like fibre glass, and the degree of reinforcement is proportional to the average length of fibre fragments within the tissue[15] (Fig. 8.8). This important property means that local damage to the collagen network does not lead rapidly to widespread failure (as it would do if the fibres provided all of the tensile strength, as in a nylon stocking, for example). The fibre-composite behaviour of the anulus also ensures that a great deal of energy is required to pull it apart completely.[22,312] This property is termed 'toughness', and the anulus is one of the toughest materials in the body.

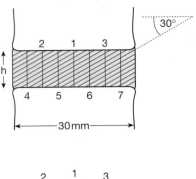
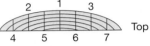

Figure 8.8 If a vertical slice of anulus and bone is taken from the lateral margin of a motion segment, as illustrated, then its tensile properties do not depend greatly on the number of collagen fibres which pass directly from bone to bone. The tensile stiffness of the anulus in the vertical direction is reduced by only 33% when vertical cut '1' is made, even though this cut would be expected to sever all collagen fibres linking the two bones.[15] Some stiffness is preserved even after 7 cuts. This suggests that fibre-matrix interactions make an important contribution to anulus integrity, just as in a fibre-composite material such as fibre glass.

NUCLEUS PULPOSUS

The high water content and loose collagen network of the nucleus give the tissue unusual mechanical properties. The water ensures that the tissue has very low rigidity, so it deforms easily in any direction and equalises any stresses applied to it.[23] In this respect, it resembles a fluid, and so it is correct to speak of a fluid 'pressure' within the nucleus, rather than a compressive 'stress' (see p. 5). When loaded rapidly, however, small samples of nucleus can withstand considerable shear stresses and behave more like a visco-elastic solid.[377] Certainly, the collagen network limits the amount of deformation that the nucleus will undergo: if two soft regions of nucleus are gripped with forceps and pulled apart, there will be negligible resistance up to the point where the collagen fibres become taut, but then considerable force is required to separate the two regions entirely. The tensile strength of the nucleus has never been measured, but may be comparable to that of the anulus when it is stretched in the

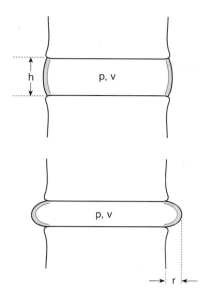

Figure 8.9   The height (h) and radial bulge (r) of an intervertebral disc depend on the pressure (P) and volume (V) of the nucleus pulposus. If the volume is reduced (lower diagram), either by water expulsion or by surgical intervention, then the nucleus pressure falls, and the anulus bulges more. This is rather like letting air out of a car tyre.

radial direction: see above. In effect, the nucleus behaves like a 'tethered fluid', and these peculiar properties blend in gradually with more conventional solid behaviour in the middle of the anulus. In old and mildly degenerated discs, the nucleus contains firm fibrous regions surrounded by a softer gel which ruptures easily when fluid is injected into it. The typical positions of fibrous and gel-like regions within the nucleus explain the 'hamburger' discograms characteristic of mature and non-degenerated discs.[19] The ease with which injected fluid can separate the fibrous nucleus from the hyaline cartilage endplates in discography argues against the theory that the creation of loose 'fragments' within the nucleus of a middle-aged disc is an important step in the process of disc protrusion.[112] In severely degenerated discs, the nucleus is a fibrous solid, often likened to 'crab meat'.[19]

The large proteoglycan molecules which attract and hold water in the nucleus also act to hinder the movements of other molecules through the matrix, even small ones such as glucose, and

water itself. There are no empty pores within the matrix for fluid to pass through quickly, so fluid flow in response to a change in mechanical loading takes place slowly over a number of hours. The precise water content of the nucleus depends on a number of factors including age and loading history,[9,542] and it has a profound effect on internal mechanics of the disc. Any increase in water content (by unopposed swelling, or by injection) increases the pressure within the nucleus[44,676] and this in turn reduces disc bulging,[110] increases disc height[110] and increases the disc's resistance to bending.[20] This is rather like pumping air into a tyre (Fig. 8.9). Conversely, a disc becomes decompressed and bulges like a flat tyre if the water content and volume of the nucleus is reduced, either by creep loading (p. 169), by degenerative changes, or by injury.[110,732]

CARTILAGE ENDPLATES

These thin layers of hyaline cartilage cover the central region of the vertebral body endplates on the disc side (see Fig. 4.3). Physically, this tissue is similar to articular cartilage near its junction with bone, but unlike articular cartilage, it is only loosely bonded to the underlying bone[22,312] presumably because it is always pressed up against the bone by the hydrostatic pressure of the nucleus. Its function appears to be to help equalise loading of the vertebral body,[728] while preventing the migration of the much softer nucleus material into the pores in the vertebral endplate. The hyaline cartilage may also act as a chemical and biological filter between the nucleus pulposus and the blood vessels in the vertebral body. It will also prevent rapid fluid loss from the nucleus into the vertebral body during sustained loading, and so will assist in maintaining the water content and internal pressurisation of the disc.

STRESS DISTRIBUTIONS WITHIN INTERVERTEBRAL DISCS

The technique of stress profilometry has revealed the internal mechanical functioning of the disc to an unprecedented extent, both in-vitro[23,29,30,544] and in-vivo.[547] Because of its importance, it is

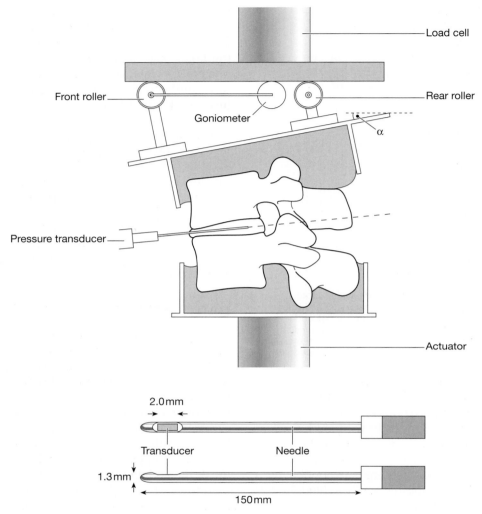

Figure 8.10 Measuring stress distributions inside cadaveric intervertebral discs. A cadaveric lumbar motion segment is secured in cups of dental plaster (shaded) and subjected to constant compressive loading by means of a hydraulic actuator. During this time, a needle-mounted pressure transducer (lower) is pulled through the disc along its mid-sagittal diameter in order to measure a 'stress profile'. Two rollers are used to load the specimen in various angles of flexion or extension, as measured by the goniometer.

appropriate to consider briefly how it is performed, and what is actually being measured.

A static compressive load of 2 kN, sufficient to simulate light manual labour, is applied to a motion segment for a period of 20 s, and during this time, the distribution of compressive stress within the disc is measured at a frequency of 25 Hz by pulling a miniature pressure transducer through it, along its sagittal mid-line, as shown in Figure 8.10. The transducer is a small 2 mm long strain-gauged membrane, mounted in the side of a 1.3 mm-diameter needle.[544,545] The anulus has excellent self-sealing properties[514] and no disc material is expressed through the needle-hole during the experiments. Rotating the needle about its long axis enables the vertical and horizontal components of compressive stress to be measured in successive tests, using the same needle track.

Validation tests have shown that the output of the transducer in most regions of the disc is approximately equal to the average compressive stress acting perpendicular to its membrane.[543] This implies that there is negligible resistance to the matrix deforming into the slight recess in the needle to press on the transducer membrane. The outer 2–4 mm of anulus is a fibrous solid in which there is unlikely to be sufficient 'coupling' between matrix and transducer membrane for reliable recordings to be made. Note that there may be high tensile forces in the collagen fibres in this region of disc, but these are not detected by the transducer. The transducer output represents an average stress acting on the 2 mm long membrane, and this may help to explain why measured compressive 'stress' usually falls steadily to zero near the disc periphery.

Typical 'stress profiles' are shown in Figure 8.11 for discs of all grades of degeneration, as defined by ourselves[19] and by others.[792] The visual appearance of similar discs is shown in Plate 1. In the young grade 1 disc, the measured vertical and horizontal compressive stresses are approximately equal to each other, and do not vary with position across most of the disc. Evidently, the whole interior region of the disc behaves like a bag of fluid, with an outer 'skin' of anulus only 2–4 mm thick. The extension of fluid-like behaviour into the anulus may explain why capillaries and nerve fibres do not grow more than a few mm into the anulus of healthy discs: fluid pressures would press on hollow blood vessels from all sides, and collapse them if the disc was heavily loaded. In the mature grade 2 disc, which is typical of non-degenerated spines aged over 35 years, the size of the hydrostatic central region shrinks to that of the histological nucleus, and small stress concentrations can be seen in the anulus, usually posterior to the nucleus. Grade 3 discs are moderately degenerated, and this is reflected by an irregular stress profile indicating variable resistance to compression from a disrupted fibrous matrix in which the central hydrostatic region is small or absent. Severely degenerated Grade 4 discs are characterised by highly irregular and variable stress profiles, and by an overall reduction in compressive stress. This suggests that such discs, which are often severely narrowed, are being shielded from compressive loading by adjacent structures such as the neural arch, or bridging vertebral body osteophytes.[23,29]

COMPRESSION OF AN INTERVERTEBRAL DISC

When a disc is compressed, the hydrostatic pressure in the nucleus rises and generates a tensile 'hoop stress' in the restraining anulus (Fig. 8.7). According to the theory of thick-walled pressure cylinders, the hoop stress decreases from the inner lamellae to the outer. The anulus also resists compression directly, causing it to bulge radially outwards, and therefore to lose height. This forces the vertebral body endplates closer together, but the central regions of the endplates cannot come much closer together because the nucleus lies between them, and its high water content makes it virtually incompressible. Therefore, the central region of the endplates bulge into the vertebral bodies.

Some of these effects have been quantified in cadaveric experiments. A compressive force of approximately 2 kN stretches the collagen fibres on the disc surface by less than 2%[761] and causes it to bulge radially by 0.4–1.0 mm. Bulging varies around the disc periphery, being greatest in the anterior anulus[762] or postero-lateral anulus[729,852] with the difference possibly being due to the age and lumbar level of specimens tested. Compared to a preload of 250 N, a compressive force of 4.5 kN reduces the height of a motion segment by 0.9 mm, but the height loss in the nucleus is only half of this, so each endplate must bulge into its vertebral body by approximately 0.25 mm.[116,361] Endplate bulging can reach 0.8 mm before failure.[116] A disc's response to compression depends very much on its precise shape and size: for example, discs which have a high ratio of height/area will exhibit higher tensile stresses in the outer anulus, and more radial bulging, for the same applied compressive force.[479] This makes it difficult to extrapolate mechanisms of disc

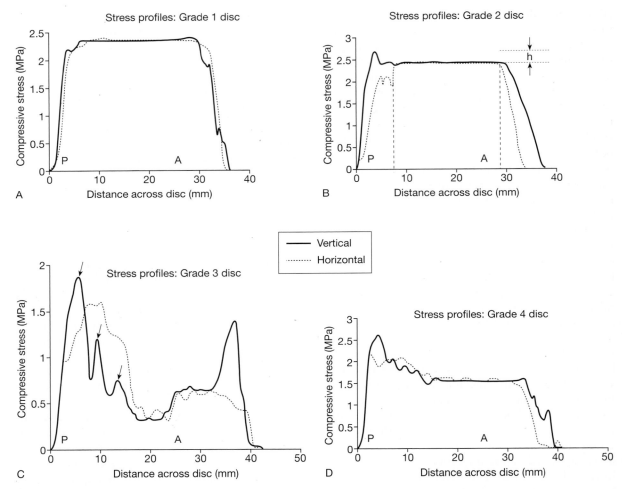

Figure 8.11 Typical 'stress profiles' for lumbar intervertebral discs. Vertical and horizontal compressive stress is plotted against position along the mid-sagittal diameter (P: posterior). (A) In a young, non-degenerated disc, there is a large 'functional nucleus' in which the horizontal and vertical stresses are equal, suggesting hydrostatic conditions. (B) With increasing age, stress concentration (peaks) appear within the anulus, and the size of the hydrostatic nucleus is reduced. (C) and (D) refer to young discs showing moderate and severe degenerative changes respectively. Note the greatly reduced hydrostatic nucleus, and high stress concentrations within the anulus. Grade 4 discs were particularly variable.

structural mechanical failure from one spinal level to another, or from animal to human discs.

BENDING OF AN INTERVERTEBRAL DISC

Flexion movements cause the lumbar discs to pivot about a centre of rotation close to the nucleus pulposus.[642] The anterior anulus becomes compressed and thickened, while the posterior anulus is stretched and thinned. Tension in the posterior anulus acts to increase the hydrostatic pressure in the nucleus.

Experiments have shown that flexion reduces the height of the anterior anulus by 25–35%[8,398] and causes it to bulge radially outwards by approximately 0.1 mm/degree of movement.[762] Concentrations of compressive stress can appear, or grow, in the matrix of the anterior anulus.[27] The posterior anulus flattens[762] and stretches by

50–90% in full flexion.[8,398,641] Crimped collagen fibres can be stretched by 14–16% before failure,[734] and direct measurements of disc surface strain indicate fibre strains of only 0.7% per degree of flexion[761] so these high vertical deformations of the anulus can be achieved only by removal of radial bulge, and by some reorientation of the fibres within each lamella,[690] as shown in Figure 2.6C. Fibre reorientation has been measured by X-ray diffraction[431] and may be facilitated by hyaluronic acid acting as a lubricant between adjacent lamellae. During flexion movements of short duration, the fluid content and volume of the posterior anulus must remain constant, so vertical stretching is accompanied by a corresponding thinning in the radial direction.[12,726] This may have important consequences for disc nutrition (p. 166).

Equivalent mechanisms must operate when the disc is bent backwards and sideways. The ratio of disc height to width is so small that angular movements of the vertebrae of only a few degrees entail large vertical deformations in the anulus. This will lead to particularly high tensile and compressive stresses in the anulus of thin discs with a large side-to-side diameter, especially when they are laterally flexed about their shorter diameter.

AXIAL ROTATION OF AN INTERVERTEBRAL DISC

Torsional movements of the spine generate most tension in half of the collagen fibres in the anulus, with the other fibres tending to become slack[443] as indicated in Figure 2.6B. It has been suggested that only 3° of axial rotation are permitted by the lumbar discs[367] but this theoretical analysis neglected the natural radial bulge of the anulus, and the crimp in its collagen fibres. When cadaveric discs are rotated to 6° by a torque of 15 Nm, collagen fibres on the disc surface are stretched by up to 7%[761] and anulus bulge is reduced by 0.2 mm.[762] Torsion raises the pressure within the nucleus of the disc, presumably because tension in the oblique collagen fibres which resist torsion act to compress the disc at the same time. A torque of 10 Nm applied to a vertebral body-disc-vertebral body unit raises intra-discal pressure in the nucleus by 0.16 MPa, whereas a bending moment of 10 Nm raises it by approximately twice that amount.[714]

SACRUM AND SACROILIAC JOINTS

SACRUM

This large wedge-shaped bone comprises five fused sacral vertebrae. Several of its features are derived from its component vertebrae, and some are more-or-less redundant. The sacrum transfers mechanical loading between the lumbar spine and pelvis by means of the sacroiliac joints, and it anchors the insertions of several back muscles (p. 34). In addition, the sacral canal and sacral foramina provide a particularly safe passage for the cauda equina and sacral nerve roots, in what would otherwise be an exposed and vulnerable location.

SACROILIAC JOINTS
Movements in-vivo

Stereo radiography has been used to visualise the position of implanted metal markers in patients with suspected sacroiliac joint problems.[234,769,770] These studies have shown that sacroiliac joint movements are small in all planes. The greatest movements occur when patients move from the upright standing position to lie prone with one leg hyperextended: in the latter position, the sacrum rotates backwards relative to the pelvis by approximately 2°, the iliac crests rotate inwards (towards each other) by up to 0.2°, and translational (gliding) movements of 0.5–0.7 mm occur between the sacrum and ilium.[769] Most rotations are approximately symmetrical in the sagittal plane, and differ little in symptomatic and pain-free joints, although small differences were observed between patients with unilateral and bilateral symptoms. Movements were 30–40% smaller in men, and tended to increase slightly with age.[769] Implanted metal wires in the sacrum and ilia have been used to demonstrate a similar small range of movement in healthy volunteers, but no significant variations with sex, age or parturition were found.[428] Interestingly, angular rotations of 6–8° and translations of 2.5 mm were observed in a single subject who reported recurrent sacroiliac joint problems.[428] However, manipulation of patients with sacroiliac joint problems failed to cause any angular or translational movement of the joint that could be detected by subsequent stereo radiography, even though there was clinical improvement.[808] Skin surface measurements made on healthy subjects and on gymnasts[746] indicate sacroiliac joint rotations of up to 18° but this probably includes skin-movement artefacts, because the accuracy of

the measurements (as opposed to their reproducibility) was not assessed.

Movements in-vitro

Large sacroiliac joint movements have been observed in five cadavers (four male, one female) aged 52–68, which were placed in extreme 'striding' positions with the legs straight, one stretched out in front, and one stretched out behind.[747] Joint movement was measured to an accuracy of 1.3 mm or 1.0° by detecting embedded lead spheres using CT scans. The total range of sacroiliac joint movement in the sagittal plane averaged 5° for

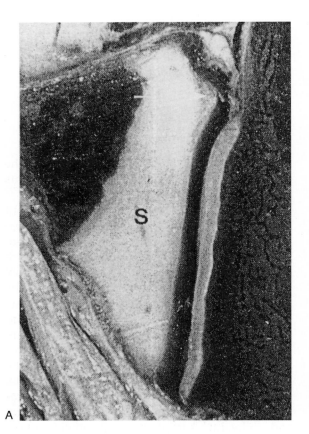 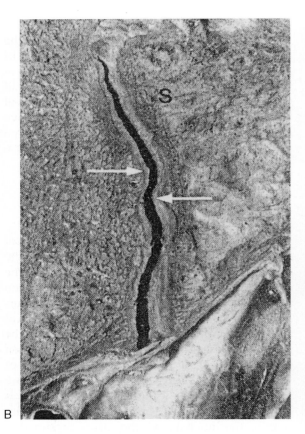

A   B

Figure 8.12 Frontal sections through the embalmed sacroiliac joints of a boy aged 12 years (left) and a man aged over 60 years (right). S indicates the sacral side. Note that the flat surfaces and abundant cartilage of the young joint are replaced with undulating surfaces (arrows) and thinner cartilage in the old joint. (From Vleeming et al.,[835] with permission of J B Lippincott, Philadelphia.)

the left joint and 8° for the right, with extreme values ranging from 3° to 17°.[747] Movements in other planes were 4° or less. Maximum linear displacements of the posterior superior iliac spines relative to the sacrum were 5–8 mm. The authors suggest that similar movements would be observed in living people during vigorous activities such as running or jumping. When eccentric forces of up to 60% body weight were applied to the sacrum of cadaveric pelvises, rotations and translations of approximately 1° and 1 mm were observed.[554,846] Rotations increased by 10% when either the posterior or anterior ligaments were cut, and by 30% when both were cut.[846]

Mechanical function

These joints allow small movements between the base of the spinal column (the sacrum) and the pelvis (ilia). Together with the pubis symphysis they also allow small relative movements of the left and right hip bones, and this could be of considerable benefit during childbirth when their movements are increased by ligament laxity. Apart from this, it is not obvious just what mechanical purpose the sacroiliac joints serve, although this uncertainty has lead to various theories. Sacroiliac joints could play some role in shock-absorption,[38] but they are too stiff to absorb much strain energy, and during locomotion most shock-absorption would come from the tendons of the leg and foot.[38] However, even a small amount of shock absorption may serve a useful function in protecting the integrity of the pelvic ring if it were subjected to a direct blow, perhaps during a fall on the buttocks or hip. Another possibility is that small movements of the sacroiliac joints somehow facilitate locomotion, but it is difficult to imagine how a few degrees of extra movement would be of much mechanical benefit to bones whose other ends are attached to such mobile joints as the hip and lumbosacral joints.

In a young person the joint surfaces are approximately flat, but with increasing age, they develop a series of undulating peaks and troughs which inter-digitate with each other (Fig. 8.12).

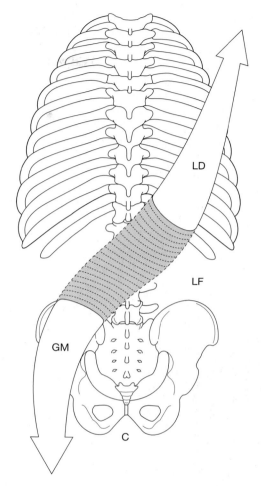

Figure 8.13   The lumbodorsal fascia (LF) forms a mechanical link between the gluteus maximus muscle (GM) on one side of the body, and the latissimus dorsi muscle (LD) on the other. The force transferred across the pelvis will act to press the surfaces of the left hand side sacroiliac joint closer together. In this way, the bilateral effects of this linkage may be to stabilise the sacroiliac joints, by the mechanism of 'force closure'.[836]

These anatomical changes greatly increase the joint's resistance to shearing movements,[834] by a mechanism which has been termed 'form closure'[836] (Fig. 8.13). The undulations suggest that a small relative displacement of the opposing surfaces might become 'locked' if two peaks were to oppose one another. Sacroiliac joint locking and slipping has not been demonstrated experimentally, although there is an extensive clinical literature on the subject.

Sacroiliac joint stability could possibly be increased by muscle action. Tension generated in the gluteal muscles on one side of the body can be transmitted diagonally across the back to the contra-lateral latissimus dorsi by means of the lumbodorsal fascia,[837] as shown in Figure 8.13. These diagonal forces will act to press the surfaces of the sacroiliac joints closer together, and may increase their stability by force closure.[836] This is an attractive hypothesis which seeks to explain how the lumbodorsal fascia can coordinate the function of some of the largest muscles in the body, whilst increasing pelvic stability. However, the size of the forces acting on the passive link – the lumbodorsal fascia – are not yet known.

9

Mechanical damage to the lumbar spine

INTRODUCTION

This chapter considers how the lumbar spine can be damaged during the activities of daily living. Mechanisms of violent trauma are dealt with only briefly because they are not of widespread interest, and there is little scientific work to support the classifications of injury that are currently accepted. On the other hand, a great deal of effort has been spent on trying to understand the origins of limited structural failure in spinal tissues, because such failure is extremely common, is linked to tissue degeneration and back pain, and may be both preventable and treatable. Mechanisms of sacroiliac joint damage are not discussed because of a lack of relevant experimental data.

Not everyone with back pain has a damaged back, and many patients have no detectable spinal pathology of any kind. Evidence is mounting that mechanical back pain can arise directly from high (but non-damaging) stress concentrations within innervated tissues. This is the underlying concept of a 'functional pathology', and is considered separately in Chapter 10.

DAMAGE, INJURY AND FATIGUE FAILURE

Damage can be defined in terms of an acquired defect to, or disruption of, a given structure. In practice, damage manifests itself as a permanent impairment of that structure's ability to withstand applied mechanical loading. An injury involves damage to a living tissue, either by mechanical loading, or by a chemical or electromagnetic influence (such as a burn). In cadaver experiments, gross damage can be detected directly by sight or sound, but the threshold of clinically relevant damage is probably the 'elastic limit' at which non-reversible deformation first occurs (p. 6). At this limit, the gradient of a force–deformation graph first decreases[18,883] as shown in Figure 1.4. If forces are applied slowly to a cadaveric specimen, then water is expelled from it and a certain amount of 'creep' occurs (p. 7). Creep is reversible and is entirely physiological, but creep deformation is not easy to distinguish from non-reversible residual deformation attributable to mechanical damage. For this reason, investigations of failure mechanisms in biological tissues require that mechanical loading be applied rapidly, in a physiologically-reasonable timescale, rather than slowly or incrementally. Quasi-static 'weights in pans' tests are unsuitable for this purpose.

'Fatigue' failure occurs by the accumulation of micro-damage caused by the repetitive application of forces which are too small to cause detectable damage if applied only once (p. 8). There is only a tenuous connection with the quite distinct metabolic process of muscle fatigue, or with 'fatigue' used to mean 'tiredness'. Note however, that fatigue failure is an engineering concept which must be interpreted with caution when applied to living tissues. Repetitive mechanical loading, and the microscopic damage resulting from it, can initiate a beneficial adaptive remodelling response within a living tissue, so that it becomes stronger rather than weaker (see Fig. 4.9). For fatigue failure to occur in a living tissue, microscopic damage must accumulate faster than the adaptive remodelling response can cope with, and this critical rate will depend upon the metabolic rate of the tissue in question, and on the age and health of the individual.[17] Clearly it would be meaningless to perform very long low-intensity fatigue tests on cadaveric tissues, because the lack of a normal biological response would ensure that the outcome could not be applied to living tissues. It would be acceptable, however, to use cadaver testing to study a tissue's response to short-term high-intensity fatigue, because this would be modified less in living tissues. For example,

in a tissue with a low metabolic rate such as the anulus fibrosus, in-vitro fatigue testing of a few thousand cycles could be used to study the effect of spinal flexion occurring in-vivo over a period of hours or weeks; but the application of millions of cycles to simulate several years' activity would be inappropriate.

COMPRESSION: ENDPLATE FRACTURES AND INTERNAL DISC DISRUPTION

As far as the vertebral column is concerned, it is conventional to speak of the 'compressive force' as being that force which acts down the long axis of the spine, at 90° to the mid-plane of the intervertebral discs (Fig. 9.1). As discussed in Chapter 7, this force arises mostly from tension in the paraspinal muscles, and from gravity acting on the mass of the upper body.

RESISTANCE TO COMPRESSION

Compressive loading is resisted mostly by the anterior column consisting of the vertebral bodies and intervertebral discs, but a variable proportion falls on the zygapophysial joints. In the simulated erect standing posture, these joints resist 16% of a typical 1 kN spinal compressive force[6] and much of this is concentrated on the inferior margins of the joint surfaces.[229,739] Intervertebral disc narrowing of 1–3 mm causes increased loading of the articular surfaces, and may also cause extra-articular impingement of the tip of the inferior facet on the lamina below.[229] If the disc height is severely reduced by degenerative change, then up to 70% of the compressive force can act on the zygapophysial joints in lordotic postures.[6] Under these circumstances, severe compressive loading may possibly damage them.

The disc is well designed to resist high compressive forces and has a higher compressive strength than the adjacent vertebrae. Even if the anulus is fissured, there is no herniation of nucleus pulposus material through the fissure in response to pure compressive loading.[109,833] This type of loading is much more likely to affect the endplate.

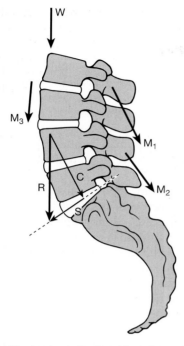

Figure 9.1 The lumbar spine is subjected to various muscle forces (M_1, M_2, etc) and to the weight of the upper body (W). All of the forces acting on a particular intervertebral disc can be represented by a single resultant force (R), and this in turn can be represented by two components (C and S) which act at 90° to each other in anatomically-meaningful directions. The component (C) which acts perpendicular to the mid-plane of the intervertebral disc is referred to as the 'compressive force', and the component (S) which acts in the mid-plane of the disc is referred to as the 'shear force'. Approximately, the compressive force acts down the long axis of the spine, but it is not necessarily vertical: indeed it could act horizontally in someone in a stooped position.

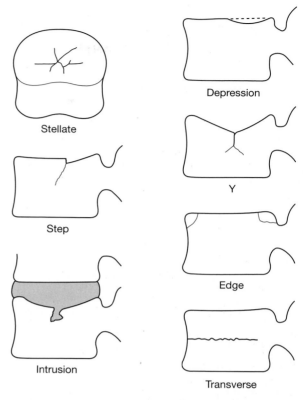

Figure 9.2 Types of vertebral compressive failure, as classified by Brinckmann.[115]

FRACTURE OF THE VERTEBRAL BODY ENDPLATE

The spine's 'weak link' in compression

The vertebral body endplate is the 'weak link' of the lumbar spine, and when the compressive force rises to high levels, the first unequivocal signs of damage always occur in the endplate, or in the trabeculae which support it.[114,371,645,884] This happens even if the postero-lateral anulus is weakened artificially prior to loading, by cutting into it from the nucleus so that a full-depth radial fissure is formed, passing from the nucleus to within 1 mm of the disc periphery.[109]

Vertebral body endplates are usually flat in young adults, but develop a marked concavity with increasing age, and this may be indicative of repeated minor injuries to the endplates themselves or to the vertically orientated trabeculae which support them.[813,824]

Mechanism of fracture

Failure is initiated by the nucleus pulposus of the adjacent disc causing the endplate to bulge into the vertebra.[116,331,361,884] The various types of vertebral compressive damage have been classified by Brinckmann[115] and are depicted in Figure 9.2. Damage can be difficult to visualise, and it is sometimes necessary to press on the bone in order to detect the fine line of fracture running through

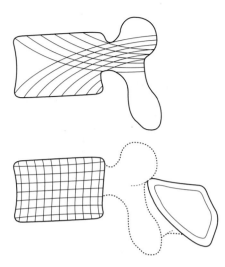

Figure 9.3 Sagittal section through a lumbar vertebra showing the orientation of trabeculae (anterior on left). The plane of the upper section passes through one of the pedicles, and it suggests how trabeculae from the pedicles can reinforce the vertebral endplates, especially the lower endplate. In the mid-sagittal plane (which does not pass through the pedicles) the trabecular architecture is more symmetrical, as shown in the lower section.

the endplate or trabecular bone. The upper endplate is more often damaged than the lower,[115,884] presumably because it is less well supported by the trabecular arcades (Fig. 9.3). In a minority of cadaveric specimens, small quantities of nucleus pulposus are expressed vertically through a damaged endplate to form an intra-osseous herniation, often referred to as a 'Schmorl's node'.[30] Nodes tend to be more irregular in older specimens with reduced bone mineral density.[331] Vertical movement of disc material probably explains why the intraosseous pressure can increase rapidly to 100 mmHg (0.013 MPa) in the damaged vertebra.[884] Adolescent vertebrae may fail in a slightly different manner: compression tests on young pig spines show that they fail by a posterior edge fracture (Fig. 9.2) running from the end-plate down to the cartilage growth plate, which appears to be a zone of weakness before skeletal maturity.[481]

It is important to realise that typical endplate fractures are difficult to detect on plain X-rays[26,116,481,884] although any displacement of nucleus pulposus can be revealed by magnetic resonance imaging (MRI).[481]

Compressive strength of lumbar vertebrae

The compressive strength of the lumbar spine ranges between 2 kN and 14 kN, depending on the sex, age and bodymass of the individual, with a typical value for a young man being 6–10 kN. The high and low extremes refer to male athletes, and old women with osteoporosis, respectively. The strength of human lumbar motion segments in different forms of loading are summarised in Table 9.1.

Vertebral compressive strength can be predicted to an accuracy of about 1 kN using quantitative computer tomography and endplate area[114,115] or from measurements of bone mineral density.[332] Endplate area, and presumably spinal compressive strength, can be estimated from certain anthropometric factors.[170] Bodyweight is a good predictor of vertebral strength in men, but not women.[371] Strength increases down the lumbar spine by approximately 0.3 kN per lumbar level.[113] Reported average strengths of motion segments from young men aged approximately 20–50 years range between 10.2 kN[371] and 6.1 kN.[115] The difference between these values may be attributable to several factors: unlike Hutton and Adams, Brinckmann tested all specimens 'fresh' without prior frozen storage (see below); he applied the compressive force only to the vertebral bodies so that the neural arches probably resisted less than if the force had been applied to the entire vertebrae; he used a sensitive definition of the first signs of failure; and many of his specimens were from patients who had prolonged bed-rest prior to death. This last difference in particular may account for the generally lower strength of his specimens. There are no systematic studies of spinal strength in powerful male athletes, but measurements of bone-mineral density suggest that it may approach 20 kN.[309] The strongest motion segments so far tested were from an athletic young coal miner (13.0 kN[660]) and from a 21-year-old male (14.1 kN[884]). A motion segment fails in compression when its height is reduced by approximately 20–50%, and this requires 4–33 J of strain energy.[884]

Additional information on vertebral strength comes from experiments on animal spines. An

Table 9.1 Strength of lumbar motion segments and intervertebral discs

	Site of failure	Average strength	Comments
A: Motion segments			
Compression	Vertebral endplate	5.2 (±1.8) kN (all specimens)	Depends on endplate area and bone
		6.1 (±1.8) kN (male, 20–50 yrs)	mineral density
		10.2 (±1.7) kN* (male, 22–46 yrs)	
Shear	Neural arch?	2.0 kN?	Strength of disc uncertain
Flexion	Posterior ligaments	73 (±18) Nm	0.5–1.0 kN compressive preload
Backwards bending	Neural arch	26–45 Nm	Disc can be damaged
Torsion	Neural arch	25–88 Nm	Strength depends on criterion of failure
Flexion + compression	Disc or vertebra	5.4 (±2.4) kN	Disc can prolapse
B: Disc + vertebral bodies			
Shear	Anulus?	0.5 kN?	Uncertain
Flexion	Posterior anulus	33 (±13) Nm	Strength unrelated to disc pressure
Torsion	Anulus?	10–31 Nm	Depends on criterion of failure

* Tested in moderate flexion.
Sources of data are given in the text. Values in brackets indicate the standard deviation, and a dash indicates a range of values. B refers to specimens tested without a neural arch.

experiment on young pig cervical spines found that vertebral strength increased if they were compressed rapidly (1 kN/s) compared to slowly (0.1 kN/s), but very rapid loading (16 kN/s) had no further strengthening effect.[881] Frozen storage has been reported to increase the compressive strength of young pig spines by 24%,[146] but it is not apparent why this should be so, or if this result can be extrapolated to mature human spines (see p. 114).

Variations in posture (angle of flexion or extension) do not influence motion segment compressive strength to any great extent.[27,310] This is probably attributable to two opposing effects: in neutral and lordotic postures, the zygapophysial joints share in the weight-bearing (p. 162), and this would be expected to increase strength; but these postures also generate concentrations of compressive stress within the posterior anulus of the disc (p. 163), and this would act to reduce strength.

ANTERIOR WEDGE FRACTURES OF THE VERTEBRAL BODY

If a motion segment is compressed while wedged in full flexion, then failure sometimes occurs in the disc rather than the vertebral body (p. 148). When failure does occur in the vertebra, it is more likely to affect the anterior cortex and a wedge-shaped region of trabeculae behind it (Fig. 9.2), rather than the endplate.[310] This is not invariably the case, however, and similar fractures are sometimes seen after pure compressive loading.[115]

In older subjects with osteoporosis, anterior wedged-shaped deformities of the vertebrae are more common than markedly concave endplates.[607] An increased preponderance of anterior vertebral damage in old people could be due to anteriorly located trabeculae losing thickness and connectivity more than posteriorly located trabeculae.[607] Changes in trabecular architecture are associated with degenerative changes in the adjacent intervertebral discs[742] suggesting that altered stress distributions in degenerated discs (p. 126) create secondary changes in the vertebral body according to Wolf's Law (p. 57). Severe disc degeneration has two major effects on loading of the vertebral body: firstly, it causes an increasing proportion of the compressive force on the spine to be resisted by the neural arch whenever the spine is in the upright position;[6,651] and secondly, degenerative changes reduce the disc's ability to distribute stress evenly, so that high concentrations of compressive stress commonly appear in the posterior anulus when the spine is upright, and in the anterior anulus when the spine is flexed (p. 163). These two effects will combine to ensure that the anterior vertebral body is habitually stress-shielded in upright postures, and so will be vulnerable to bone loss, and yet is heavily loaded whenever the spine is flexed.[651] This could explain why anterior wedge fractures are so common in elderly people, and why vertebral fractures in the elderly are often associated with bending forwards or falling.[573] It can be assumed that any fall on the buttocks will involve high compressive loading of the spine combined with substantial lumbar flexion.[597]

FATIGUE FAILURE OF THE VERTEBRAL BODY

Compressive failure occurs at lower loads during fatigue loading,[113,334,471] as shown in Table 9.2. Typically, compressive strength is reduced by 30–40% if 100 loading cycles are applied, and by 50–60% if 5000 cycles are applied. Damage is reported to be similar to that which occurs during a single loading cycle (Fig. 9.2). However, some slight differences might be expected, because sustained or cyclic loading expels water from the central region of the intervertebral discs,[542] causing them to concentrate more of the loading on to the periphery of the endplate (p. 169). Compressive fatigue damage is probably a common event in life, because micro-fractures and healing trabeculae are found in most cadaveric vertebral bodies.[824]

Table 9.2 Cyclic loading reduces the compressive strength of the lumbar spine

Relative load (%)	Number of loading cycles				
	10	100	500	1000	5000
60–70	10%	55%	80%	95%	100%
50–60	0%	40%	65%	80%	90%
40–50	0%	25%	45%	60%	70%
30–40	0%	0%	10%	20%	25%
20–30	0%	0%	0%	0%	10%

Values in the table indicate the *probability* of compressive failure if a motion segment is loaded for the specified number of cycles at the specified relative load. Relative load is the actual compressive load expressed as a percentage of the load required to cause compressive failure in a single loading cycle. From Brinckmann et al. (1988).[113]

VIBRATIONS

Fatigue damage may accumulate rapidly if the spine is exposed to mechanical vibrations, for example, by sitting on a tractor seat. Vibration frequencies close to the natural resonant frequency of the seated human spine (4–5 Hz) cause the largest vertical accelerations[631,856] and the largest intervertebral movements.[654] Considerable muscle tension is then required to hold the upper body steady.[725,771] In erect standing, the resonant frequency can rise to 5.5–7 Hz, depending on posture, but a distinct resonance is lost when the knees are flexed.[653] Increased muscle tension associated with vibrations would increase disc creep, and cause back muscle fatigue, both of which could lead indirectly to back pain, as discussed in Chapter 10.

INTERNAL DISC DISRUPTION

The idea that compressive overload can directly damage lumbar discs has been disproved by the experiments described above, but compression may lead indirectly to intervertebral disc failure. Compressive damage to the vertebra allows the endplate to bulge into the vertebral body to a greater extent.[110] This effectively increases the volume available for the nucleus, and causes a large and immediate drop in nucleus pressure.[26,30] (A similar pressure drop would occur in any closed hydraulic system if its volume was suddenly increased.) The decompressed nucleus resists less of the applied compressive force, so more of it falls upon the anulus fibrosus, where it generates large peaks of compressive stress within the tissue, particularly posterior to the nucleus (Fig. 9.4). This makes the anulus unstable: the approximately vertical lamellae are more severely compressed than before, and yet receive less lateral support from the decompressed nucleus. It might be expected that the inner lamellae would buckle and collapse into the nucleus as shown in Figure 9.5, and there is recent evidence from cadaveric experiments that this does in fact happen.[30] The inner lamellae also bulge inwards when the nucleus is decompressed by experimental removal of nucleus material.[726] Internal derangements of intervertebral discs are more common than disc prolapse,[178] and reverse bulging of the inner lamellae is found in approximately 35% of severely degenerated discs[321,786] (Plates 1C and 2C).

The effect of endplate damage on internal disc function depends greatly on age, with young discs being less affected than those aged 50–70 years.[26,30] This is probably because the inner anulus of a young disc behaves like a fluid which can deform readily to accommodate the altered shape of the endplates. Hence, the pressure in the nucleus does not fall so much, and stress gradients within the anulus are smaller. Nevertheless, a recent MRI study has shown that vertebral damage in adolescents does often lead on to disc degeneration in the following few years, although this is not often symptomatic.[421] Old and severely degenerated discs may also be less affected by endplate damage than middle-aged discs, but for a quite different reason: they may be narrowed and therefore stress-shielded by the zygapophysial joints, so that decompression of the nucleus leads to extra compressive loading of the neural arch rather than the anulus.[29]

Cadaveric experiments can indicate only the short-term effects of endplate damage on disc function. Longer term effects would be dominated by the reaction of disc cells to changes in their mechanical environment. Paradoxically, this could make matters worse, because disc cell metabolism is impaired by very high and very low matrix compressive stresses.[382] Therefore, the irregular stress distributions created by endplate damage (Fig. 9.4) would probably inhibit metabolism throughout the disc. Reduced proteoglycan synthesis in the nucleus would serve only to reduce nuclear volume and pressure further, so that a vicious cycle of decompression

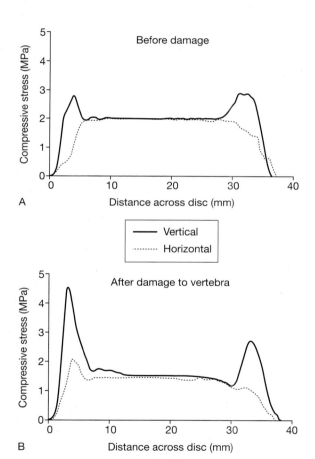

Figure 9.4 The distribution of compressive stress along the sagittal mid-plane of a cadaveric intervertebral disc is greatly affected by damage to an adjacent vertebral endplate. (A) A normal distribution of horizontal and vertical stress for a 46-year-old disc (anterior on right). (B) Endplate damage, caused by overloading the motion segment in compression, reduces the pressure in the nucleus, and generates high stress peaks in the anulus. ('Stress profiles' are explained on p. 124.)

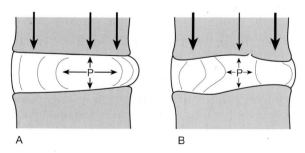

Figure 9.5 Diagrams of a mid-sagittal section through an intervertebral disc (anterior on left). (A) In a normal disc, the pressure (P) in the nucleus pulposus prevents the lamellae of the anulus from collapsing inwards in response to high compressive loading. (B) Endplate damage decompresses the nucleus and increases the direct compressive loading on the anulus. Under these circumstances, the inner lamellae can buckle and collapse into the nucleus.

and cell inactivity could be initiated. Stress peaks in the anulus greater than 3 MPa, such as those in Figure 9.4, would stimulate the production of matrix-degrading enzymes[329] so the anulus might suffer progressive mechanical and enzymatic disruption.

The mechanism just outlined shows how an initial compressive injury to a vertebral body endplate could lead to internal collapse of the anulus, followed by cell-mediated enzymatic degradation of the matrix. It is not necessary to invoke more elaborate biological events, such as inflammatory or auto-immune reactions of the nucleus cells to blood from the vertebral body,[93] although these could occur nonetheless.

Endplate disruption may threaten the adjacent discs in yet another way: healing of the damaged bone may block the nutrient pathways which appear to be essential for normal cell function in the nucleus.[516] Endplate impermeability is closely associated with degeneration of the adjacent disc.[579] (Disc nutrition is discussed on page 166.)

ACTIVITIES WHICH COULD INJURE THE SPINE IN COMPRESSION

During normal living, most of the compressive force acting on the spine is generated by tension in the muscles of the back and trunk (p. 97), and any activity which requires maximal contraction of these muscles can threaten the spine with compressive overload. Vertebrae are frequently crushed during grand epileptic seizures, when normal neurological inhibition of muscle contraction force is lacking.[822] (Many of these injuries occur with the subject lying in bed, so they can not be attributed to falls.) Alarming events, or emergencies during manual handling, could have a similar effect on muscle action and spinal loading. Lifting heavy or bulky objects in a rapid or awkward manner can generate compressive forces higher than the fatigue threshold[217] so fatigue failure would occur if such activities were performed sufficiently often that microdamage accumulated at a faster rate than the body's adaptive remodelling response could cope with. Accidents involving falls and collisions could also injure the lumbar spine in compression.

SHEAR: IMPACTION OF ZYGAPOPHYSIAL JOINTS, AND SPONDYLOLYSIS

It is convenient to define a 'shear' force on the vertebral column as that force which acts parallel to the mid-plane of the intervertebral disc, at 90° to the compressive force discussed above. (This is not quite what engineers usually mean by shear when discussing stress analysis, but there is little scope for confusion.) The shear force arises mostly from gravity acting on the upper body, and so is greater in the lower lumbar spine where the discs are inclined at a steep angle to the horizontal (Fig. 9.1), and in forward stooping postures.

RESISTANCE TO SHEAR

The collagen fibres of the disc and intervertebral ligaments are poorly orientated to resist shear, and indeed the disc just 'creeps away' from it during repetitive loading.[187] It can therefore be assumed that, under most circumstances in life, most or all of the shear force acting on the lumbar spine is resisted by the neural arch. If the zygapophysial joints are asymmetrical in the horizontal plane ('articular tropism') then the intervertebral shear force tends to cause the upper vertebra to rotate towards the side of the facet which is orientated more in the frontal plane.[186] The erector spinae muscles have many fascicles which pass in an inferior–posterior direction from the neural arch to the sacrum and ilium (p. 39), and these are capable of resisting most of the intervertebral shear force.[664] However, it is not certain whether or not they do this in practice. In the upright posture, the muscles of the trunk exert a net anterior shear force on the lumbar spine.[98]

DAMAGE IN SHEAR

The orientation of the lower lumbar zygapophysial joints suits them well for resisting shear (see Fig. 8.5), and when loaded perpendicular to the pars interarticularis, the inferior articular processes can resist approximately 2 kN (range 0.6–2.8 kN) before fracture occurs in the pars, or pedicle.[189] Fracture of the pars can also occur in response to cyclic forces oscillating between 380 N and 760 N.[184] Fractures resemble the pars defects seen in spondylolysis, and this may indeed be one cause of spondylolysis. (Other causes probably include repeated flexion and extension movements, as discussed on p. 156.) Shear damage would be more likely to occur if the zygapophysial joint surfaces were orientated more medially (see Fig. 8.5), or if they were so asymmetrical that one or other of them was called upon to resist most of the shear force by itself. If the zygapophysial joints are removed, then repetitive loading in compression and shear causes the disc to slip forwards by several mm, with a greater slip occurring when the disc is degenerated.[187] More than 20 mm of forward slip can occur if the loading is severe.[187] This may explain why spondylolysthesis often follows bi-lateral spondylolysis.

ACTIVITIES WHICH COULD INJURE THE SPINE IN SHEAR

Vertical gravitational loading creates a forwards shear force on the L4 and L5 vertebrae, because these tend to be inclined forwards to the horizontal (Fig. 9.1). The forward shear force would increase if the trunk was inclined forwards, and if its weight was increased, so marching long distances with a heavy back pack could be a common cause of shear failure of the neural arch.[372] Standing with the abdomen distended in an excessively lordotic posture would increase the inclination of the sacrum, and therefore increase the shear force acting on L5 and S1.

TORSION: IMPACTION OF ZYGAPOPHYSIAL JOINTS, AND ANTERIOR ANULUS TEARS

CENTRE OF ROTATION

The lumbar spine does not have a clearly defined axis for axial rotation (torsion) movements. It probably lies somewhere in the posterior anulus fibrosus, because this is where the axis of minimal torsional stiffness lies[7] and where a motion

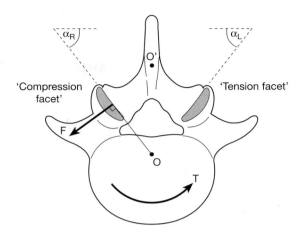

Figure 9.6   Superior view of a lumbar vertebra, showing how the orientation of the zygapophysial joint surfaces restricts axial rotation (torsion) movements. An applied torque (T) causes a superior vertebra to rotate about an axis (O) within the posterior anulus fibrosus, rather than about a posterior axis representing the centre of curvature of the joint surfaces (O'). This brings the articulating surfaces of the 'compression facet' into firm contact and generates a high compressive force (F) on those surfaces. The capsule and ligaments of the opposite 'tension facet' provide little resistance. Note that the orientation of the zygapophysial joints, represented by the angles α_L and α_R, is often asymmetrical, a condition referred to as 'facet tropism'.

segment appears to rotate around if it is subjected to a pure torque.[176] However, small rotational movements bring one of the zygapophysial joints into firm contact (Fig. 9.6) and this probably causes the axis to migrate towards that joint as the applied torque increases. Note that the axis does not lie near the centre of curvature of the zygapophysial joint surfaces (Fig. 9.6). Such a location would minimise the resistance to torsion from these joints, but their function is to limit and guide movement, not merely facilitate it.

RESISTANCE TO TORSION

Lumbar motion segments offer little resistance to very small angles of axial rotation. Collagen fibres in the anulus simply straighten out their 'crimp' waveform (p. 63). Further movement then brings the articular surfaces firmly together in one of the two zygapophysial joints (the 'compression joint') and this restricts movement to 1–2° in young and healthy spines.[7,623] A similarly restricted range of movement has been measured in-vivo (p. 109). The range of axial rotation increases with increasing disc degeneration,[623] and old lumbar motion segments can be axially rotated up to 8° without apparent damage.[7] This could be because age-related degenerative changes reduce the thickness of articular cartilage in the zygapophysial joints, allowing more 'free play'. If a torque of 8.5 Nm is applied to a motion segment, without any compressive loading, then the anterior and lateral anulus resist torsion more strongly than the zygapophysial joints.[443] However, the resistance from the latter increases at higher torques, and when high compressive preloads press the vertebrae closer together: typically, at the limit of the physiological range of movement, 30–70% of the applied torque is resisted by the zygapophysial joint in compression, 20–50% by the disc, and only 0–15% by all of the intervertebral ligaments combined.[7] Of the ligaments, only those associated with the zygapophysial joint capsule are stretched more than 5% when the applied torque reaches 15 Nm.[627]

The fact that torsion is resisted more by bony surfaces than by ligaments or anulus fibrosus may explain why torsion has less effect than bending on intradiscal pressure: the measured increase in pressure in response to an applied torque is less than 15% of that which occurs when an equivalent bending moment is applied.[714]

TORSIONAL DAMAGE

Damage is initiated when the applied torque rises to approximately 10–30 Nm, which is equivalent to a force of 250–500 N acting on the compressed zygapophysial joint.[7] The precise nature of the initial torsional damage is uncertain, but probably involves the articular cartilage or subchondral bone of the compressed zygapophysial joint.

The effects of torsional loading on the disc have long been controversial, but the experimental evidence appears simple enough: in the small range of movement permitted by the lumbar zygapophysial joints, no disc damage has been demonstrated, and none would be expected. Several authors have repeated the suggestion of Farfan[247] that a change in torsional stiffness which

occurs at approximately 3° of rotation represents 'micro-damage' to the disc. However, similar changes in stiffness with increasing displacement are seen in all other disc movements, and is attributable to the opening out of the 'crimp' structure of the disc's collagen fibres (see Fig. 1.4). This is not evidence of damage. Collagen fibres in discs, ligaments and tendons all show this initial region of low stiffness before entering a linear region, up to approximately 10% strain, at which damage really does occur. No evidence of torsional damage to the disc can be detected in the range of movement 1–9°.[10] It would be difficult to reconcile the suggestion that lumbar discs suffer microscopic damage at 3° of rotation with the fact that thoracic discs, which receive less torsional protection from the zygapophysial joints, can be rotated by an average of 3° to each side in-vivo, and by up to 10° at T12–L1, without apparent harm.[314] If motion segments are subjected to cyclic torsional loading, then the only demonstrable damage occurs in the zygapophysial joints rather than the disc.[472] Finite element modelling of the lumbar spine also suggests that disc failure in pure axial rotation is unlikely.[738]

It has been proposed that the range of axial rotation, and the consequent risk of disc injury, depends on the obliquity of the zygapophysial joint surfaces, or on asymmetry in the obliquity of the two joints at a given level ('facet tropism') as shown in Figure 9.6. However, the experimental evidence does not support this theory[34,320] not even when coupled movements are taken into account.[228] Associations between facet tropism and disc degeneration[91,245,605] can be explained by a mechanism involving bending rather than torsion, because tropism could lead to asymmetrical bending and increased stretching of the postero-lateral anulus (Fig. 9.7).

The precise range of torsional movement, and the risk of disc injury, will also be influenced by other components of spinal loading. For example, in a forward 'stooped' posture, the intervertebral shear force rises[372] and presses the zygapophysial joint surfaces closely together, reducing the small range of axial rotation even more.[320] It has been proposed that the tapered shape of the articular facets allows them more free play in certain flexed postures, and this may explain why sitting with the lumbar spine flexed and the legs stretched out in front appears to increase the range of axial rotation.[639] However, the skin-surface measurements offered in support of this mechanism greatly over-estimate the true axial rotation movements of the vertebral column; they may also be influenced by the posteriorly directed shear force which acts on the lumbar spine in this peculiar sitting posture, and which may 'open up' the space between the articular surfaces.

If the zygapophysial joints are cut away, then forced axial rotation damages the disc at approximately 10–20° of rotation, with ultimate failure occurring at 11–32°.[247] Circumferential tears appear in the outer anulus, but there is no formation of radial fissures or displacement of nucleus pulposus.[247] Torsional stresses would be greatest in that region of the disc which lies furthest from the centre of rotation, and this region is always the antero-lateral anulus, even when the centre of rotation moves towards the zygapophysial joint in compression. In life, this mechanism might explain the 'rim tears' which commonly affect the antero-lateral anulus[321,825] and its attachments to bone.[349] Usually, however, torsional damage must be inflicted on the zygapophysial joints (a 'crumpled neural arch'[772]) before lumbar discs are adversely affected.

ACTIVITIES WHICH COULD INJURE THE SPINE IN TORSION

The lumbar spine would be subjected to a large torque if a force were exerted on an outstretched arm, perhaps during a fall, or during some contact sport such as rugby football. Activities such as hurling a discus would generate substantial angular momentum in the upper body, and this would have to be resisted by the spine and trunk muscles in order to bring the body to rest. Serving in tennis, fast bowling in cricket, and driving in golf similarly twist the lumbar spine, but the effects of torsion are difficult to distinguish from those of backwards and lateral bending, which accompany these movements (see p. 111). The back muscles are poorly positioned to oppose any dynamically applied torque (p. 42) but axial torques of up to 100 Nm can be generated by a combination of other muscles, particularly the external obliques and latissimus dorsi.[530] A certain amount of torque would be generated on the lumbar spine when someone bends forwards and twists round to one side. Such awkward twisting movements are closely related to disc prolapse and back pain,[419,523] but it is likely that the main movements of the lumbar spine are forward and lateral bending, rather than torsion (Fig. 9.8).

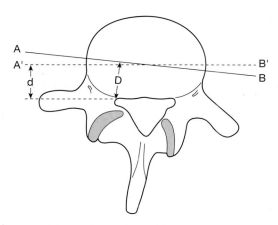

Figure 9.7 Asymmetrical zygapophysial joints could possibly contribute to disc degeneration by causing the disc to flex about an oblique axis (solid line, AB) rather than about a symmetrical axis (dashed line A'B'). In this example, the left postero-lateral corner of the disc lies farther from the oblique axis (D), than from the symmetric axis (d) and so would be stretched more during bending movements.

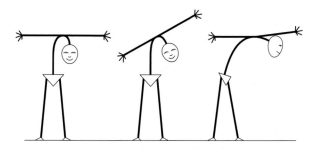

Figure 9.8 Left: bending directly forwards flexes the lumbar spine. Middle: if the lumbar spine is axially rotated at the same time as it is flexed, then the upper body will be rotated as shown. This is not a common movement in life. Right: adding lateral bending to the forward flexion produces the asymmetrical bending which is common in manual handling. This asymmetrical bending may also involve some coupled axial rotation, but axial rotation is not a primary movement.

BACKWARDS BENDING: IMPACTION OF NEURAL ARCHES, AND POSTERIOR DISC BULGING

CENTRE OF ROTATION

During flexion and extension movements in the sagittal plane, the axis of rotation is not fixed, but moves slightly within the nucleus pulposus of the intervertebral disc (Fig. 9.9). In effect, the superior vertebra glides anteriorly and posteriorly, respectively, as it flexes and extends about the nucleus.

RESISTANCE TO BACKWARDS BENDING

The neural arch resists approximately 60–70% of the applied bending moment when a motion segment is extended right up to its elastic limit. On average, damage can be detected after 3–8° of movement (mean 5°) with a bending moment of 28 Nm[21] or 45 Nm,[313] depending on the criterion

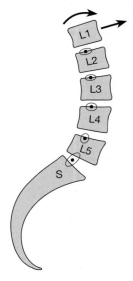

Figure 9.9 When the lumbar spine moves from extension to flexion, the axis of rotation between adjacent vertebrae (shown by black dots), move around the centre of the intervertebral disc, normally within the limits shown by the ellipses. This causes each vertebra to move by a combination of rotation and translation (as shown for L1) rather than by pure rotation. (From Pearcy and Bogduk.[642])

of damage and the accompanying compressive force. Typically, an extension moment of 10 Nm combined with a compressive load of 190 N creates an zygapophysial joint force of 200 N.[707] Forces on the neural arch increase further if compressive loading is high, as would often be the case in-vivo. For example, if a normal motion segment were subjected to 3 kN of compression while positioned in 4° of extension, the neural arches would resist approximately 570 N (calculated from [27]). Such a high force would generate very high stress concentrations in the lower margins of these joints, or adjacent laminae.[229]

The rest of the resistance to backwards bending must come from the intervertebral disc, and from the anterior longitudinal ligament.[627,707] Concentrations of compressive stress appear in the posterior anulus after just 2° of extension and increase considerably at 4° of extension.[27] The posterior anulus bulges into the vertebral canal, reducing its diameter by 2 mm.[712] Stress concentrations within the neural arch and disc may explain why so many people find it uncomfortable to fully-extend their lumbar spine while in the erect standing position. Although backward bending usually develops high stress concentrations within the posterior anulus, there are exceptions to this 'rule'. In a recent study, several motion segments showed a reduction in peak compressive stress within the posterior anulus in 2° and 4° of extension, compared to the neutral posture.[29] This is discussed on pages 164–165.

DAMAGE IN BACKWARDS BENDING

It is not easy to identify the first structure to be damaged in hyperextension, and it may depend on anatomical details such as the height of the disc, and the spacing and shape of adjacent spinous processes.[21] Most likely, the zygapophysial joints would be damaged first, but the interspinous ligament may be squashed between opposing spinous processes, and primary disc damage can not be ruled out. A combination of full backwards bending and 1 kN of compressive loading can cause the inferior articular processes to be deflected posteriorly by approximately 2° (Fig. 9.10), presumably because they make contact with the lamina below, and pivot about the pars interarticularis.[313] The deformation is not entirely elastic,[27,313] so it could involve damage to the joint capsule, as suggested in Figure 9.10. This was first proposed as a mechanism for back pain by Yang and King.[878] Rapid lumbar extension movements, which occur in

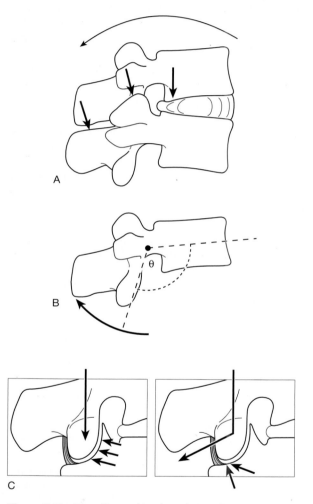

A

B

C

Figure 9.10 The effects of backwards bending on a lumbar motion segment. (A) Concentrations of compressive stress appear in the posterior anulus, the zygapophysial joints, and between the spinous processes. (B) The inferior articular facets bend backwards about the pars interarticularis by several degrees. (C) Moderate extension generates high contact forces in the lower margins of the articular surfaces (right) and hyperextension can lead to extra-articular impingement, backwards rotation of the inferior facet, and stretching of the joint capsule (left).

sports such as gymnastics, athletics, tennis and cricket, could conceivably force the neural arches together with sufficient violence to fracture the pars interarticularis, and cause spondylolysis (p. 156).

If a motion segment is positioned in hyperextension and compressed rapidly to failure, then in certain cases the nucleus pulposus of the intervertebral disc can herniate through the anterior anulus.[21] The mechanism is probably similar to that for posterior disc herniation (p. 148) but anterior prolapse is harder to achieve (at least in the laboratory) because the anterior anulus is thicker than the posterior (Plate 1). If the neural arches are removed from cadaveric motion segments, then severe repetitive loading in backwards bending and compression leads to posterior bulging of the posterior anulus. Extreme 'hairpin bending' of individual lamellae can persist after cessation of loading (Plate 2E). This mechanism probably explains why backwards bending leads to posterior disc protrusion in the tails of experimental rats[466] and mice.[477] In living humans, prior or accompanying damage to the neural arch may be necessary in order to deform the disc sufficiently. If a complete radial fissure exists already in the posterior anulus, then repeated extension movements can force injected radiographic contrast fluid down the fissure and into the vertebral canal.[288] It is unclear if nucleus pulposus material can migrate as easily as contrast fluid.

ACTIVITIES WHICH COULD INJURE THE SPINE IN BACKWARDS BENDING

Full backwards bending movements of the lumbar spine can occur during overhead manual work, such as painting a ceiling. It is difficult to measure lumbar extension accurately using skin-surface techniques, because skin wrinkling interferes with the measurements,[25] but approximate measures of thoraco-lumbar extension obtained from large electro-mechanical devices do indicate that lumbar extension movements are not uncommon in industry, and that they are closely associated with back pain.[523] Exertions in the upright or extended postures are also likely to generate substantial antagonistic activity of the trunk muscles, and lead to high compressive loading of the spine.[305] Sporting activities such as serving in tennis, and fast bowling at cricket, subject the lumbar spine to combinations of backwards bending, lateral bending and torsion, and could cause a variety of injuries to the neural arch, including spondylolysis (p. 156).

FORWARD BENDING: INTERVERTEBRAL LIGAMENT SPRAINS

CENTRE OF ROTATION

As indicated in Figure 9.9, the centre of rotation for sagittal plane flexion and extension movements moves around the nucleus pulposus, as the vertebrae simultaneously pivot and glide past each other.[642] It is difficult to locate this centre accurately, and experimental errors may partly explain the long and tortuous path taken by the centre of rotation in degenerated discs.[283] Alternatively, a moving centre of rotation may reflect differing amounts of coupling between translation and rotation at different phases of the motion. Also, of course, living subjects bend forwards in an individual manner, and variations in muscle activation patterns may affect both the centre of rotation, and the size and direction of any coupled movements.

RESISTANCE TO FORWARD BENDING

When motion segments are subjected to complex loading in bending, compression and shear in order to simulate flexion of the lumbar spine in-vivo, the intervertebral ligaments provide most of the resistance to movement.

During the first few degrees of flexion, there is slight resistance from the intervertebral disc and ligamentum flavum.[14,18] Reference is sometimes made to a 'neutral zone' in which the motion segment has zero resistance to bending,[627] but this is an artefact due to applying discrete weights to

cadaveric spines, and then allowing creep to occur before measuring the flexion angle. During dynamic activities, the lumbar vertebral column provides some resistance even to small movements. The concept of a 'neutral zone' as a region of low bending stiffness is still useful.

Half way to full flexion, the disc resists more strongly than the posterior intervertebral ligaments, and this is attributable to tension in the outer posterior anulus, and compression of the anterior anulus, which bulges anteriorly by approximately 0.1 mm per degree of flexion.[762] Ligament tension rises rapidly over the last few degrees of movement, so that in full flexion, 39% of the resistance comes from the capsular ligaments of the zygapophysial joint, 29% from the disc, 19% from the interspinous and supraspinous ligaments, and 13% from the ligamentum flavum.[18] The bending moment resisted by the spine is almost doubled during the final 2–3° of movement (Fig. 9.11). Tension in the intervertebral

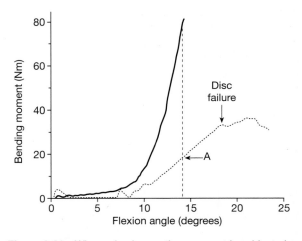

Figure 9.11 When a lumbar motion segment is subjected to a combination of bending and compression, to simulate forward flexion in life, its resistance to bending is initially slight, but increases rapidly as the ligamentous limit of movement is approached (solid curve). This particular specimen (male, 28 years, L45), has a 'neutral zone' of 7° and a full range of flexion of 14°. When the neural arch and ligaments were removed, then the remaining disc could be flexed to 18° before damage (dashed curve). The bending moment resisted by the disc at the limit of flexion (A) is usually much less than that required to injure the disc, indicating that the ligaments protect the disc in flexion. (After Adams et al.[22])

ligaments can be sufficient to bend the inferior articular processes forwards by several degrees about the pars interarticularis[313] and it increases pressure in the nucleus by up to 110% in full flexion,[22] even if the applied compressive load stays the same. It has been suggested that the articular surfaces of the zygapophysial joints resist flexion,[812] but this is based on experiments which actually measured the joints' resistance to combined bending and shear, and it is the latter that is resisted by the zygapophysial joints. There is experimental and theoretical evidence that the articular surfaces play a negligible role in resisting lumbar flexion.[18,737]

There is an interesting diurnal variation in the spine's resistance to flexion: prolonged loading expels water from the disc, reducing its height and allowing some slack to the short collagen fibres of the anulus and intervertebral ligaments. This has the effect of increasing the range of flexion, and reducing the proportion of bending moment resisted by the disc (p. 170). On the other hand, a high compressive preload removes any slack from collagen fibres in the anulus, and therefore increases the disc's resistance to bending.[14,386,861]

Comparisons between in-vivo and in-vitro measurements show that the back muscles do not normally permit the vertebral column to be flexed right up to its elastic limit.[13] The margin of safety for the whole lumbar spine increases from the early morning to later in the day.[20]

DAMAGE IN FORWARD BENDING
Rapid bending

Injury in flexion typically occurs when the bending moment rises to 50–80 Nm, but the spine's strength in bending can be as high as 124 Nm in strong young men.[14,18,22] The flexion angle at which injury occurs is usually between 5–9° per motion segment for the upper lumbar spine, and 10–16° for the lower lumbar spine. The similarity in mobility between cadaveric motion segments and living joints (see Fig. 8.3) suggests that the range of movement in life is influenced strongly by the mechanical properties of discs and ligaments, rather than by the length of the back muscles. This makes it feasible to estimate the bending moment acting on the lumbar spine of living subjects by comparing spinal movements with the bending stiffness properties of cadaveric spines (p. 102).

The first structure to sustain damage beyond the elastic limit (50–80 Nm) is the interspinous/supraspinous ligament complex.[6] If forwards bending is combined with lateral bending, then the capsular ligaments of the contra-lateral zygapophysial joint are put to an additional stretch because they lie at some distance from the sagittal midline.[593] They could then sustain damage before the interspinous ligament (Fig. 9.12). In normal forward bending, however, a further 2° of hyperflexion is required to overstretch the capsular ligaments.[3]

In more violent flexion injuries, 'overt' damage has been reported when the bending moment exceeds 70 Nm.[556] Gross damage is evident at 120 Nm[593] and complete failure of the tissues occurs at 140–185 Nm, with a flexion angle of

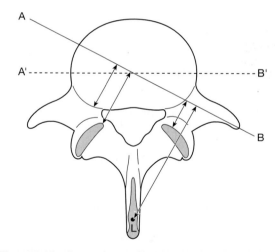

Figure 9.12 Superior view of a lumbar vertebra, illustrating the dangers of bending forwards and to one side.
The oblique axis of bending (AB) then lies close to one zygapophysial joint, but far from one postero-lateral corner of the disc. Stretching of ligaments and anulus is proportional to their distance from the axis, so in this example, the left postero-lateral anulus will be stretched more than in normal flexion about A'B'. This region of anulus must also resist a higher proportion of the applied bending moment, because the right zygapophysial joint lies so close to the bending axis (AB) that its resistance to bending will be negligible. Furthermore, stretching of the interspinous/supraspinous ligament (L) will be reduced, so its apparent function as the 'check' on forward bending would be jeopardised.

approximately 20°.[619,620] The last structure to fail is the outer posterior anulus fibrosus. Its strong fibres either pull a fragment of the vertebra away from the rest of the bone,[8] or else pull out of their vertebral anchorages, or rupture and pull out of the disc matrix at mid-disc height.[312] These latter two mechanisms, which require a great deal of energy, indicate how well the collagen 'cross-weave' of the anulus is able to reinforce the matrix in the manner of a fibre-composite material, and prevent the propagation of tensile damage throughout the anulus. Once the outer 'ligamentous' portion of the anulus has failed in hyperflexion, it is easy for the inner anulus to pull the cartilaginous endplate away from subchondral bone.[22] Discs tested to destruction in forward bending, without any ligamentous protection, resist 15–50 Nm before failing in this manner, at a typical flexion angle of 18°.[22] Strength in bending appears to be independent of nucleus pressure[22] suggesting that, in extreme flexion, the posterior anulus behaves like a simple ligament. The role of intervertebral ligaments in protecting the disc in flexion is illustrated in Figure 9.11.

Slow and sustained bending

The spine's strength and stiffness in bending depend on the speed of movement.[16,620,875] The visco-elastic properties of ligaments and discs cause their resistance to flexion to increase by 12% if the duration of the movement is reduced from 10 s to 1 s; conversely, sustained flexion reduces motion segment resistance to bending by 42% in just 5 minutes, and 67% in 1 hour.[16] Most of the 5-minutes effect is probably due to rapid 'stress relaxation' in stretched spinal ligaments[875] and this effect would probably be even quicker in living tissues at 37°C. Visco-elastic deformations of the disc are slower because they involve fluid movements over long distances (p. 169). Because of these effects, rapid flexion movements are more likely to injure the discs and ligaments than slow movements to the same end position, and sustained flexion may reduce ligamentous protection of the discs during dynamic movements. Sustained bending also reduces the protective action of the back muscles (p. 172).

INTERACTIONS BETWEEN BENDING AND COMPRESSION

Bending stiffness also increases in the presence of a substantial compressive preload[14,386] presumably because a pre-stressed anulus resists deformation more strongly. Typically, raising the preload from 400 N to 1300 N increases motion segment resistance to flexion by 30%,[14] emphasising the importance of a realistic compressive preload in cadaveric experiments.

ACTIVITIES WHICH COULD INJURE THE SPINE IN FORWARD BENDING

As discussed on page 95, healthy people flex their lumbar spine by 80–100% whenever they bend forwards to lift objects up from the floor. 'Awkward' bending movements (forwards and to one side) require some lateral flexion of the lumbar spine,[425] and this would increase stretching of the contra-lateral zygapophysial joint capsule. Full flexion right up to or beyond the normal static limit can occur in simple tasks such as putting on a sock or shoe, especially in people with a low range of sagittal plane movement in the lumbar spine and hips, who tend to lunge forwards in order to accomplish the task.[210] Risks would increase following a long period of flexed posture (for example, driving a car) because stress-relaxation will occur in ligaments and other collagenous tissues which have been stretched for a long time. This presents a double risk to the spine: firstly, it allows the spine to creep into more and more flexion[535] so that conditions are then more favourable for disc prolapse (see next section). Secondly, stress-relaxation of ligaments and tendons de-sensitises their mechano-receptors, and greatly diminishes reflex muscular protection of the spine (p. 172).[751] During repetitive bending and lifting activities, this loss of reflex muscular protection is exacerbated by muscle fatigue[211] which reduces the muscles' ability to generate maximum force in an emergency.[503] Gross ruptures of the interspinous ligament have been reported in 20% of all cadaveric spines examined,[681] suggesting that hyperflexion injuries to the lumbar spine are not uncommon in life.

LATERAL BENDING: LIGAMENT SPRAINS, AND ZYGAPOPHYSIAL JOINT IMPACTION

Lateral bending of the lumbar spine has not been studied in much detail. By itself it is an uncommon movement, but a component of lateral flexion frequently accompanies forwards flexion when people bend to reach objects which are not directly in front of them (Fig. 9.8). Small lateral bending movements can also accompany axial rotation, although this effect is variable, and may be under muscular control.[640] Symmetry suggests that the axis of lateral bending lies along the mid-sagittal plane of the disc, so that most of the spine's resistance to lateral bending probably comes from compression of the apophyseal joint on the side towards which the spine is bent,[707] and from stretching of the contralateral anulus fibrosus and capsular ligaments (Fig. 9.13). The intertransverse ligaments are stretched most by lateral bending,[627] but they are not strong (p. 119) and would be unable to protect the disc mechanically.

A lateral bending moment of 10 Nm causes 4–6° of lateral bending, with most of the resistance coming from the disc.[623,714] If the disc is degenerated, then the range of movement falls to 3–4°, and the 'neutral zone' is almost eliminated[623] suggesting that zygapophysial joints are becoming impacted. The rise in nucleus pressure generated by a lateral bending moment is greater than when the same moment is applied in forward bending.[714] This is probably because much of the resistance to lateral bending comes from collagen fibres in the lateral anulus, and they lie closer to the axis of bending than do the posterior intervertebral ligaments which resist forward bending, and so they exert a greater compressive 'penalty' on the nucleus for the same resistance to bending (p. 95). When a lateral bending moment of 60 Nm was applied to three young motion segments, 12–15° of angular movement was observed, and two of the specimens were damaged.[556] Unfortunately, the method of gripping the specimen contributed to the damage, and may have influenced the mode of failure (the superior endplate was pulled away from the vertebral body).

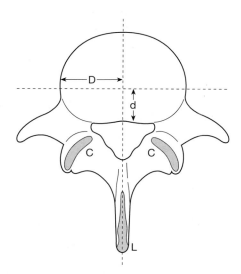

Figure 9.13 Superior view of a lumbar vertebra, showing that lateral bending stretches the peripheral anulus fibrosus more than the same angular movement in flexion. Stretching of a region of anulus is proportional to its distance from the axis of bending, and this can be much higher in lateral bending (D) compared to forward bending (d). The effect is greatest in lower lumbar discs where the ratio D/d is highest. The interspinous/supraspinous ligament (L) and zygapophysial joint capsular ligaments (C) lie close to the axis of lateral bending and so do not offer much resistance to movement.

BENDING AND COMPRESSION: DISC PROLAPSE AND RADIAL FISSURES

Direct compressive loading of a lumbar motion segment does not cause direct damage to the disc.[114,235,371] The disc has a higher compressive strength than the vertebral bodies on either side of it, regardless of whether the disc is healthy or degenerated, or if the compression is applied rapidly or slowly[645] or repetitively.[113,471] Even if the disc is deliberately weakened before testing, by cutting into the postero-lateral anulus from the outside[833] or from the nucleus,[109] the disc does not prolapse when loaded in compression. As described on page 133, the thin plate of perforated cortical bone which constitutes the vertebral body endplate is the 'weak link' of the lumbar spine in compression. Torsional loading also does not generate radial fissures, or cause discs to prolapse, not even if the zygapophysial joints are first destroyed, and the disc twisted to angles ten times greater than its normal range in life (p. 141).

The only proven method of inducing disc prolapse in response to mechanical loading is to bend the disc so much that the stretched and thinned posterior anulus becomes weaker than the vertebral endplate (Fig. 9.14). Two large cadaveric experiments have provided well-documented evidence that disc prolapse can occur in response to severe or repetitive loading in bending and compression, without artificial weakening of the anulus.[8,11]

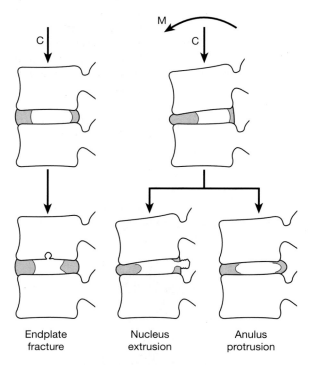

| Endplate | Nucleus | Anulus |
| fracture | extrusion | protrusion |

Figure 9.14 Left: compressive loading (C) damages the vertebral endplate before the intervertebral disc. Right: a bending moment (M) acting on the spine stretches and thins the anulus on the contra-lateral side, reducing its strength compared to the endplate. The simultaneous application of a high compressive force (C) raises the pressure in the nucleus pulposus, and the disc can then prolapse: either nucleus pulposus herniates through the weakened anulus ('nucleus extrusion') or else it causes the anulus to collapse outwards ('anulus protrusion').

DISC PROLAPSE BY SUDDEN LOADING[8]

When lumbar motion segments were positioned in antero-lateral flexion or hyperflexion, and then compressed rapidly to failure, approximately half of them failed by posterior prolapse of the intervertebral disc.[8] Discs which appeared to prolapse most readily were non-degenerated, lower lumbar discs from cadavers aged 40–50 years. Severely degenerated discs (grade 4 on a scale of 1–4: Plate 1D) could not be made to prolapse.

The applied compressive force required to cause prolapse was 5.4 kN on average (range 2.8–13.0 kN) and the average flexion angle was 15.8° (range 9–21°). (Flexion angles reported in the original paper were 3° too low, because of a calibration error in the goniometer used to measure them.) Each motion segment would have been flexed several degrees beyond its normal range of motion defined by the interspinous ligament (p. 145), but this could not be verified because the neural arches were removed before testing in order to reveal the posterior anulus more clearly. This interference could have had little influence on whether the discs prolapsed or not, because in several subsequent experiments, the same technique has been used as a matter of routine to cause disc prolapse in intact motion segments.[213,546,660] These later experiments have clarified one important detail: it is not absolutely necessary for the flexion angle to be high, provided that *either* the flexion angle *or* the compressive force exceeds normal everyday limits. The large prolapse shown in Plate 3F occurred in an intact motion segment flexed only 6°, which was well within the elastic range of its ligaments.

Some details of these experimental prolapses may be of clinical interest. Prolapse occurred in approximately 1 second, sometimes with an audible 'pop', and in one specimen the displaced nucleus material was projected through the air for a considerable distance! A complete radial fissure was created to allow posterior migration of nuclear material, but the excellent 'self-sealing' properties of the anulus[109,514] made these fissures difficult to visualise when the disc was sectioned horizontally (Plate 3A). In the sagittal plane, however, they are quite obvious (Plate 3F). In a minority of specimens, prolapse appeared as a localised outwards collapse of the posterior anulus, but usually it involved the extrusion, or sequestration, of nucleus pulposus material, sometimes with harder material attached to it (Plate 3D). The displaced material either emerged from the postero-lateral corner of the disc which was stretched most by the component of lateral bending (Plate 3A), or else it was more midline and trapped behind, or displaced by, the posterior longitudinal ligament (Plate 3F). Manual pulling of the vertebrae into flexion caused some of the nucleus material to be sucked back into the disc, but it was always expelled again as soon as the 'manipulation' stopped. In contrast, it was a simple matter to push the material sideways away from the site of extrusion.

A later experiment showed that discs which prolapsed were more likely to exhibit peaks of compressive stress in the matrix of the posterior anulus when loaded in bending and compression.[546] The origin of these stress concentrations is unclear: they may indicate focal damage to the collagen network, causing a localised loss of proteoglycans and water, and resulting in a loss of hydrostatic properties in that region of the disc. Alternatively, they may reflect normal ageing processes in discs aged between 30 and 50 years.[23]

In another experiment on mostly non-degenerated motion segments aged 20–52 years, posterior disc prolapse was simulated using up to 8° of flexion, and between 1 kN and 6 kN of compression.[112] However, it was necessary to weaken these discs before testing began by cutting a 10 mm × 10 mm channel into the posterior anulus from the nucleus, so that only the outermost 1 mm of anulus was intact. Also, the nucleus was replaced by chopped pieces of anulus taken from another disc. This experiment explains how a severely degenerated disc could prolapse at low flexion angles after a large radial fissure and fragmented nucleus have been created by other means.

It is not surprising that disc prolapse should occur most easily in discs which show age-related weakening of the anulus, and yet still retain the large pressurised nucleus of youth. Severely degenerated discs do not prolapse in the laboratory,[8,546]

presumably because the nucleus is too fibrous and dehydrated to exert a hydrostatic pressure on the anulus (see Fig. 8.11). Similarly, discs which have been dehydrated by several hours of creep loading exhibit a reduced nuclear pressure (see Fig. 10.15) and a greatly reduced propensity to prolapse when loaded severely.[20] Mathematical models suggest that prolapse is more likely to occur when the loading is applied rapidly to a fully hydrated disc, and when some axial rotation is added to the bending and compression.[478,757]

DISC PROLAPSE BY REPETITIVE LOADING[11]

The same combination of compression, bending and lateral bending can create disc prolapse at lower load levels during cyclic 'fatigue' loading.[11] This type of injury has been produced in-vitro only in young non-degenerated discs, and it is typified by a large postero-lateral radial fissure which allows extrusion of small quantities of soft nuclear pulp (Fig. 9.15 and Plate 3E).

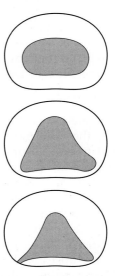

Figure 9.15 Superior view of intervertebral discs showing how postero-lateral radial fissures develop. Top: normal disc, with nucleus (shaded) having a similar shape to the peripheral anulus. Middle: repetitive loading in bending and compression can cause the anulus to be deformed into a typical 'bell' shape. Bottom: lamellae of the anulus eventually rupture in one or both postero-lateral corners.

Motion segments with an intact neural arch were positioned in full flexion, with an additional component of lateral flexion, and subjected to 40 cycles of compressive loading per minute for up to 6 hours. An initial injection of radiopaque fluid (including blue dye) into the nucleus enabled a discogram to be taken to demonstrate the absence of radial fissures prior to testing. Cyclic loading was gentle at first, in order to expel the extra fluid associated with discography, but the peak compressive force increased gradually to a maximum value which depended on specimen age and body mass. As the experiment progressed, water expulsion from the disc increased its range of flexion (p. 170), and the flexion angle was increased accordingly, without exceeding the elastic limit of the ligaments. Of 29 specimens tested in this manner, six developed a complete radial fissure, and these were all grade 1 discs (Plate 3E), aged under 44 years, from the L4–L5 and L5–S1 levels. Fissures were confirmed after testing by a second discogram, and the expulsion of small quantities of blue-stained nucleus pulp was plain to see. For the six discs which prolapsed, peak cyclic compressive force was 3.5 kN on average (range 2.5 kN–4.5 kN) and peak flexion angle was 14° (range 8–16°). The other 23 specimens either sustained vertebral fractures, or remained undamaged, but many showed 'bell-shaped' distortions of the anulus which resembled incomplete radial fissures (Fig. 9.15).

Again, some details may be of clinical interest. In several discs, the outermost lamella of the anulus appeared to halt fissure progression by bulging outwards, and allowing nucleus pulp to accumulate behind it rather than penetrate it (Fig. 9.16). If this outermost 1–2 mm of anulus was removed with a scalpel during the period of cyclic loading, an immediate herniation of nuclear pulp occurred. (These were not included among the six 'prolapses'.) The pre-test discogram revealed pre-existing radial fissures in 13 older discs, but none of these allowed posterior herniation of nucleus pulposus material during cyclic loading. Either old fissures heal efficiently, or else the nucleus becomes too fibrous to be expelled down the fissure, in the absence of

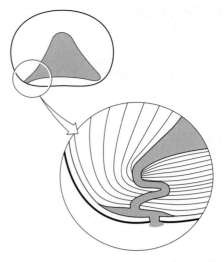

Figure 9.16 Upper: superior view of an intervertebral disc, showing nucleus pulposus material (shaded) migrating down a postero-lateral radial fissure. Lower: inset shows nucleus pulposus material breaking through the peripheral anulus, and accumulating behind the outermost lamella, which is reinforced on the outside by the posterior longitudinal ligament, before finally escaping from the disc. Compare with Fig. 9.15. This gradual migration of nucleus pulposus has been demonstrated in-vitro by applying cyclic loading to young discs with a soft nucleus.

severe bending or compression. One 33-year-old L5–S1 disc was cyclically loaded for 3 hours before being compressed rapidly to failure, at 17° of flexion and 5.9 kN of compression. The disc prolapsed suddenly, as described above, but it was probably weakened already by the cyclic loading.[11]

Adding torsion to bending, lateral bending and compression increases compressive stresses in the inner postero-lateral anulus[757] and enables prolapse to occur at lower flexion angles during repetitive loading,[299] although the evidence that prolapse occurred during the course of the latter experiment is not compelling. Of 14 discs that prolapsed during cyclic loading, four involved extrusion of nucleus pulposus, and 10 failed by anular protrusion. The relative importance of bending, lateral bending, torsion and compression in causing disc prolapse during repetitive loading has been analysed in a finite element model.[734]

CONSEQUENCES OF DISC PROLAPSE

Mechanical consequences

When disc prolapse is simulated on cadaveric specimens, it causes an immediate drop in nuclear pressure (Fig. 9.17) which probably explains why only a small quantity of nuclear material is extruded during subsequent cyclic loading.[11] This decompression must persist in living patients, because the average pressure in the nucleus of herniated discs in-vivo is 45% lower than that of healthy control discs (calculated from: Sato et al.[702]). A decompressed disc has a reduced resistance to bending, and the affected motion segment may well exhibit 'instability' (p. 152). Radial fissures in the anulus following disc prolapse have good self-sealing properties[11] but they impair the disc's resistance to bending and torsion[710] and increase shear stresses between adjacent lamellae,[291] so they probably pre-dispose the motion segment to further mechanical disruption.

Once released from the pressurised confines of a (cadaveric) disc, any displaced nucleus material can swell up in saline to approximately 2–3 times its size in just a few hours (Plates 3B and 3C).[213] During the following 96 hours, gradual leaching

of proteoglycans from the swollen tissue causes it to shrink again to its original size. If similar processes occur in-vivo (and it would be difficult to imagine why they would not) then they could explain why some patients report a worsening of symptoms several hours after an incident during which they felt their back 'give way'.

Biological consequences

Inflammatory-like responses within nerve roots are probably more important in the aetiology of sciatica than mechanical compression[410,615,616] although the contribution of the latter should not be disregarded.[870] Inflammation could be triggered by proteoglycans leaching from herniated disc tissue, together with the matrix-degrading enzymes and cytokines which are produced in quantity in this tissue.[401] Animal experiments have shown that nerve root morphology can be altered after only 3 hours' contact with nucleus pulposus tissue.[144] Changes in nerve function (decreased conduction velocity) are not so rapid, and were found to be reversible after 2 months in one animal model.[621] If an extruded fragment of nucleus pulposus is not removed surgically, it can shrink markedly over several months, and sometimes disappear entirely from the MRI image.[435]

Longer term consequences of disc prolapse will be dominated by cell-mediated biological changes. In young animals, the nucleus pulposus is able to regenerate itself to a limited extent following chymopapain-induced injury,[107,774] and this could help restore nucleus pressure and function. It could also lead to repeated prolapse down the same fissure, and explain the recurrent sciatica which can be such a problem in young humans. In older individuals, nucleus regeneration is not so apparent[635] and the initial decompression following prolapse is likely to be more severe.[30] Tissue culture experiments suggest that a large pressure drop will actually inhibit proteoglycan synthesis in the nucleus.[382] Abnormally large stress concentrations in the anulus which accompany nucleus decompression would also be expected to inhibit proteoglycan synthesis,[382] and stimulate production of the matrix-degrading enzyme MMP3.[329] Clearly, disc prolapse sets up

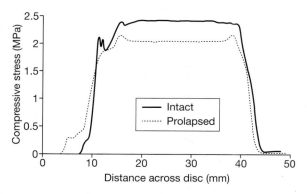

Figure 9.17 Distribution of vertical compressive stress along the sagittal mid-line of a cadaveric intervertebral disc, before and after the disc was induced to prolapse by loading in bending and compression. (Anterior on right. Specimen: male, 40 years L23.) Prolapse reduces the pressure in the nucleus, and in some discs, can generate stress peaks in the anulus. Note the increased diameter of the disc after prolapse, which can be attributed to increased posterior bulging. ('Stress profiles' are explained on p. 124.)

the potential for a 'vicious circle' of structural disruption, cell-mediated weakening of the matrix, and further disruption. In this way, disc prolapse may cause disc degeneration (rather than the other way round).

ACTIVITIES WHICH COULD CAUSE DISC PROLAPSE

Most intervertebral disc herniations removed at surgery are composed primarily of nucleus pulposus tissue, as in the above experiments, and none contains only anulus fibrosus,[569] so 'real life' disc prolapses are probably similar to those shown in Plate 3. Many manual handling activities load the lumbar spine simultaneously in compression, bending and lateral bending, and so might be expected to cause disc prolapse if the severity of just one of these components rose to damaging levels.

Circumstances which could lead to excessive bending or excessive compression in-vivo have been discussed above. Disc prolapse is most likely to occur when these circumstances are combined. For example, falling on the buttocks with the legs stretched out in front, or stumbling while carrying a heavy weight, or lifting a heavy object while alarmed, could combine excessive compression with high bending. Excessive bending with high compression could occur when lunging to catch or retain a falling object, or when attempting a heavy lift after the spine has been allowed to 'creep' into excessive flexion. Any event involving the trunk being dragged forwards into a flexed posture is likely to be particularly dangerous because forces in the back muscles are highest when the muscles are stretched, and when contracting eccentrically (resisting further stretching). A great deal of biomechanical evidence suggests that disc prolapse is more likely to occur in the early morning, when the discs are swollen with water (p. 170), although there is currently no epidemiological evidence to confirm this.

Many repetitive manual handling tasks generate peak compressive forces on the spine greater than the 2.5–4.5 kN used in the fatigue experiments described above, and at the same time, these tasks

frequently involve full lumbar flexion.[217] It appears therefore that discs could prolapse in-vivo whenever the number of loading cycles per day is sufficiently high that fatigue damage accumulates faster than the discs' adaptive remodelling response can deal with (p. 70). It is difficult to predict when this might occur, because it depends on the age, health and work experience of the individual, as well as the work environment.

SEGMENTAL 'INSTABILITY'

WHAT IS 'INSTABILITY'?

This vague term is used to describe some spinal dysfunction which involves excessive or otherwise abnormal movements of the lumbar spine. In engineering terms, a system is stable, unstable or 'neutral' according to criteria depicted in (Fig. 9.18). An unstable system, or 'instability', implies some lack of restraint which allows movements to be excessive or abnormal. Evidently this

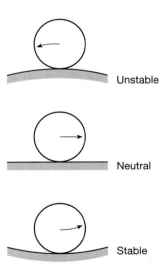

Figure 9.18   Mechanical criteria of 'stability' as illustrated by a sphere on a surface. Top: in this unstable system, any displacement of the sphere will progress to further displacements, and the 'system' will collapse. Middle: in this neutral system, any displacement of the sphere will neither progress nor be reversed. Bottom: in this stable system, any displacement will be reversed as soon as the perturbing force is removed.

engineering usage is close to the clinical uses of the term, and although small differences remain, they should be tolerated so that potentially valuable clinical perceptions of 'instability' are not distorted in order to conform to strict engineering concepts which were developed for quite different purposes.

It is not easy to decide which type (or types) of spinal dysfunction should be labelled 'segmental instability'. It does need to be defined, or else one clinician's experience of 'instability' cannot be equated with another's, and it should be defined in such a manner that it can be measured. Only then can experiments be performed to evaluate the usefulness of the definition. For example, if segmental instability were defined in terms of maximum translational (gliding) movements between adjacent vertebrae, and if such measurements then failed to predict which patients respond well to various treatments, then clearly, the definition should be abandoned, and another tried. If no definitions of segmental instability lead to clinically useful measurements, then the whole concept should be abandoned.

One simple definition is that segmental instability represents an excessive range of movement at a particular spinal level. Another is that it represents a tendency for small abnormal intervertebral movements within a normal range of movement. The causes and possible consequences of these types of instability will be considered next. Other definitions of instability could be analysed in a similar manner.

WHAT CAUSES INSTABILITY?

The simplest explanation for an excessive range of segmental movement is that the structure or structures which normally limit that movement have been damaged. Likely mechanisms of damage have been described above. Abnormal intervertebral movements within a normal range could conceivably be caused by a structure such as an osteophyte causing a temporary block or 'catch' at a particular point during an otherwise smooth movement. This concept is supported by the subjective experiences of many people with

back pain, and by the small flexion/extension oscillations which can be measured in cadaveric motion segments which are moved rapidly in the sagittal plane.[610] Alternatively, small inappropriate movements may simply reflect a negligible resistance to small movements, so that the motion segment 'wobbles' within an enlarged neutral zone. Small angular movements between vertebrae are resisted by the intervertebral discs and ligamentum flavum.[18] The following sections suggest two mechanisms which could reduce the bending stiffness of the disc to very low levels, so that the motion segment can 'wobble'.

Instability following disc degeneration

If a disc loses water as a result of disc degeneration or sustained loading, then the volume and pressure of the nucleus are decreased, and the anulus and intervertebral ligaments become slack (Fig. 10.17). Resistance to bending is therefore reduced, especially in the anulus because its bony attachments are closer together than those of the intervertebral ligaments, and so are more affected by small reductions in disc height.[20] The permanent changes associated with disc degeneration lead to a permanent joint laxity, so that the motion segment develops an increased 'neutral zone' in bending and torsion.[558] However, other degenerative changes, such as vertebral osteophytes, may have the opposite effect, and increase the motion segment's bending stiffness. Perhaps these events occur in sequence: first the nucleus loses volume and pressure, causing the anulus to resist bending less; then more advanced degeneration leads to osteophyte formation and restores stability? According to this scheme, the 'wobbling' unstable disc represents a transitional stage between a normal disc, and a grossly degenerated and stable one.

Instability following injury to endplate or anulus

As discussed above, disc prolapse or endplate fracture both decompress the nucleus pulposus,

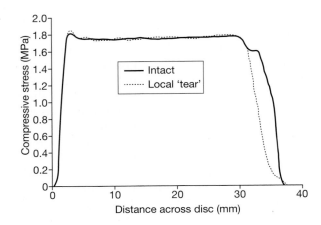

Figure 9.19 The distribution of vertical compressive stress along the sagittal mid-line of a cadaveric intervertebral disc, before (thick line) and after (thin line) a 'rim tear' was created in the anulus. A horizontal incision, 10 mm wide and 10 mm deep, was created by means of a scalpel in the anterior anulus, at the exact location where the pressure-sensitive needle exited the disc. The incision removed the compressive stress from the outermost 3 mm of anulus, but only in the immediate vicinity of the cut: stress distributions in the rest of the disc were unaffected. (Anterior on right. Specimen: male, 60 years, T12–L1) ('Stress profiles' are explained on p. 124.)

thereby reducing motion segment height, and creating slack in the intervertebral ligaments. The motion segment's resistance to bending is therefore greatly reduced (see Fig. 10.16). This type of instability would probably be exacerbated by cell-mediated degenerative changes in the disc which usually follow such injuries. Simulated 'rim tears' in the peripheral anterior anulus, created by means of a scalpel, have little direct effect on nuclear pressure (Fig. 9.19) or on the disc's resistance to bending and torsion.[628] In living animals, such injuries gradually increase the motion segment's range of motion and neutral zone over a period of several weeks, until the healing process reduces it again.[33] However, long-term experiments on sheep show that rim tears eventually cause degenerative changes to progress throughout the entire disc.[567,568,617] These secondary degenerative changes will affect nucleus pressure, and hence disc bending stiffness, more than the initial damage to the anulus, and could lead to segmental instability.

WHIPLASH

WHAT IS 'WHIPLASH'?

'Whiplash' is typified by low-velocity car crashes in which the upper body is thrown forwards and then back, or vice versa. Whiplash injuries are commonly associated with the neck, but similar events can probably injure the lumbar spine, even if a seat belt is worn, because sitting down causes the lower lumbar spine to be almost fully flexed,[46] so only a modest forward movement is required to throw the lumbar spine into hyperflexion. For this reason, a brief account of whiplash is given in a book primarily devoted to the lumbar spine. There are good anatomical reasons, however, to be wary of equating the two regions of the spine.[552]

WHAT IS INJURED IN WHIPLASH?

Practically every tissue and structure in the neck can be injured in cervical whiplash,[677] although increasing evidence points towards the zygapophysial joints as being the major source of chronic pain.[64] The purpose of the following sections is to apply some of the mechanical principles outlined in this book to help identify the site of whiplash injury, both to the neck and lumbar spine.

Firstly, the site and severity of injury must depend on how much warning (and alarm) the victim received just prior to impact. Any screech of brakes, or flashing image in the driver's mirror, would allow time for the back or neck muscles to contract in a reflex manner to protect the spine. In mechanical terms, this reflex muscle action may be sufficient to reduce the peak bending moment acting on the spine (provided that the impact was not extremely violent) but only at the expense of increasing greatly the spinal compressive force.[507] The resulting injury would more likely be 'compressive' in nature and involve the discs and vertebral bodies (as well as the muscles themselves), rather than intervertebral ligaments or the neural arch (Fig. 9.20). On the other hand, if an impact occurred without warning, then the neck muscles would have insufficient time to prevent the spine

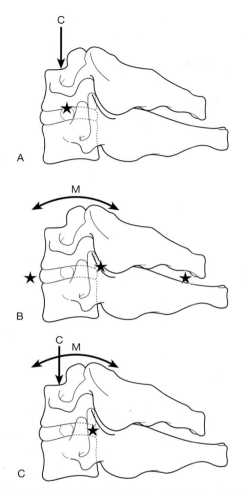

Figure 9.20   Diagrams illustrating the likely sites of injury (★) when the cervical spine is loaded in bending (M) and/or compression (C). (Interpretations are based on experimental results from lumbar motion segments.) (A) Excessive compression damages the vertebral endplate. (B) Bending damages peripheral structures, including intervertebral ligaments. (C) Combined bending and compression can cause disc prolapse.

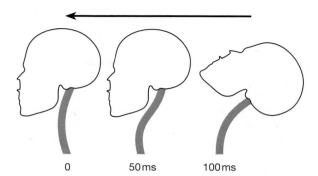

Figure 9.21   Movements of the skull and neck during whiplash. The orientation of the cervical vertebral bodies are represented by thick black lines, and the arrow indicates the direction of the impacting force applied to the shoulders. Approximately 50–75 ms after impact, the cervical spine develops an exaggerated 'S-shaped' curvature, and maximal extension at all cervical levels occurs after 100 ms. Data from experiments on cadaveric cervical spines.[632]

from being injured in bending, although stretch reflexes[399] may cause them to generate enough force to influence the outcome to a certain extent.[494] Bending injuries would probably involve the posterior intervertebral ligaments (in the hyperflexion stage of whiplash) or the neural arch (in the hyperextension phase). Clearly, to assume that the forces acting on the spine during whiplash are small just because the vehicle impacts are usually of low velocity would be a serious mistake. Muscle forces can be magnified in alarming situations, and if the muscles do not have time to react, then the underlying spine is extremely vulnerable to bending.

A second aspect of whiplash may also be applicable to the cervical and lumbar spines: the site of injury will be affected by any axial rotation of the head or torso. If the victim was turning round at the moment of impact, then the spine could suffer a bending injury about an oblique plane. This would be more likely to involve structures which lie away from the mid-sagittal plane, such as the zygapophysial joints and iliolumbar ligaments.

Whiplash injury mechanisms have recently been investigated in a variety of 'models'. When whole human cadaveric cervical spines were subjected to a simulated rear-end collision[632] a biphasic response was noted. In the first phase (50–75 ms after impact), the cervical spine formed an exaggerated 'S-shaped' curve as the lower cervical levels extended, and the upper ones flexed. In the second phase (>75 ms), all levels were extended, with overall maximum extension of the head occurring after 100 ms (Fig. 9.21). Injuries were most likely to occur by hyperextension in the C5–C7 region during the first phase of neck movement, and involved both anterior and posterior structures. These experiments neglected the effects of muscle activation, as did several earlier 'crash test dummy' tests, and so they reproduced only the bending-type injuries which represent one end of a spectrum of injuries involving varying amounts of bending and compression. When living volunteers were subjected to mild rear-end collisions,[399] they also showed early 'S-shaped' deformations of the cervical spine associated with abnormal and large extension movements of the lower cervical vertebrae. Radiographic movement data suggested particularly high stretching of the anterior anulus, and compression of the zygapophysial joints, at C5–C6.

Very different types of injury could result from rapid extension of the neck: an experiment on anaesthetised pigs showed that a 'shock wave' developed within the cerebro-spinal fluid which could possibly damage nerve cell membranes.[776]

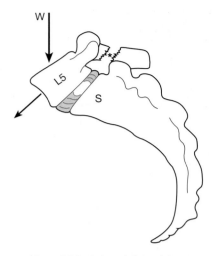

Figure 9.22   Spondylolysis is a defect of the pars interarticularis (∗), which occurs either unilaterally or bilaterally. L5 is most commonly affected. Gravitational forces (W) sometimes cause a forward slipping of the upper (damaged) vertebra upon the one below, a condition known as spondylolysthesis. Fractures of the pars which resemble spondylolysis can be simulated by repeatedly applying a posteriorly directed force to the inferior articular processes of cadaveric lumbar vertebrae.

SPONDYLOLYSIS AND SPONDYLOLYSTHESIS

Fractures of the pars interarticularis resembling spondylolysis can be reproduced by applying posteriorly-directed forces to the inferior articular processes of cadaveric lumbar vertebrae (Fig. 9.22). A single loading cycle causes fracture at a force of approximately 2 kN,[189] and cyclic loading oscillating between 380 N and 760 N can cause fatigue failure.[184] In life, the forces required for fatigue failure could arise when marching with a heavy backpack,[372] and also during hyperflexion or hyperextension movements.[384,449] Alternating flexion and extension movements of the lumbar spine may be particularly dangerous, because they cause the inferior articular processes to bend about the pars by 2–3° in the antero-inferior direction (in flexion) and postero-superior direction (in extension) as shown in Figure 9.10. Alternating movements would therefore cause large and potentially damaging stress reversals in the pars, and pose the greatest threat of spondylolysis.[313] This may explain the high incidence of spondylolysis in gymnasts[384] and cricket fast bowlers.[336]

Genetic pre-disposition must also be important in spondylolysis, because 26% of the close relatives of those with spondylolysis have a similar problem themselves.[869] The inherited factor may simply be a small cross-sectional area of bone in the pars interarticularis.[185] Higher incidences of spondylolysis in Alaskan natives[760] may depend partly upon (inherited) differences in lifestyle.[237]

Spondylolysis usually affects the lower lumbar vertebrae which are inclined at a steep angle to the vertical during many upright postures (Fig. 9.1). Not surprisingly, the loss of the normal resistance of the zygapophysial joints to shear often results in a forwards slip of L4 or L5 relative to the vertebra below, under the influence of gravity (pp. 138–139). This forwards slip, spondylolysthesis, can in theory be opposed by the action of the erector spinae muscles resisting the forward shear force[664] but only in stooped postures, and not in standing. Spondylolysthesis is associated with more sagittally-oriented zygapophysial joints rather than with asymmetrical facets, and this probably represents a predisposing weakness rather than secondary remodelling.[91]

SPINAL TRAUMA

Several classifications of spinal trauma have been published for the benefit of orthopaedic surgeons.[197,359] Much of the information appears to be based upon experience and conjecture rather than experiment, but nevertheless is consistent with the principles outlined in this chapter. Two particular types of injury have been investigated more methodically.

FLEXION-DISTRACTION ('SEAT BELT') INJURIES

When a car occupant is thrown forwards on to a lap-type seat belt, the lumbar spine is loaded in combined flexion, forward shear, and compression. Gross damage is evident at 120 Nm (p. 145) and complete failure of the tissues occurs at 140–185 Nm, with a flexion angle of 20°.[619,620] Interpreting these and other experiments, Neumann et al. (1995) suggested that total instability occurs when flexion exceeds 19°, and spinous process separation increases by more than 33 mm.[591]

BURST FRACTURES OF THE VERTEBRAL BODY

These can be defined as comminuted vertebral body fractures with disruption of the anterior and posterior walls of the vertebral body,[197] and they are characterised by an increased interpedicular distance.[733] They can cause severe neurological problems from the retropulsion of bone into the spinal canal. The name 'burst fracture' suggests some involvement from tissue fluid trapped within a rapidly loaded vertebra, and there is some evidence that rapid loading is more likely to damage the vertebral body cortex rather than the endplates.[881] However, the involvement of trapped fluid may not be great, because the compressive strength of cadaveric lumbar vertebrae is little affected by preventing fluid egress using paraffin wax.[373] Burst fractures can be simulated in the laboratory by dropping a heavy weight on to a section of thoraco-lumbar spine.[261,630] The resulting severe compression injuries resemble the transverse fractures described by Brinckmann (Fig. 9.2) but also involve damage to both of the adjacent intervertebral discs[261] with disc material being forced into the vertebral bodies. The loss of vertebral height creates severe rotational instability in the affected motion segment[630] presumably because of the consequent loss of tension in the intervertebral ligaments and anulus. Burst fractures are less common in the lumbar spine than in the thoracic, and they are less likely to occur if the intervertebral discs are degenerated.[733]

10

Functional pathology

INTRODUCTION

Mechanical loading does not have to be severe to cause pain. Small forces can give rise to pain if they are concentrated into a sufficiently small area of innervated tissue, and if you doubt this, try pricking yourself gently with a pin! The extent to which loading is distributed across and between different spinal structures is sensitive to the manner in which the spine is used during everyday activities. In this chapter on 'functional pathology' we analyse several mechanisms that can generate abnormally high stress concentrations in undamaged spinal tissues.

The first mechanism to be considered is posture, which is interpreted in terms of the orientation of adjacent vertebrae. If vertebrae are pressed together at an unusual angle, then high stress concentrations can arise in the intervertebral discs, ligaments and zygapophysial joints. The second mechanism to be considered is sustained 'creep' loading, which can reduce the stress-equalising ability of intervertebral discs, and reduce the separation of adjacent neural arches. Thirdly, excessive or asymmetrical muscle activity can impose abnormal stresses on the underlying spine, and normal muscle protection of the spine can be reduced following sustained or repetitive bending movements. The final section summarises the evidence concerning stress concentrations in the lumbar spine, and suggests a rational basis for the concept of 'good' posture.

POSTURE AND THE LUMBAR SPINE

Spinal 'posture' can be characterised in various ways, depending on the shape or curvature of the spinal column, and the orientation of the entire column to the vertical. The 'moment arm analysis' described on page 94 explains why inclining the spinal column to the vertical requires trunk muscle activity to balance the external moment generated by gravity acting on the mass of the upper body. Any tendency to lean forwards or backwards therefore increases the spinal compressive force (Fig. 10.1), and spinal loading is minimised when the vertebral column is balanced vertically on the pelvis. The following sections consider some mechanical implications of the other aspect of posture: changes in spinal curvature.

POSTURE AND LUMBAR CURVATURE IN THE SAGITTAL PLANE

It is useful and convenient to define spinal posture in terms of the angle subtended in the sagittal plane by the upper surface of the L1 vertebral body and the top of the sacrum (Fig. 10.2). This angle is referred to as the 'lumbar curvature', or 'lumbar lordosis', and typical values are 49–61° in erect standing, and 22–34° in unsupported sitting.[46,385,475] In full flexion, the angle is reversed and can be denoted by a negative value. For cadaveric lumbar spines, cut free from all muscle attachments and therefore entirely unloaded, the lumbar curvature is typically 41–45°.[21,246] We will refer to this as the 'neutral' configuration of the lumbar spine. Evidently, upright standing increases lumbar curvature by 8–16° compared to the neutral configuration (approximately 2° for each motion segment), whereas upright sitting decreases it by about 10–21°. Neither standing nor sitting corresponds to the neutral configuration, so neither should be considered a more 'natural' or 'normal' posture than the other.

The precise amount of lumbar flexion or extension in a given posture can be quantified from

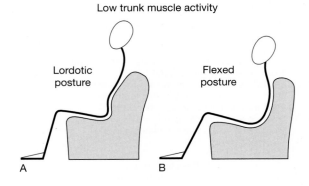

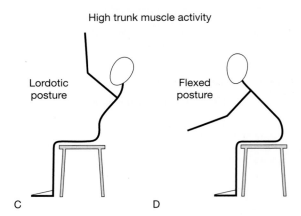

Figure 10.1 Trunk muscle activity is minimal when the spinal column is vertical (A and B), and high when it is inclined to the vertical (C and D). The actual shape of the lumbar spine, either lordotic or flexed, has much less effect on muscle activity.

changes in lumbar curvature, as shown in Figure 10.3. Lumbar curvature as defined above should really be measured from X-rays, but it can be estimated by measuring the angle between the tangents to the surface of the back at L1 and S2. There is no fundamental reason why these two measures of lumbar curvature should be the same, but they are similar because the skin surface lies at approximately 90° to the top surface of the lumbar vertebral bodies and sacrum. Changes in lumbar curvature defined in Figure 10.2 should correspond exactly to changes measured at the skin surface (Fig. 10.3), although skin-movement artefacts can lead to small differences, especially in lordotic postures.[25]

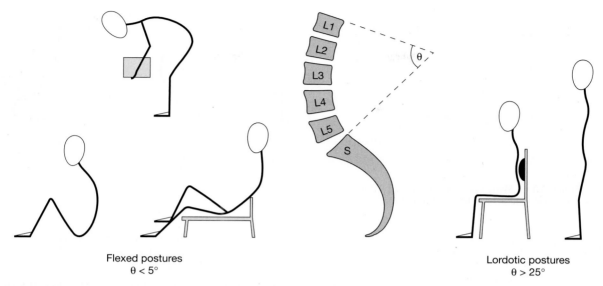

Figure 10.2 Lumbar posture can be categorised as 'lordotic' or 'flexed' depending on the size of the lumbar curvature (θ) as defined in the figure. The 'neutral' configuration refers to the shape of an unloaded cadaveric lumbar spine (centre).

Flexed postures
θ < 5°

Lordotic postures
θ > 25°

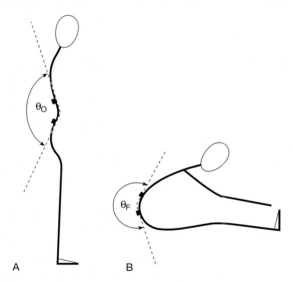

Figure 10.3 If the lumbar curvature in a particular posture was measured to be θ, then this represents a lumbar flexion angle of $(\theta - \theta_o)$ degrees. This can be expressed as a % of the full range of movement between the erect standing position (A) and full flexion (B) using the formula:
% flexion = $100 \times (\theta - \theta_o)/(\theta_F - \theta_o)$.

When referring to living subjects, it is convenient to consider the upright standing position to represent zero flexion. The fully flexed toe-touching posture is then 100% flexion. Typical values of lumbar flexion obtained with skin-mounted inclinometers are shown in Figure 10.4 for a wide range of postures. Note that common postural habits such as crossing the legs while sitting, or standing with one foot slightly raised, serve to reduce lumbar curvature by a small amount.[214] Nearly all sitting postures flex the lumbar spine, often substantially, and the L4–5 and L5–S1 levels are almost fully flexed.[46] Indeed, lumbar flexion is one of the defining characteristics of sitting, together with weight transfer through the ischial tuberosities.[36] Walking appears to involve a slight flattening of the lumbar lordosis compared to standing still.[782] Lordosis increases during the early stages of pregnancy.[227] Standing lordosis is largely unrelated to age or gender, although lordosis in the lower lumbar spine is reduced slightly in older people.[282] Patients with back pain show reduced lordosis, especially in the lower lumbar spine[385] and a particularly flat back is a risk factor for future low back pain.[24]

POSTURE AND LOAD-SHARING IN THE LUMBAR SPINE

Flexed postures stretch the posterior intervertebral ligaments, and tension in these ligaments

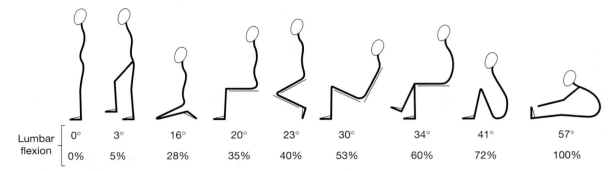

Lumbar flexion	0°	3°	16°	20°	23°	30°	34°	41°	57°
	0%	5%	28%	35%	40%	53%	60%	72%	100%

Figure 10.4 Many commonly adopted postures flex the lumbar spine to a greater or lesser extent. '% flexion' is defined in Figure 10.3. (After Dolan et al.[214])

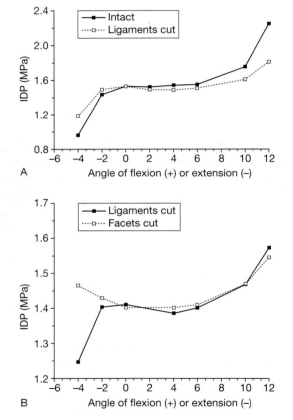

Figure 10.5 Intradiscal pressure (IDP), which is the hydrostatic pressure within the nucleus pulposus, is a good indicator of the overall compressive force acting on an intervertebral disc. (A) IDP increases in flexion, because of ligament tension. (B) IDP is reduced in extension because of load bearing by the zygapophysial joint surfaces (facets). Data for a cadaveric motion segment (male, 49 years, L23) which was subjected to a constant compressive force of 2 kN in each posture.

increases the compressive force acting on the intervertebral disc. Lordotic postures cause these ligaments to become slack, and increase loading of the neural arch, so that compressive loading of the disc is reduced. These effects are demonstrated in Figure 10.5, and are discussed in more detail below.

POSTURE AND THE NEURAL ARCH

The bony neural arches of adjacent vertebrae make sliding contact with each other in the zygapophysial joints, and their spinous processes are separated by only a few millimetres of interspinous ligament. Not surprisingly, small changes in posture can lead to high stress concentrations at these points of contact.

The proportion of the compressive force acting on the spine which is transmitted through the zygapophysial joints rises from 1% in the 'neutral' posture to 16% in 2° of lordosis.[6] Furthermore, lordosis causes this increased force to be concentrated on the inferior margins of the articular surfaces, and on the very tips of the inferior processes as they impinge on the lamina below[229,735] (Fig. 10.6). There is no articular cartilage to soften this extra-articular impingement, so it could give rise to particularly high stress concentrations. Moderately flexed postures, on the other hand, cause the articular surfaces to be orientated parallel to each other, and contact stresses are low and evenly distributed. Extra-articular impingement does not then occur. 'Kissing' spinous

Lordotic posture   Flexed posture

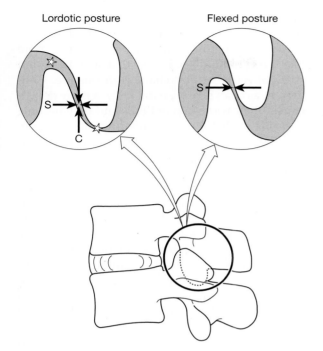

Figure 10.6 Lordotic postures (left) increase the compressive force (C) acting on the zygapophysial joints, and concentrate stresses in the inferior margins of the articular surfaces. Direct bone–bone contact (indicated by stars) can also occur. Flexed postures (right) remove the compressive loading from these joints, and cause the shear force (S) to be resisted by the middle and upper margins of the articular surfaces.

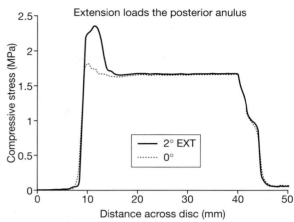

Figure 10.7 The distribution of vertical compressive stress along the sagittal mid-plane of a cadaveric intervertebral disc, compressed in the neutral configuration (0 deg) and in a lordotic posture (2° EXT). (Specimen: male, 19 years, L45, anterior on right. Compressive force = 2 kN.) Lordotic postures tend to increase the peak compressive stress in the posterior anulus. ('Stress profiles' are explained on p. 124.)

processes can also transmit considerable compressive forces down the spine if the vertebrae are orientated in several degrees of extension.[21] However, the resulting stress concentrations have not been measured.

POSTURE AND INTERVERTEBRAL DISC MECHANICS

Small changes in posture can have large effects on the distribution of compressive stress inside the anulus fibrosus of intervertebral discs. When discs are subjected to compressive loading in the 'neutral' posture (i.e. without any bending being applied) they generally exhibit a small 'peak' of compressive stress in the posterior anulus, and a fairly even compressive stress throughout the nucleus and anterior anulus (see Fig. 8.11B). In a simulated lordotic posture such as erect standing (i.e. in 2° of backwards bending) the size of this stress peak usually increases (Fig. 10.7), whereas moderately flexed postures usually distribute stresses evenly across the disc (Fig. 10.8). In full flexion, stress peaks can appear in the anterior anulus, but they are rarely as high as those in the posterior anulus in full extension.[27] These stress concentrations can be explained in terms of the elastic properties of the anulus fibrosus which is deformed vertically during flexion/extension movements (Fig. 10.9).

Posture also affects the hydrostatic pressure in the nucleus pulposus. For an applied compressive force of 500 N, the nucleus pressure is 40% less in 4° of extension than in the neutral configuration because the neural arches of adjacent vertebrae are pressed more firmly together and resist more of the compressive force.[27] On the other hand, nucleus pressure rises by 100% in full flexion because flexion stretches the ligaments of the neural arch, and ligament tension acts to compress the disc. If the neural arch is removed from a motion segment, then lumbar extension and flexion both increase nucleus pressure, by 8% and

38% respectively.[27] This shows that a stretched anulus can act like a ligament to compress the adjacent nucleus. High compressive forces (up to 3 kN) increase the compressive stiffness of the

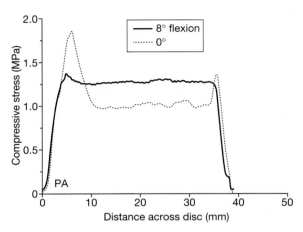

Figure 10.8 The distribution of vertical compressive stress along the sagittal mid-plane of a cadaveric intervertebral disc, compressed in the neutral configuration (0°) and in moderate flexion (8° FLX). (Specimen: male, 55 years, L45, anterior on right. Compressive force = 1 kN.) Moderate flexion tends to distribute compressive stress evenly across the disc, although it usually increases the pressure in the nucleus pulposus. ('Stress profiles' are explained on p. 124.)

disc, and these postural effects on nucleus pressure are then diminished (Table 10.1).

A young highly hydrated disc behaves more like a 'bag of fluid' (p. 125) so that stresses within it are affected less by changes in posture. Conversely, as discs become older and/or more degenerated, their water content falls and they become less able to distribute compressive stress evenly (p. 125). The effects of posture are then magnified, so that just 2° of bending can substantially increase stress peaks in the anulus (Fig. 10.10).

Increased sensitivity to posture in degenerated discs has been demonstrated in cadaveric specimens by damaging the endplate, and then expelling water from the disc by means of cyclic loading.[29] This treatment simulates two biomechanical consequences of advanced disc degeneration (structural disruption and dehydration) rather than the degenerative process itself, and it results in intra-discal stress profiles similar to those seen in severely-degenerated discs in-vivo.[547] On average, 'degenerated' cadaveric discs showed stress peaks (over and above the nucleus pressure) of 1.9 MPa in the posterior anulus in 2° of extension. This was reduced to 0.6 MPa in moderate flexion. However, a minority of discs behaved quite differently from the average (Fig. 10.11): in these discs, extension reduced the

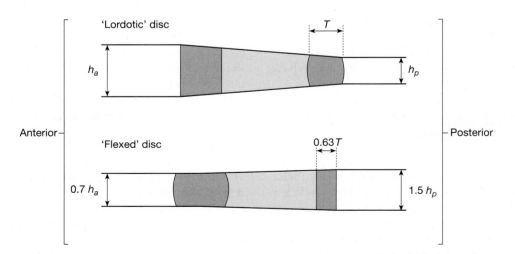

Figure 10.9 Diagram showing how an intervertebral disc deforms in the sagittal plane when the lumbar spine is in a flexed posture (lower) and a lordotic posture (upper). Changes in anulus height can be measured directly from radiographs.

Table 10.1 The effect of flexion and extension on intradiscal pressure (IDP), for isolated discs (below) and intact motion segments (above). Average data for 5–8 specimens.[27]

Compression (N)	% increase (+) or decrease (−) in IDP					
	−4°	−2°	0°	50% flx	75% flx	100% flx
Motion segments						
500	−40	−10	0	+12	+45	+110
1000	−30	−6	0	+4	+23	+79
3000	−15	−4	0	+1	+6	+30
Disc-vertebral body						
500	+8	+3	0	+3	+12	+38
1000	+3	+4	0	0	+5	+12
3000	0	+2	0	−1	+1	+4

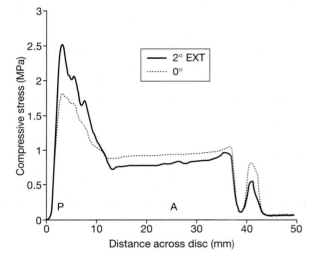

Figure 10.10 The distribution of vertical compressive stress along the sagittal mid-plane of a cadaveric intervertebral disc, compressed in the neutral configuration (0°) and in a lordotic posture (2° EXT). (Specimen: male, 54 years, L34, anterior on right. Compressive force = 2 kN.) This disc was damaged in compression prior to testing, and structural failure makes the stress distribution very sensitive to small changes in posture. ('Stress profiles' are explained on p. 124.) Data from Adams et al.[29]

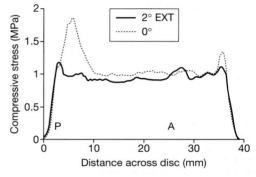

Figure 10.11 The distribution of vertical compressive stress along the sagittal mid-plane of a cadaveric intervertebral disc, compressed in the neutral configuration (0°) and in a lordotic posture (2° EXT). (Specimen: 55-year-old male, L45, anterior on right. Compressive force = 2 kN.) In a minority of discs tested, lordotic posture reduced the stress peak in the posterior anulus, presumably because of stress-shielding by the neural arch. ('Stress profiles' are explained on p. 124.) Data from Adams et al.[29]

stress peaks in the posterior anulus, by as much as 40%, and the hydrostatic pressure in the nucleus was also reduced.[29] Discs which appeared to benefit in this way from backwards bending tended to be more 'degenerated' than the others in terms of their stress-profiles recorded in the neutral posture. This suggests that when a disc is narrowed, it is possible for the neural arch to 'stress-shield' the posterior anulus in full extension, so that much of the compressive force on the spine is transmitted through the neural arch and anterior anulus. The detailed results also illustrate two dangers of in-vitro experimentation: the tendency to assume average results are generally true of all spines, and the tendency to extrapolate results on essentially 'normal' cadaveric material to the often-degenerated spines of patients with back pain.

The above discussion has considered only the compressive stress within the disc matrix, but it should be remembered that the outer anulus behaves like a ligamentous structure, in tension. Tensile stresses in the outer anulus are not detected by the pressure transducer used to record 'stress profiles' (p. 124). However, the presence of tension in the outer anulus can be inferred from its effect of increasing the pressure within the nucleus. Tensile stresses in the outer posterior anulus rise rapidly as the limit of flexion is approached, but the data in Table 10.1 suggest that they are unlikely to exceed 190 N (i.e. 38% of 500 N).

POSTURE AND INTERVERTEBRAL DISC NUTRITION

The supply of metabolites to cells within the intervertebral disc is barely adequate for normal requirements[516,756,819] and impaired metabolite transport is associated with disc degeneration.[360,579] Recent cell-culture experiments suggest that nucleus pulposus cells are tolerant of low oxygen concentrations, but die if the extracellular concentration of glucose falls below a critical level for a period of several days.[364] Any influence of posture on disc metabolism may therefore be important, and in fact, posture appears to have large effects on both of the two transport mechanisms, diffusion and fluid flow.

The amount of a metabolite that can diffuse into a given region of the disc depends critically on the diffusion path length, which is the distance to the nearest blood vessel on the disc's surface or in the vertebral body. Compared to erect standing, flexed postures stretch the posterior anulus by 50%, and compress the anterior anulus by 30%.[8,641] In order to maintain constant tissue volume, the thickness (and hence diffusion path length) of the anterior and posterior anulus must be correspondingly increased and decreased respectively (Fig. 10.9). Flexion therefore reduces the diffusion path length into the posterior anulus. In cadaveric experiments, flexion enhances metabolite diffusion into the inner posterior anulus,[12] which is the region of the disc with the most precarious nutrient supply.[516] Similar events would occur in living discs because diffusion is a physical process, and measurements of diffusion into living discs agree with calculations based on

cadaveric experiments.[819] The beneficial effects of flexion would be compounded by the fact that the stretched posterior anulus has an increased surface area, so that a greater flux of metabolites could be 'funnelled' into the inner posterior anulus.[12] Flexion causes a corresponding decrease of metabolite diffusion into the thickened anterior anulus,[12] but this is the last region of the disc to show degenerative changes.

Posture also affects fluid flow within discs, and this is particularly important for the transport of high molecular weight metabolites which diffuse very slowly.[611] Flexion increases intradiscal stresses, while at the same time thinning the posterior anulus and increasing its surface area, so fluid expulsion from the loaded disc is increased.[9] Fluid expelled under high load returns when loading is reduced, bringing metabolites with it. Flexion and extension tend to generate the highest compressive stresses in the anterior and posterior anulus, respectively (p. 163), so changes in posture will move the position of maximum compressive stress within the disc, and therefore enhance intra-discal fluid flow. These cadaveric experiments suggest that metabolite transport by fluid flow, both into and within the disc, is enhanced when flexed postures are alternated with lordotic postures. Figure 10.12 summarises the evidence concerning posture and disc metabolite transport.

POSTURE AND SPINAL NERVE ROOTS

Compared to the neutral (unloaded) position of a cadaveric lumbar spine, moderate flexion increases the cross-sectional area of the vertebral foramen by 12%, and extension reduces it by 15%.[381] In the same specimens, nerve root compression was judged to occur in the intervertebral foramen in 15%, 21% and 33% of specimens which were sectioned in the flexed, neutral and lordotic postures respectively. Extension decreases the volume and sagittal diameter of the neural sac when it is visualised by myelograms in cadaveric spines.[473] These changes are mostly due to lordotic postures pressing the neural arches more closely together, but it is possible that in

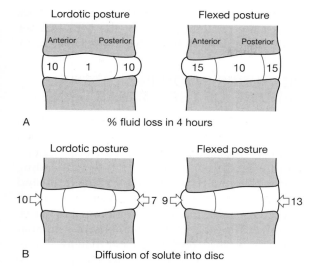

A   % fluid loss in 4 hours

B   Diffusion of solute into disc

Figure 10.12   The influence of posture on metabolite transport into lumbar intervertebral discs. (A) Numbers indicate the % water loss from the anterior anulus, nucleus and posterior anulus of a cadaveric disc loaded at bodyweight during a 4 h experiment.[9] (B) Numbers represent the average density of a small solute that has diffused into the anterior and posterior half of cadaveric intervertebral discs during a 4 h experiment.[12]

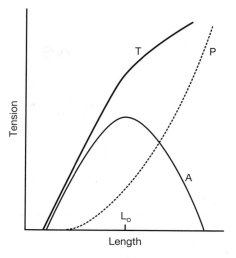

Figure 10.13   The length of a muscle affects the maximum active tension it can produce (A), as well as the passive tension (P) in stretched collagenous tissue within the muscle. Overall tension in the muscle (T) is greatest when the muscle is stretched compared to its resting length (L_o). (After Wilkie.[859])

full extension, the ligamentum flavum could bulge anteriorly and contribute to the 'postural' stenosis.

Although lumbar flexion would reduce the effects of nerve root compression, it would increase any effects of nerve root tension, especially if the nerve root were tethered to underlying structures by scar tissue.

POSTURE AND MUSCLE ACTION

Posture affects three properties of the back and abdominal muscles: their length, the angles at which they pull on vertebrae, and their lever arms relative to centres of rotation. The most important of these influences is on muscle length. Muscles generate maximum active tension when stretched to approximately 100–110% of 'resting muscle length', and active tension falls when the muscle is shortened and cross-bridge formation is impaired. In addition to this, muscles can generate substantial passive tension in their non-contractile collagenous components, and this passive tension increases greatly as the muscle is stretched[668] (Fig. 10.13). Trunk muscles are probably at their 'resting length' when the spine is in the neutral configuration (Fig. 10.2). Therefore, erect standing, which extends the lumbar spine by approximately 12°,[21] will shorten the back muscles slightly, whereas flexed postures will stretch them. Not surprisingly, overall back muscle strength is substantially higher in flexed postures[216,217] compared to the erect standing posture,[549] and maximum strength increases by approximately 18% between 30% lumbar flexion and 60% flexion.[504] Although back muscle strength in more flexed postures has not been investigated thoroughly, it appears that strength is not diminished at 70% flexion.[216]

Above 80% lumbar flexion, the back muscles receive substantial help from the lumbodorsal fascia and stretched intervertebral ligaments. This has been demonstrated in a large study which measured the maximum extensor moment that could be generated across the lumbosacral joint while the lumbar and thoracic back muscles remained electrically silent.[216] Extensor moment must therefore have been generated by more distant muscles, perhaps the gluteals and latissimus dorsi, and transmitted across the lumbar spine by the lumbodorsal fascia. Stretched supraspinous and intervertebral ligaments would also have generated some 'passive' extensor moment, but their contribution becomes substantial only when full flexion is approached (see Fig. 7.4). The hypothesis that tension in the lumbodorsal fascia can be elevated substantially by the action of the abdominal muscles has been disproved by anatomically precise calculations,[485] so it appears that flexing the lumbar spine is the most effective way of employing the fascia to assist in heavy lifting. This assistance is beneficial in two ways: it increases the maximum load that can be lifted; and because the fascia has a long lever arm relative to the centre of rotation in the disc, it also reduces the 'compressive penalty' of lifting, as discussed on page 95. The mechanics of weight lifting is considered in more detail in Chapter 7.

Lordotic postures enable the erector spinae to pull backwards at an increasing angle on the lower lumbar vertebrae and help them to limit the gravitational forward shearing force acting on these vertebrae to approximately 200 N.[664] This may be of some benefit, although the apophyseal joints are able to resist 2 kN of shear without this assistance.[189] Full flexion reduces the posteriorly directed shear force exerted by muscles on the upper lumbar vertebrae, and changes the net shear force acting on L5/S1 from an anteriorly directed force to a posteriorly directed one.[487]

Lumbar curvature has little effect on the lever arms of the back muscles relative to the flexion–extension axis of rotation, and so does not greatly influence the compressive force acting on the lower lumbar spine. This has been demonstrated using bi-lateral X-rays to compare the attachment points of the back muscles (including multifidus) in the erect standing and fully flexed postures.[487] This study concluded that flexion increased the lever arms of some muscles, but reduced them in others, so that there was no overall difference in the muscles' ability to generate extensor moment. A magnetic resonance imaging (MRI) study has claimed that flexed postures reduce the lever arm of the erector spinae,[809] but this may be an artefact caused by subjects squashing their back muscles against the confining walls of the MRI scanner whilst attempting to flex in a confined space.

POSTURES INVOLVING LATERAL BENDING OF THE LUMBAR SPINE

Lateral bending has received little attention from biomechanists, presumably because it is not a common movement in life. However, lateral bending is often combined with forward bending during asymmetrical manual handling tasks, and in awkward postures, so it is important to understand the significance of the component of lateral bending. The side-to-side diameter of a lumbar disc is approximately 50% greater than its antero-posterior diameter, so a given angular movement between two vertebrae in the frontal plane will cause 50% greater vertical deformations of the peripheral anulus than the same movement in the sagittal plane (see Fig. 9.13). Intradiscal stress distributions should therefore be more sensitive to lateral bending than to flexion or extension, and the stress peaks shown in Figures 10.7 and 10.10 would probably be larger if the 2° angulation was in the frontal plane rather than the sagittal plane. Similarly, small angles of spinal bending in the frontal plane could possibly generate high compressive stresses in the ipsilateral zygapophysial joint, and high tensile stresses in the capsule of the contralateral joint. By implication, postures which involve angular movements in both the sagittal and frontal planes will be capable of generating particularly high stress concentrations in the disc, zygapophysial joints and intervertebral ligaments.

These possibilities have not been tested by experiment, but antero-lateral bending does indeed create large concentrations of compressive stress in the lateral and posterior anulus fibrosus, and these stress concentrations are linked with the disc's susceptibility to prolapse under the influence of combined bending and compression.[546] Lateral bending is usually coupled with axial rotation (p. 111), and a combination of compression, bending and axial rotation generates particularly high intra-discal stresses in the inner postero-lateral anulus.[757]

'CREEP' IN SPINAL TISSUES

COMPRESSIVE 'CREEP' OF THE INTERVERTEBRAL DISC

Sustained loading of intervertebral discs causes them to lose height gradually, a process known as 'creep' (Fig. 10.14). Most disc creep is due to the expulsion of water,[9,440,542] but about 25% of the height loss may be due to viscoelastic (time-dependent) deformation in the collagenous matrix of the anulus fibrosus.[120] Anulus tissue becomes more elastic as a result.[432,744] After 6 hours of creep loading at 1.5 kN, creep slows down markedly. The volume and hydration of the nucleus and inner anulus are then reduced by approximately 20%,[542] an increasing proportion of the inner anulus loses its ability to behave as a hydrostatic fluid (Fig. 10.15), and concentrations of compressive stress appear within the anulus, usually posterior to the nucleus.[23,56] Pressure in the nucleus is typically reduced by 30–40%, allowing the anulus to bulge radially outwards, rather like a 'flat tyre'[111,448] and causing the inner lamellae to bulge into the nucleus.[736] The disc's resistance to shear is reduced.[187] Eventually, water expulsion causes the swelling pressure of the disc's proteoglycan-rich matrix to increase until it approaches a balance with the external mechanical pressure, and then water expulsion stops, or is greatly reduced.[818]

DIURNAL CHANGES IN HUMAN STATURE

During the course of each day, physical activity reduces the height and volume of intervertebral discs by about 20%.[104] There is a corresponding reduction in human stature of 15–25 mm,[194,441,815] much of which occurs during the first hour after rising. During the night, when the spine

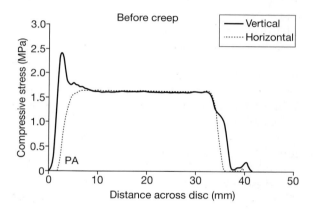

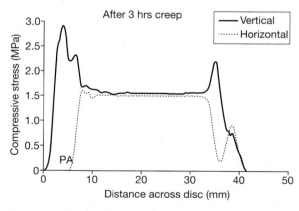

Figure 10.15 Distribution of vertical and horizontal compressive stress along the sagittal mid-plane of a cadaveric intervertebral disc, before and after a 3 h period of compressive creep loading in a lordotic posture (2° of extension). (Specimen: male, 59 years, L34, anterior on right. Compressive force = 2 kN.) Creep increases stress concentrations in the anulus, and reduces the size of the region that exhibits a hydrostatic pressure. ('Stress profiles' are explained on p. 124.)

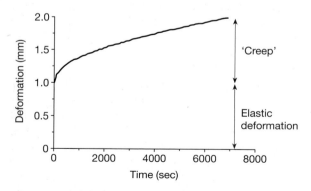

Figure 10.14 Typical 'creep curve' for a cadaveric intervertebral disc (male, 55 years, L23). When a compressive force (1.7 kN) is first applied, the disc deforms immediately, but this 'elastic deformation' is followed by a slow 'creep' deformation over a period of hours as water is expelled from the disc.

is relatively unloaded, the disc's elevated swelling pressure sucks in water from surrounding tissues, causing tissue hydration to increase, and swelling pressure to fall, until it approaches equilibrium once more with external mechanical load. In this way, the disc's water content exhibits a cyclic diurnal variation, which is modified by periods of hard work or rest. Three hours of carrying a backpack weighing 20 kg, for example, reduces disc volume by 4.5%.[499] There is no evidence that the disc's water content ever achieves an equilibrium with applied load – only that it approaches equilibrium after several hours of constant loading – so there is no such thing as a precise 'physiological' disc hydration, just a physiological range which depends on loading history. Measurements of spinal shrinkage during discrete time intervals can be used to infer the approximate magnitude of spinal loading (p. 98).

DIURNAL CHANGES IN SPINAL MECHANICS

Any loss of disc height brings adjacent vertebrae closer together and increases loading of the zygapophysial joints: approximately, a 1 mm height loss can increase their load-bearing from 4% to 16% of an applied compressive force of 1 kN.[6] As disc height is lost, compressive stresses become concentrated in the inferior margins of the zygapophysial joints, especially in lordotic postures, and extra-articular (bone–bone) impingement of the inferior facets on the subjacent lamina can occur.[229] The height of the intervertebral foramen is reduced directly by disc creep, and its anteroposterior diameter is reduced also by the concomitant increase in disc radial bulging, so the space available for the spinal nerve roots is reduced considerably as the day progresses.

Loss of disc height slackens the intervertebral ligaments and fibres of the anulus fibrosus, so that they resist bending movements less.[16,20,213] On average, 2 hours of compressive creep loading at 1.5 kN reduces disc height by 1.1 mm, reduces the bending moment resisted at full flexion by 41%, and increases the range of flexion by 12%,[16] as shown in Figure 10.16. The effect of disc creep is relatively greater for the short fibres of the anulus

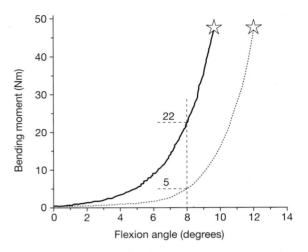

Figure 10.16 The resistance to flexion of a cadaveric lumbar motion segment before (solid line) and after (broken line) 2 hours of compressive creep loading at 1.5 kN. (Specimen: male, 52 years, L23, height loss = 1.0 mm.) Creep reduced this specimen's resistance at 8° of flexion by 77%, and increased its range of flexion by 2°. Stars indicate the elastic limit of flexion.

than for the longer fibres of most intervertebral ligaments, so the disc becomes better protected in bending.[20] After creep, it becomes more difficult to cause discs to prolapse posteriorly (see p. 148) presumably because creep loading decompresses the nucleus and reduces tension in the posterior anulus in flexion.[20,478] Increasing the volume of the nucleus by injecting water into it has the opposite effect: the pressure increases[44,676] and so does the motion segment's resistance to bending.[44]

Some of these changes have been measured in living people. The range of lumbar flexion increases by approximately 5° during the course of a day,[20] with 77% of the increase occurring during the first hour after rising.[215] This explains the common experience that it is easier to touch your toes in the evening, when all of the intervertebral ligaments (and the spinal cord!) have more slack. Similarly, the range of straight leg raising increases as the day progresses.[659] Diurnal loss of disc height and approximation of the neural arches should make spinal extension movements more difficult in the evening, although this has not been quantified. Diurnal changes in spinal mechanics are summarised in Figure 10.17.

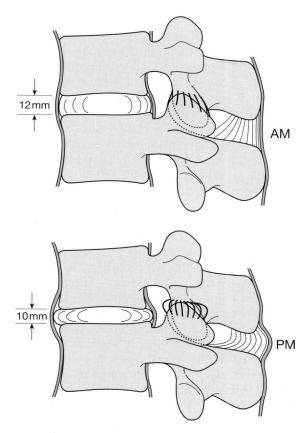

Figure 10.17 Representation of diurnal changes in spinal mechanics. In the early morning (AM), the discs are swollen with fluid, and collagen fibres in the discs and ligaments have no slack. Later in the day (PM), fluid expulsion from the discs causes them to lose height and bulge radially, giving slack to the intervertebral ligaments and increasing the load-bearing function of the zygapophysial joints.

SPINAL 'CREEP' IN FLEXION AND EXTENSION

Sitting in a slumped position causes the lumbar spine to 'creep' into more and more flexion.[535] This is not simply due to changes in the back muscles, because flexion creep has been measured in cadaveric spines subjected to sustained or repetitive bending.[16,810] Typically, 5 minutes in full flexion reduces a motion segment's resistance to flexion by 42%, whereas 100 full flexion movements during the same period reduces it by 17%.[16] Experiments on isolated ligaments[875] show that they creep substantially in a few minutes, whereas

disc creep involves fluid redistribution over long distances and takes hours to approach equilibrium.[542] Therefore, sustained or repetitive lumbar flexion will have a relatively greater relaxation effect on the posterior intervertebral ligaments than on the disc, so that ligamentous protection of the discs will be reduced. Sustained backwards bending also causes creep in cadaveric specimens, but extension creep during 20 minutes amounts to less than 10% of the normal full range of movement, presumably because of bony impaction between the neural arches.[614]

MUSCLE FUNCTION AND DYSFUNCTION

ANTAGONISTIC MUSCLE ACTIVITY

Muscles which flex the spine normally work antagonistically with those that extend it. Antagonistic muscle activity stabilises the vertebral column in the sense that it reduces the need to recruit additional muscles to deal with some unexpected event.[765] However, antagonistic muscle tension increases the compressive force acting on the spine, as described on page 100. For each posture or activity, there must be an optimum level of antagonistic muscle activity which achieves adequate spinal stability, while minimising spinal loading and metabolic cost. When stability is a major concern, as in upright and rotated postures, then antagonistic muscle activity is relatively high, and can increase spinal compressive loading by up to 45%.[162,305,456,530] Conversely, when high compressive loading of the spine is more of a problem, as when lifting heavy objects from the ground, then antagonistic muscle activity is low, accounting for approximately 10% of spinal compressive loading.[426]

Antagonistic muscle activity is often increased in people with back pain[31] although this is not necessarily the case in chronic sufferers.[155] Evidently, trunk muscles can increase their activity in order to 'splint' a painful spinal segment, and so reduce the risk of sudden movements deforming injured tissues. Alternatively, high antagonistic muscle forces could possibly cause pain by subjecting the underlying spine to high chronic loading, leading to accelerated creep and high stress concentrations. To the authors' knowledge, this possibility remains unsupported by experimental evidence.

Muscle 'spasm' represents an extreme form of muscle splinting, in which a vigorous reflex contraction of a muscle is induced by stimulated nociceptors in some adjacent tissue.[751] Muscle spasm ensures that a painful spinal segment is effectively splinted, but muscle tension imposes high compressive forces on that segment, and the affected muscle can probably become a source of pain in its own right,[66] possibly because of high intramuscular pressure.

FLEXION RELAXATION

A similar problem is the loss of the normal 'flexion–relaxation' phenomenon. When someone bends forwards, it is normal for the back muscles to fall electrically silent and allow the forward bending moment of the inclined trunk to be supported by stretched, non-contractile, tissue within the muscles[668] and by adjacent structures such as the lumbo-dorsal fascia and intervertebral ligaments.[255,536,715] If the spine is sufficiently flexed, then the thoracic erector spinae fall silent as well.[216] Skin surface electrodes used in these investigations are capable of picking up signals from the deep muscles of the trunk as well as from superficial muscles.[529] The flexion–relaxation response is often lost in people with back pain,[32,848] but there is no evidence that the response is lost before the pain starts. The simplest explanation is that the back muscles are attempting to 'splint' a painful spinal segment during a potentially threatening movement into full flexion.

MOTOR CONTROL

So many muscles are capable of moving the human torso that any particular task can be achieved by many different combinations of activated muscles. This inherent 'redundancy' in the problem of trunk muscle activation means that mathematical models of muscle function are unable to predict which is the optimum muscle strategy for a particular task, unless they introduce somewhat arbitrary 'minimising principles' in order to obtain a unique solution.[162,292] For example, it might be decided to minimise muscle force per unit cross-sectional area, or minimise shear loading of the spine. However, a variety of muscle activation patterns can be explained simply in terms of anatomical diversity, combined with personal preferences, perhaps even a preference for variety. Asymptomatic people with considerable experience in manual handling actually show more variability in spinal loading when repeating a lifting task than do novice workers.[308] This argues against the physical importance of 'optimum' muscle strategies. There is no reliable evidence that unusual muscle activation patterns cause back pain, although a tendency to load the spine heavily during laboratory lifting tasks is associated with future back pain.[506]

However, asymmetrical muscle activation could possibly be of clinical significance. As described above, spinal posture has a marked effect on stresses within the disc and neural arch, and on the dimensions of the intervertebral foramen. Therefore it is conceivable that back pain could arise from gross left–right asymmetries in the back muscles, or from an imbalance in flexor/extensor muscle strength, if the asymmetry was sufficiently marked to change the angulation of adjacent lumbar vertebrae by 2° or more. Large asymmetries have been detected in the electromyographic (EMG) signals from the back muscles of patients with back pain[155] (Fig. 10.18) but there is currently no evidence to suggest that they cause the pain. Asymmetrical muscle activation may represent an attempt by muscles on one side of the back to 'splint' a painful spinal segment, or they may occur as a result of selective muscle atrophy, or following reflex inhibition (see below).

SPINAL REFLEXES

Rapid forward bending movements of the spine cause the back muscles to contract vigorously in order to decelerate the upper body and prevent hyperflexion injury.[209] This back muscle activation may be at least partly reflex in nature (Fig. 10.19) and true reflex activity of multifidus

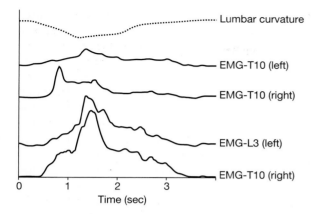

---- Lumbar curvature

---- EMG-T10 (left)

---- EMG-T10 (right)

---- EMG-L3 (left)

---- EMG-T10 (right)

Time (sec)

Figure 10.18 Evidence of asymmetrical back muscle activity in a patient with acute back pain, who flexed forwards to lift a 10 kg weight from the ground. The top curve shows that peak lumbar flexion occurred after 1.2 s. The other curves indicate the EMG signal recorded from four sites on the surface of the back, at the levels of T10 and L3. Note the early activation of the muscle at T10 on the right hand side of the back. (Dolan 2000, unpublished data.)

has been demonstrated in similar circumstances in anaesthetised cats.[768] Prolonged or repeated stretching of the interspinous ligament causes the normal reflex activation of multifidus to diminish, and then disappear entirely,[751] and several hours of recovery time are required for the reflex to be fully restored.[752] These phenomena can probably be explained in terms of time-dependent changes in the immediate vicinity of stretch receptors in ligaments and tendons, so that the receptors are either de-sensitised from overuse, or else fooled by the manner in which creep stretching removes the normal close correspondence between tissue stress and strain (see p. 171). Whatever the explanation, any loss of stretch reflexes will reduce the ability of the back muscles to protect the lumbar spine by contracting vigorously as the limit of flexion is approached. This protective action has been demonstrated when subjects bend forwards to lift an object from the ground: a sudden burst of back muscle activity decelerates the upper body, and prevents excessive lumbar flexion (see Fig. 7.6).

A failure of spinal reflexes could explain why people tend to apply much higher bending moments to their lumbar spine when bending

forwards during the early morning compared to later in the day.[20] Overnight swelling of the intervertebral discs makes them stiffer in bending (Fig. 10.16), whereas the small concomitant increase in disc height (less than 2 mm) may be insufficient to have much influence on stretch receptors in adjacent ligaments and tendons. Therefore, the spine can be flexed almost as much during the early morning as later in the day, even though this entails a 300% increase in the bending moment acting on the swollen intervertebral discs.[20] This could explain why avoiding lumbar flexion in the early morning reduces the recurrence of back pain.[750]

A similar argument could explain why people with only a small range of lumbar flexion tend to apply higher bending moments to their lumbar spine than do more supple people during forward bending movement.[210] Spinal mobility shows a similar age-related decline in living people[70,128] and in cadaveric spines[13,351] so it is reasonable to assume that particularly 'stiff' individuals are stiff because they have a relatively inflexible vertebral column, possibly because their discs have a low ratio of height to antero-posterior diameter. If this intrinsic spinal stiffness was not adequately detected by stretch receptors in adjacent ligaments and tendons, then this could explain why peak bending moments acting on the osteoligamentous spine can be up to twice as high in stiff people compared to supple people.[210]

Spinal reflexes may have direct links with back pain. Chronic joint pain and swelling are known to inhibit the recruitment of specific muscles near the joint via a 'short loop' spinal reflex (Fig. 10.19). This process of 'reflex inhibition' has been described for the knee joint,[766] but it could also operate to reduce back muscle protection in patients with chronic back pain. Inhibition of specific back muscles may also arise from a 'long loop' reflex, involving perceived pain,[348] and generalised muscle disuse atrophy can result from any chronic pain. Studies of back muscle cross-sectional area, fibre types, and EMG characteristics have attempted to explain selective and generalised back muscle changes in back pain patients in terms of these various interacting mechanisms.[31,348,508,511,767]

'GOOD' AND 'BAD' POSTURE FOR THE LUMBAR SPINE

SITTING AND STANDING

Recommendations concerning 'good' or 'bad' posture should not be based on experimental data concerning only one or two structures: the whole lumbar spine must be considered, including muscles and fascia. Unfortunately, early investigations of the biomechanical effects of spinal posture concerned only the hydrostatic pressure in the nucleus pulposus of the intervertebral disc, which was measured in cadaveric specimens,[581] and subsequently in living people.[41,575,582] These studies found that lordotic postures reduce the pressure in the nucleus pulposus compared to flexed postures, and they concluded that lordotic postures reduce spinal loading. We now know that lordotic postures reduce nucleus pressure only because they transfer load-bearing to the posterior anulus fibrous and zygapophysial joints (see above). These latter structures are frequent sources of back pain,[446] whereas the nucleus is not, so the concept of 'good' posture needs to be re-evaluated.

The relative merits of a flexed and lordotic lumbar spine are summarized in Table 10.2. These statements suggest that moderate flexion is preferable in static postures, whereas a slight lordosis has certain advantages during locomotion.

Table 10.2 Advantages of moderately flexed and lordotic postures

Advantages of moderately flexed postures:
1. Even distribution of stress in the intervertebral discs
2. Increased supply of metabolites to vulnerable regions of discs
3. Reduced loading of the zygapophysial joints
4. Increased volume of intervertebral foramen and spinal canal
5. Lumbodorsal fascia is able to resist lumbar flexion

Advantages of lordotic postures:
1. Reduced pressure in the nucleus pulposus
2. Reduced compressive stresses in the anterior anulus
3. Zygapophysial joints contribute to spinal compressive strength
4. Improved shock absorption during locomotion
5. Spinal stretch reflexes preserved

Too much lumbar flexion is worse than too little, because prolonged full flexion severely compromises the ability of the back muscles to protect the lumbar spine, as described above. The evident dangers of excessive flexion may have been apparent before the benefits of moderate flexion were understood, and this could explain why the advocacy of lordotic postures was so readily accepted. But now that a more complete picture is emerging, it is time to recognise the benefits of moderation: not too much flexion, and not too much lordosis either.

On a practical level, it is reassuring that the biomechanical and nutritional benefits of moderate flexion are matched by a perception that a flattened lumbar spine is also more comfortable. Common postural habits such as standing with one foot raised on a bar rail, or sitting with the legs crossed, all tend to move the lumbar spine from lordosis to slight flexion (p. 161). However, there is no ideal sitting or standing posture, because no single posture can be comfortably maintained for a long period of time, presumably because of blood flow restrictions in compressed or contracted tissues. Therefore, any recommendations on 'good' sitting or standing postures must incorporate the need for intermittent postural adjustments. Recommendations should also pay attention to the additional stress concentrations which arise from lateral bending of the lumbar spine, and to the benefits of minimising muscle activity. According to these criteria, the ideal posture would be the foetal position! Realistically, it would be better to advocate a straight (moderately flexed) back, with the head and vertebral column finely balanced so as to allow the supporting muscles to relax.

MANUAL HANDLING

The benefits of moderate lumbar flexion can also be realised during vigorous activities such as lifting heavy weights. In fact, when spinal compressive loading rises to high levels, the only clear advantage of lordotic postures (reduced nucleus pressure) becomes insignificant.[27] The compressive strength of cadaveric lumbar motion segments appears to vary little in the range between the neutral position and moderate (4–10°) flexion[27] presumably because two opposing effects cancel each other: flexed postures probably strengthen the disc-vertebral body unit by equalizing the distribution of compressive stress within the disc, whereas lordotic postures will strengthen motion segments by sharing load-bearing between the disc and neural arch. In full flexion, tensile forces in the posterior intervertebral ligaments act to compress the disc, but this effect becomes smaller when the compressive force rises to high levels (Table 10.1). There is some slight evidence that motion segments are weaker when flexed to 15°, which is beyond the physiological limit of many specimens, and failure is then more likely to involve the anterior vertebral body rather than the endplate.[310] Also, in full flexion and hyperflexion, stretching of the posterior anulus fibrosus increases the risk of posterior disc prolapse (p. 148).

When heavy lifting is viewed in a wider perspective, it can be seen that a flat, moderately flexed lumbar spine has the additional advantage of stretching passive tissues, including the lumbodorsal fascia, so that the 'compressive penalty' of lifting is reduced (p. 95). Flexion also reduces the metabolic cost of lifting by causing elastic energy to be stored in stretched tissues (p. 95). A recent finite element model predicted that 'slight to moderate' flattening of the lumbar curvature was beneficial during lifting because it reduced peak collagen fibre strains in the intervertebral discs, and decreased the muscle activity required to stabilise the lumbar spine.[740] It is not surprising, therefore, that healthy people flex their lumbar spine by approximately 80% when lifting weights from the ground, regardless of whether they adopt a 'bent-knees' style (see Fig. 7.7),[217] or lift in a manner of their own choosing.[216] Even when they attempted to maintain a lordosis throughout the lift, a group of experienced lifters found it impossible to avoid flexing their lumbar spine by less than 57% on average.[216] The widely held belief that weight lifters should, or even can, maintain a normal (standing?) lumbar lordosis is evidently mistaken, and may arise from a quite proper appreciation of the dangers of too much

flexion during lifting. It may be of practical benefit to instruct novices to lift with a lordosis in order to reduce the risk of them lifting with a fully flexed or hyperflexed back, but the instructor should know that the lumbar spine will in fact be moderately flexed, and that this is beneficial to the spine.

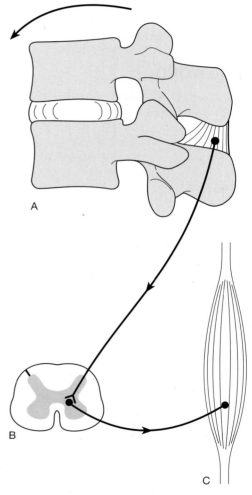

Figure 10.19 In a spinal reflex, stimulation of receptors in a stretched ligament or tendon (A) sends a signal to the spinal cord (B), which directly sends a signal to the muscle (C). In this case, the muscle will contract in order to counter the initial stimulus. In a 'long-loop' or long-latency reflex, the incoming signal from the stimulated tissue reaches the spinal cord in the same manner, but is then reflected from the brain stem, before a modulated response is sent to the muscle.

POSTURE AND BACK PAIN

The above discussion has considered how 'good posture' should be interpreted for people with a healthy back, but these arguments can not necessarily be extended to those with an injured or painful back. Obviously, the need to avoid pain and to minimise loading of damaged tissues would take precedence. Maintaining an exaggerated lordosis may help some patients, but this is an expedient for particular individuals which should not be applied to healthy people.

A FINAL WORD

The final word on 'good posture' should be reserved for unambiguous epidemiological evidence concerning living people, rather than the interpretation of laboratory experiments. Intervertebral disc degeneration is less common in populations who habitually adopt squatting postures which flex the lumbar spine, than it is in industrialised populations who generally prefer chairs[243,244] and who have a reduced range of lumbar flexion.[79,392] Although several factors may contribute to the relative health of the discs of those who squat, this evidence makes it difficult to argue that flexed postures are harmful to the back.

11

Preventing and treating back pain

INTRODUCTION

This chapter serves to complete the picture of the biomechanics of back pain by presenting a brief overview of the current status in prevention and treatment.

As discussed in Chapter 6, low back pain is a highly prevalent disorder which shows little sign of reduction, despite considerable scientific research across numerous biomedical disciplines. The high rate of disability due to back pain is evidence that we have singularly failed either to prevent or treat the problem satisfactorily.[129] Human beings have had back pain throughout recorded history, but it is only since the late 19th century that it has become (with few exceptions) a disabling problem requiring substantial health care resources; indeed, it is possible that health care may have contributed to the problem.[840] In recent years we have, however, begun to understand a great deal more about how to deal with back pain. This chapter reviews the evidence for the efficacy and potential benefits of current interventions.

Because the range of preventive strategies and treatment methods is so vast, the discussion adopts the principles of evidence-based medicine and concentrates on existing systematic reviews and clinical guidelines, with some reference to individual scientific studies where necessary. The rationale for this approach is discussed on page 81, where some of the limitations of systematic reviews are pointed out. Inevitably, some management strategies will be omitted because of a lack of 'scientific' evidence for their efficacy in preventing or treating low back pain (LBP), though others will be discussed because they are of particular biomechanical interest.

PREVENTION

The epidemiology of back pain (see Ch. 6) indicates that primary prevention is an unrealistic goal;[129] there is no single factor (or collection of factors) that, if removed from life, would result in the abolition of back disorders. Reducing physical loading, particularly at work, would be expected to lead to a reduction in new episodes of back pain, but this does not appear to be happening despite a general reduction of physical job characteristics in modern industrialised societies. Evidently, much back pain is not caused by work, so the impact of any further ergonomic improvements is likely to be small. That is not to say that ergonomic considerations should not be applied to the design of work: they should – but not in a vain hope that such action will make any appreciable difference to the development of back pain in the majority. Rather, accepting that people with back pain find biomechanical demands challenging (or even impossible) until their back pain improves, workplaces should be provided that are 'comfortable when we are well and accommodating when we are ill'.[323] This approach, whilst not offering anything substantial for primary prevention, has the potential to contribute to reductions in sick leave, compensation, and chronic disability.[129]

Scientists are moving away from a narrow view of 'mechanical' back pain towards a broader 'mechanistic' understanding of tissue injury and degeneration, including cellular responses to changes in tissue stress.[30,476] The focus of research remains on disorders of the intervertebral disc, perhaps because it is tempting to associate the unique characteristics of back pain with a unique anatomical structure, but only time will tell if this endeavour will lead to practical measures to prevent back pain.

Many studies report the apparent success of various interventions in reducing back pain. However, few of them are conducted as randomised controlled trials, so strong scientific evidence for their effectiveness is often scarce or inconsistent.[841] Even when an intervention has a beneficial effect in 'small area' scenarios,[319,871] it may not be obvious to what extent the results can be generalised.

Viewed overall, interventions to reduce physical workload have an inconsistent impact on occupational back pain: where there has been an effect it remains unclear if the interventions actually reduced 'symptoms' or 'injuries', or simply modified reporting patterns and altered what workers do about their back pain.[841] Stated simply, there is as yet no scientific evidence for the efficacy of ergonomic interventions.[469] It is convenient to quote from the UK Occupational Health Guidelines for the Management of Low Back Pain at Work,[152] which embodies a systematic review that considered prevention among other matters.[841,842] The star rating against each evidence statement below represents the strength of the evidence: *** = strong evidence; ** = moderate evidence; * = limited or contradictory evidence; – = no scientific evidence. (The full text of the guidelines and accompanying review can be found at www.facoccmed.ac.uk).

* There is contradictory evidence that various general exercise/physical fitness programmes can reduce future LBP and work loss; any effect size appears to be modest.[208,280,403,447,655,838]

*** There is strong evidence that traditional biomedical education based on an injury model does not reduce future LBP and work loss.[190,208,259,403,447,655]

– There is preliminary evidence that educational interventions which specifically address beliefs and attitudes may reduce future work loss due to low back pain.[784]

*** There is strong evidence that lumbar belts or supports do not reduce work-related LBP and work loss.[447,655,656,847]

* There is limited evidence but general consensus that joint employer–worker initiatives (generally involving organisational culture and high stakeholder

commitment to identify and control occupational risk factors and improve safety, surveillance measures and 'safety culture') can reduce the number of reported back 'injuries' and sickness absences, but there is no clear evidence on the optimum strategies, and inconsistent evidence on the effect size.[208,251,369,411,618,652,730,854]

In respect of the first of the above statements, it should be noted that a recent systematic review (not available at the time the guidelines were produced) concluded that there is consistent evidence that exercise has a moderate utility in prevention of back pain.[469]

Of interest is a recent, particularly focused study. It suggested that a simple mechanical intervention can help to prevent back pain: avoiding forward bending movements of the lumbar spine during the first 3 hours of the day reduces the incidence of recurrent attacks of LBP.[750] Presumably this is because it reduces the risk of bending injury to intervertebral discs and ligaments at a time when the discs are swollen with fluid (p. 149).

It should, perhaps, be pointed out that the concern of the guidelines was 'secondary' prevention of recurrent pain and disability (which was considered to be of particular importance in the occupational health setting). This is quite different from consideration of therapeutic effects, usually measured in terms of reduction of symptoms/disability related to the presenting spell, which is discussed in the following section.

TREATMENT

Clinicians involved in the treatment of back pain face a significant challenge, namely that the cause of the pain cannot often be determined.[95] Clinicians are uncomfortable with uncertainty (as indeed are patients!), so it is not surprising that the various clinical professions that treat back pain have adopted their own theories about the origin of back pain, and have developed their treatments accordingly.[840] It could be argued that the origins of symptoms are irrelevant if the

treatment works, but such an attitude is intellectually unsatisfactory, and makes it difficult to develop and improve the treatment.

What is the best way to determine if a treatment is effective? The currently-accepted 'gold-standard' scientific test of efficacy is the randomised controlled trial (RCT).[583] A treatment that outperforms both a competing treatment and the placebo effect in respect of the chosen outcome measure (reduction of symptoms or disability) and over a chosen time frame can be accepted as preferred practice until a more effective treatment is developed.

It is against this background that clinical guidelines for the management of back pain have been developed. The developers of guidelines take the RCT as their primary source of evidence, and generally rely on systematic reviews that synthesise the published research. The Cochrane Collaboration is the major source of systematic reviews in the field of back pain (www.update-software.com/ccweb) and much useful information has come from that source.

It is appropriate to breakdown the treatment of back pain into two broad areas: surgical and non-surgical. The historical and practical reasons for this have been discussed elsewhere.[840] In principle, surgery should be restricted to those cases where there is an identifiable lesion that (a) is the likely cause of the symptoms and (b) is amenable to surgical correction. That this principle is not always followed in practice is evident from the dramatically different surgery rates across countries or localities.[333] Surgical intervention is generally considered to be appropriate in cases of sciatica due to lumbar disc herniation, but is regularly performed for back pain in the presence of other lumbar pathologies such as disc degeneration (and associated spinal stenosis), spondylosis, spondylolisthesis and so-called 'instability'. As indicated in Chapter 6, the correlation between symptoms and these pathologies is uncertain, added to which their diagnosis can be difficult.[49] Taking the case of instability, the very concept may be spurious (p. 152) and even when diagnosed clinically, it cannot be confirmed biomechanically.[131] Similar arguments can be raised about some other types of apparently symptomatic lumbar pathology, with the result that it is often treated conservatively, thus blurring the distinction between surgically amenable disorders and other sources of back pain.

In recognition of the move towards evidence-based medicine, many countries have produced clinical guidelines for the treatment/management of back pain, though the extent to which these have been implemented is uncertain. A summary of the state of the evidence relating to the various treatment options for back pain and related symptoms is presented below. The starting point is the existing clinical guidelines, most of which are aimed at primary care, followed by more novel approaches and surgical intervention.

EXISTING CLINICAL GUIDELINES

The various existing national guidelines have themselves recently been subjected to critical review.[130,434] A major, highly influential synthesis of the evidence on back pain diagnosis and treatment was undertaken by the Quebec Task Force and published in 1987,[754] but strictly this did not comprise the development of a clinical guideline. The first true guidelines were produced by the Agency for Health Care Policy and Research in the USA in 1994.[50] Since then at least 10 countries have published clinical guidelines for the management of LBP, in the English, German and Dutch languages.[434] These are listed below, together with the UK occupational Health Guidelines (which were excluded from that review because they were not produced specifically for primary care).

Dutch College of General Practice (NHG), Netherlands.[242]
Israeli Low Back Pain Guideline Group, Israel.[103]
National Advisory Committee on Health and Disability, New Zealand.[51]
Finnish Medical Association (Duodecim), Finland.[500]
National Health and Medical Research Council, Australia.[96]
Royal College of General Practitioners (RCGP), United Kingdom.[53]

Swiss Medical Society (FMH), Switzerland.[412]
Drug Committee of the German Medical Society.[52]
Danish Institute for Health Technology Assessment, Denmark.[501]
The Swedish Council on Technology Assessment in Health Care.[54]
Faculty of Occupational Medicine, United Kingdom.[152]

The composition of the guidelines development groups, the way they addressed the subject, and the target populations differ somewhat between countries. For example, some countries have focused on acute back pain whilst others have given recommendations for chronic back pain of more than 12 weeks duration, though generally they did not clearly differentiate between 12 weeks from onset, or 12 weeks from presentation to a health care professional. Since the literature available to the guideline developers was international, the various guidelines should give similar recommendations regarding treatment. By and large this is the case,[130,434] but differences do occur, and these have been indicated in the following summary of existing guidelines.

Diagnostic triage

All guidelines propose some form of diagnostic triage into (1) non-specific back pain; (2) sciatica/radicular syndrome; and (3) specific back pain due to a 'red flag' condition such as tumour, infection or fracture. Sciatica was not always categorised separately but was variously included as specific or non-specific back pain.

Primary care

There appears to be a consensus that the vast majority of LBP can be managed adequately in primary care, and that X-rays are not a useful investigation in non-specific LBP (although they may reassure patient and clinician alike). Therapeutic recommendations are reasonably consistent for acute LBP, and focused on maintenance or promotion of activity as opposed to passive interventions. Bed-rest is discouraged, and advocated only if the pain is severe, and then only for a couple of days.

Advice to patients

There are consistent recommendations that patients should be reassured that they do not have a serious disease, and that the prognosis is generally favourable, though there may be recurrences. The form that the advice should take was not always consistent, but the UK guidelines in particular suggest a format for the messages to be given to patients, and specifically recommended a novel educational booklet, *The Back Book*,[689] which is one of very few to have been subjected to a randomised controlled trial and shown to have a modest beneficial effect on clinical outcomes in primary care.[138] However, that effect may be dependent on the target population and method of delivery, since a pamphlet giving somewhat similar (but much briefer) messages was ineffective for reducing work loss when mailed to American workers filing claims for occupational back injury.[341]

Medication

The prescription of medication (perhaps on a time-contingent basis) is essentially for pain control to facilitate return to normal activity. Simple analgesics were recommended by all guidelines as a first choice, with resort to non-steroidal anti-inflammatory preparations where analgesics were not sufficient. The use of muscle relaxants and opioids was inconsistently recommended.

Exercise

Recommendations for back-specific exercise therapy varied between the guidelines. Some considered they were not useful (Dutch and UK). Low stress aerobic exercise (USA) and McKenzie exercises (Dutch) were considered to be a therapeutic option. Guidelines that included chronic LBP were consistent in the recommendation that exercise therapy was a useful intervention (Dutch, German and Danish), but the suggested type and intensity was inconsistent.

Manipulative therapy

Recommendations regarding the use of manipulative therapy showed some variation. In most guidelines, manipulation was considered to be a therapeutic option in the early weeks of an episode, but in some (Dutch, Australian and Israeli) manipulation was not recommended for acute LBP. It was, however, considered useful for chronic LBP (Dutch and Danish).

RECENT EVIDENCE

A number of recent trials of physical and exercise therapies were not available to the guidelines development groups. For example, group aerobic/stretching classes were found to be as effective as modern (active) physiotherapy, and as effective as muscle strengthening/coordination using training devices, in terms of reducing pain and disability in chronic LBP patients.[509] Furthermore, a general lack of treatment specificity was considered to suggest that the main effects of the therapies came not through the reversal of physical weakness, but rather through some 'central' effect, perhaps involving perceptions of pain disability.[509] This suggestion was supported by subsequent analyses of the data which showed that improved performance in back muscle endurance tests was unrelated to improvements in electromyographic (EMG) measures of fatiguability.[510] Also, improvements in back muscle strength were only weakly correlated with changes in erector spinae size in these patients.[405] Two further RCTs, one in patients with chronic LBP[402] and another in patients following microdiscectomy[219] showed that programmes involving graded active exercise aimed at improving spinal mobility and trunk muscle function brought about improvements in pain and disability which were still evident 12 months later. Furthermore, both of these studies showed that early improvements in objective EMG measures of back muscle endurance after completion of the exercise programme were followed by more significant changes in pain and disability at the 12-month follow-up when compared to patients in the control groups. A somewhat unusual exercise therapy that has been shown to be effective in post-discectomy patients is 'orthopaedic hippo-therapy',[691] which uses horse riding as a rehabilitation program. The effect may be a combination of small multi-directional movements of the spine, exerting an eccentric training effect on the inter-segmental muscles.

There have been at least three recent trials of manipulation. A comparison of osteopathic manipulation with standard care for back pain over a duration of 3–6 weeks found that both groups improved over the following 12 weeks, and that clinical outcomes were similar, but medication use was greater in the standard care group.[47] Curtis et al.[183] took the unusual step of training physicians in manipulative techniques, and compared enhanced physician-care (essentially a guidelines approach) with enhanced care plus manipulation. The limited training in manipulative techniques had a very modest benefit compared with the enhanced care for acute LBP. A further trial compared osteopathic manipulation with chemonucleolysis for sciatica due to confirmed disc herniation. Clinical outcomes at 1 year did not differ between the treatments, but manipulation offered more rapid improvement for back pain and disability (although not for leg pain) during the first few weeks.[136] These studies all involved relatively small numbers of subjects and their results cannot necessarily be generalised. The results of the large, ongoing primary care randomised controlled trial in the UK of exercise classes and manipulative treatment (the UK BEAM trial – www.york.ac.uk/depts/hsce/ukbeam.htm) are eagerly awaited. Basic science investigations into the mechanisms and biomechanical influences of spinal manipulation are few, but recent work has shown that while no consistent kinematic or EMG changes occur following manipulation, short-term individual changes have been observed.[458]

Evidence-based and evidence-linked guidelines specifically oriented to the management of LBP in occupational health care have been issued only in the UK.[152] Their recommendations for managing acute LBP followed closely the Royal College of General Practitioners guidelines,[53] but these were extended to cover management of patients having difficulty returning to normal activities, including work, at 4–12 weeks. The recommendations and accompanying evidence statements are reproduced in Table 11.1. Rehabilitative interventions were seen as important to reduce the risk of chronicity for those patients not improving within the first month or two, but there remains limited information on their optimal form; the guidelines offered an outline of the key issues that might usefully be incorporated, and this is shown in Table 11.2.

Compliance with guideline recommendations will be variable, and dependent on implementation strategies,[60] so there is likely to be a time lag from publication before changes in practice are evident. There is little information on the efficacy of clinical guidelines for LBP, but GPs in the UK have increasingly recommended activity (and not rest) since the original UK guidelines were produced in 1996, though considerable variations in practice still exist.[260] Training medical practitioners to use the guidelines can help (McGuirk et al., Spine 2001, in press).

CHRONIC BACK PAIN

Most of the evidence discussed above concerns back pain of variable duration, but some other studies have concentrated on chronic pain. Specific guidelines for the management of chronic LBP are not currently available, but an international, multidisciplinary group, under the European COST Action B13, is addressing this topic. A systematic review of treatment for chronic LBP has concluded that the evidence for the effectiveness of most of the interventions is limited.[804] Nevertheless, strong evidence was found for the effectiveness of manual therapy, exercise therapy, multidisciplinary pain treatment programmes and spa therapy, especially for short-term outcomes.[804] In patients with chronic LBP, several well-designed randomised controlled trials have shown that active exercise improves outcome when compared to a placebo therapy,[330,755] or less active exercise[330,402,502] or self-exercise programmes.[266,796] Improvements in pain, disability and spinal function have also been reported in

Table 11.1 Management of the worker having difficulty returning to normal occupational duties at approximately 4–12 weeks (After Carter and Birrell[152])

Recommendation	Evidence	
Ensure that workers, employers and primary care health professionals understand that the longer anyone is off work with LBP, the greater the risk of chronic pain and disability, and the lower their chances of ever returning to work.	***	The longer a worker is off work with LBP, the lower their chances of ever returning to work. Once a worker is off work for 4–12 weeks they have a 10–40% risk (depending on the setting) of still being off work at 1 year; after 1–2 years absence it is unlikely they will return to any form of work in the foreseeable future, irrespective of further treatment.
Address the common misconception among workers and employers of the need to be pain-free before return to work. Some pain is to be expected and the early resumption of work activity improves the prognosis.	***	Various treatments for chronic LBP may produce some clinical improvement, but most clinical interventions are quite ineffective at returning people to work once they have been off work for a protracted period with LBP.
Encourage the employer to establish a surveillance system to identify those off work with LBP for over 4 weeks so that appropriate action can be taken. Intervention at this stage is more effective than delaying and having to deal with established intractable chronic pain and disability.	**	From an organisational perspective, the temporary provision of lighter or modified duties facilitates return to work and reduces time off work.
Advise employers on ways in which the physical demands of the job can be temporarily modified to facilitate return to work.	–	Conversely, there is some suggestion that clinical advice to return only to restricted duties may act as a barrier to return to normal work, particularly if no lighter or modified duties are available.
If medical treatment fails to produce recovery and return to work by 4–12 weeks, communicate and collaborate with primary health care professionals to shift the emphasis from dependence on symptomatic treatment to rehabilitation and self-management strategies.	**	Changing the focus from purely symptomatic treatment to an 'active rehabilitation programme' can produce faster return to work, less chronic disability and less sickness absence. There is no clear evidence on the optimum content or intensity of such packages, but there is generally consistent evidence on certain basic elements. Such interventions are more effective in an occupational setting than in a health care setting.
Where practicable, refer the worker who is having difficulty returning to normal occupational duties at 4–12 weeks to an active rehabilitation programme. Such a rehabilitation programme needs to be carefully designed to fit local circumstances and should consist of a multidisciplinary 'package' of interventions.	**	A combination of optimum clinical management, a rehabilitation programme, and organisational interventions designed to assist the worker with LBP return to work, is more effective than single elements alone.

*** = strong evidence; ** = moderate evidence; * = limited or contradictory evidence; – = no scientific evidence.

Table 11.2 Components of an active rehabilitation programme (After Carter and Birrell[152])

Education:
Directed primarily at overcoming fear avoidance beliefs and encouraging patients to learn to manage and take responsibility for their own self-care (for example *The Back Book*).

Reassurance and advice:
Strong reassurance and advice to stay active.

Exercise:
An active, progressive exercise and physical fitness programme.

Pain management:
Behavioural principles of pain management.

Work:
A programme should be delivered in an occupational setting and directed strongly towards return to work.

Rehabilitation:
May also include some symptomatic relief measures, but if so these should supplement and reinforce, and must not interfere with the primary goal of rehabilitation.

two RCTs which assessed the effects of an early graded exercise programme following lumbar discectomy.[219,429]

Non-steroidal anti-inflammatory agents may be effective for return to work/normal activities outcomes, but interventions such as transcutaneous electrical nerve stimulation, EMG feedback, acupuncture and orthoses do not seem to be.[804] No evidence has been found to support any form of long-term maintenance therapy.[804] A recent report on a prospective cohort study of common treatments for chronic sick-listed LBP across six countries, found that almost none of the treatments (GP care, physiotherapy, manipulation, back school) had any positive effects on clinical outcomes or work resumption; an exception being the use of surgery in Sweden.[333]

Longer-lasting intractable back pain is an altogether more complex matter and will not be discussed here, other than to say that interdisciplinary pain management programmes[497] are now the preferred approach.

NOVEL TREATMENTS FOR BACK PAIN

Psychosocial

Psychosocial interventions for back pain are primarily aimed at influencing factors known to be associated with chronicity; that is, removal/reduction of 'obstacles to recovery' (p. 90). The scientific evidence concerning these approaches is rather limited, but two recent systematic reviews suggest some effectiveness. It has been concluded (albeit based on just two methodologically low quality trials) that multidisciplinary rehabilitation for subacute LBP in adults may be effective.[404] Behavioural treatment for chronic LBP seems to be an effective treatment (based on six high quality trials), but it is still unknown which type of patients benefit most from which type of behavioural treatment.[806,807] More recently, a brief (two session) cognitive–behavioural intervention for chronic back pain in primary care found greater reductions in back-related worry and fear avoidance beliefs than a usual care group, together with modest effects on pain and disability.[565]

Education

The potential for patient educational interventions has been mentioned above. One radical approach has been implemented in the state of Victoria, Australia, which used an ongoing statewide media campaign including television commercials, outdoor and print advertising, seminars, and workplace visits.[125] Also, a patient educational booklet (*The Back Book*) was supplied to all clinicians likely to treat back pain, with a recommendation that it should be given to patients. Essentially this intervention promoted, at a population level, the positive messages embodied in *The Back Book*.[689] The intervention improved beliefs about back pain in the general population, and knowledge and attitudes in general practitioners, and seemed to influence medical management and reduce disability and workers' compensation costs related to back pain.[125] As mentioned above, the uncompromising messages used in the Australian study have been found to be effective in changing beliefs and clinical outcomes in primary care[138] as well as reducing extended absence in an industrial sample.[784] This can be viewed against a lack of effectiveness for more traditional messages in other back pain educational booklets.[160]

Acupuncture

Though hardly novel in temporal terms, acupuncture is considered under this heading for convenience. A systematic review of acupuncture for LBP did not find evidence to clearly indicate that it is an effective treatment for either acute or chronic back pain.[805]

SURGICAL TREATMENT

The most common surgical treatments can be divided into two categories: surgery for lumbar disc prolapse, and surgery for degenerative disc disorders. Since there is no evidence that back pathology differs between countries (see Ch. 6), it would be expected that the number of patients coming to surgery would be broadly comparable, but wide variations are found in practice.[333]

There remains uncertainty over the indications for surgery, and non-medical factors doubtless have some influence on decision-making.

Disc prolapse

There are numerous surgical techniques for treating lumbar disc prolapse, but the goal is the same: removal of herniated/extruded nuclear material to relieve nerve root compromise. It is a treatment for leg symptoms, not back pain. An alternative, less invasive procedure is chemonucleolysis, which involves the injection of an enzyme such as chymopapain to dissolve nuclear material (again to relieve leg pain). Surprisingly, only one RCT has compared surgical treatment of lumbar disc prolapse with conservative treatment, but several have compared surgery with chemonucleolysis. A systematic review of this evidence concluded that there was limited direct evidence on the efficacy of surgical discectomy, and strong indirect evidence that it is more effective than chemonucleolysis, which in turn is more effective than placebo.[286] Clinical series suggest that 70% to 95% of carefully selected patients can expect a good or excellent relief of sciatica from discectomy.[158,253,354,439] However, a recent review of 3544 patients who had undergone surgery for disc herniation showed that only 70% were fit to return to work within 12 months.[222] It is interesting to reflect on the biomechanical 'cost' of these procedures; discectomy will reduce disc height and lower intradiscal pressure,[111] and a permanent lowering of disc height occurs after chemonucleolysis.[460]

Disc degeneration

Surgical intervention for degenerative disc disease is less common. It may involve intervertebral fusion (to relieve zygapophysial joint or discogenic pain) or decompression procedures (to relieve neurogenic claudication and other symptoms of spinal stenosis). Sometime these two procedures are used together. Fusion procedures – with or without instrumentation – are also used for symptoms (including back pain) which are believed to arise from spinal instability. A systematic review

found that there was no acceptable evidence on the efficacy of any form of fusion for back pain or 'instability'.[286] Similarly there was no acceptable evidence on the efficacy of any form of decompression for degenerative lumbar disc disease or spinal stenosis.[286] Note, however, that a lack of evidence should not be confused with negative evidence.

A large RCT of surgical fusion has recently been reported from Sweden.[263] Ostensibly this compared surgical fusion with nonsurgical management for patients who had chronic LBP and degenerative changes in the lower lumbar spine. In practice, it compared fusion with natural history. Back pain and disability improved to a significantly greater extent in the surgical fusion group, though there was no difference in the return to work rate. The authors concluded that it could now be considered consistent with evidence-based treatment to use lumbar fusion for severe chronic LBP in carefully selected patients where nonsurgical treatment has failed. Whether this conclusion can be generalised to other countries remains to be seen. A similar trial in the UK is due to report within a few years. Some surgical techniques can be effective in a biomechanical sense (for example, instrumented fusion produces a higher fusion rate), but the complexity of instrumentation has little effect on clinical outcomes.[264]

Novel surgical approaches such as prosthetic intervertebral discs,[461] vertebroplasty,[81] and intradiscal electrotherapy (IDET)[695] have not yet been subjected to controlled clinical trials, whilst other novel procedures such as gene therapy[563] are still in the development stage.

SUMMARY

The epidemiology of LBP (see Ch. 6) suggests that the concept of primary prevention is an unrealistic dream for all but a minority of cases. Whilst reductions in the physical requirements of work have apparently reduced demonstrable mechanical overload damage to the spine,[117] a corresponding reduction in the prevalence of symptoms and disability has not followed.

Conventional ergonomic and biomechanical interventions have the potential to reduce the incidence of back problems, but that potential has not been demonstrated and the overall impact is unlikely to be large.

So far as therapeutic interventions are concerned, there is strong evidence to support a conservative management strategy based on early activation (or reactivation) in primary care. Specific therapies appear to add only modest benefits when their efficacy is assessed in a statistical sense, although the pain relief is doubtless appreciated by those individuals who do respond to treatment. The potential for early psychological interventions to reduce the burden of chronic disability due to back pain has been demonstrated, albeit in a limited number of studies. There is also evidence from several recent studies that exercise therapy is effective in the treatment of chronic LBP. The value of surgical interventions can be accepted only for a small proportion of patients presenting with highly specific conditions, the selection of whom remains a challenge.

It is quite striking that no single form of treatment for LBP, either physical, psychological or surgical, is able to improve greatly on the natural history of the phenomenon. This is doubtless largely due to the extremely heterogeneous nature of LBP, the complex relationships between pathology, pain and pain behaviour (p. 201), and the practical difficulties of patient selection.

The situation can change rapidly, however, as results from controlled clinical trials are continually being added to the literature. The Cochrane Collaboration provides an international database to support evidence-based medicine, and produces systematic reviews of treatment options for LBP which are updated at regular intervals (www.update-software.com/ccweb).

POSTSCRIPT: PRACTICAL ADVICE

The authors of this book strongly endorse the principles of evidence-based medicine, but recognize that systematic reviews (the stuff of evidence-based medicine) can be somewhat nihilistic (p. 81) and can reduce the impact of new ideas. As an aid to the uncertainty likely to be felt by many clinicians over what advice they might give, the authors present some practical steps that could conceivably be of help for individuals.

ADVICE FOR PREVENTING BACK PROBLEMS

The biomechanical literature reviewed in this book indicates that numerous simple strategies could be helpful in the prevention of back pain. This advice, based on theoretical considerations, has not yet been scientifically validated but it should certainly do no harm!

- **Keep your spine supple**
  This will reduce peak bending stresses on the spine[210] and could reduce the risk of future back pain.[24]
- **Keep your back muscles strong and fatigue-resistant**
  Fatigued back muscles allow increased bending stresses to act on the spine.[211] Fatigue-resistant back muscles protect from future first-time back pain.[508] Having strong muscles does not reduce the risk of future back pain, but training the muscles you already have could be beneficial (p. 172).
- **Avoid spending long periods of time in lordotic or fully flexed postures**
  Lordotic postures concentrate compressive stresses in the zygapophysial joints and posterior anulus (p. 162). Sustained full flexion can impair the reflexes that enable the back muscles to protect the spine in bending (p. 172). Lumbar lordosis can be reduced by sitting, or by relaxing the knees when standing.
- **Sleep on your side rather than on your back**
  The foetal position maintains the lumbar spine in moderate flexion, whereas lying supine preserves the lumbar lordosis. Cadaver experiments suggest that flexion aids metabolite transport into the intervertebral discs (p. 166), and equalises stress distributions in the disc and neural arch (p. 162). Flexion may also help to keep the spine and back muscles supple.

- **Avoid rapid and awkward bending movements, especially in the early morning**
  Bending injuries to intervertebral discs and ligaments are most easily simulated in-vitro when the intervertebral discs are swollen with fluid (p. 144) and when there is a component of lateral bending. Rapid movements increase internal muscle forces (p. 101).
- **Lift slowly, with the spine balanced, the muscles relaxed, and the weight close to the body**
  These factors reduce the peak compressive forces acting on the spine (p. 101).
- **When starting an arduous job or sporting activity, build up your back strength slowly**
  Muscles can strengthen much faster than the underlying spine, and may cause problems for the latter (p. 70).

ADVICE FOR COPING WITH BACK PAIN

The following advice (taken from the messages given in *The Back Book*[689]) is likely to help patients cope with a spell of back pain. Verbal reinforcement of such messages is believed to enhance, though not replace, the effect of giving patients the booklet.

- 'There is no sign of any serious disease.'
- 'The spine is strong. There is no suggestion of any permanent damage. Even when it is very painful, hurt does not mean harm.'
- 'Back pain is a symptom that your back is simply not moving and working quite as it should.'
- 'There are a number of treatments that can help to control the pain, but lasting relief depends on your own effort.'
- 'Recovery depends on getting your back moving and working again and restoring normal function and fitness. The sooner you get active, the sooner your back will feel better.'
- 'Positive attitudes are important. Do not let your back take over your life. 'Copers' suffer less at the time, get better quicker, and have less trouble in the long run.'

For patients with back pain associated with a whiplash injury to the neck, *The Whiplash Book* may be more appropriate. (The Stationery Office, Norwich – (www.clicktso.com))

12

Medico-legal considerations

INTRODUCTION

Low back pain (LBP) frequently gives rise to litigation concerning medical negligence or occupational causation. Litigation and compensation issues in turn influence the outcomes of LBP, and any resulting disability. The aim of this chapter is simply to raise some biomechanical issues and consider the available scientific evidence concerning three common medico-legal questions:

1. Can a given incident or work practice be held responsible for an individual's back disorder?
2. In the absence of such an incident or work practice, would that individual's back be likely to develop the disorder?
3. Would the disorder be likely to place the individual at a disadvantage on the open labour market?

The generic label 'disorder' is used deliberately to encompass both spinal pathology and the pain and disability that may result. This is a tall order, and there is no intention here to provide definitive answers, partly because science has no absolute answers, and partly because there will inevitably be a need for legal interpretation of the facts. However, the Court often does require expert or professional opinion in order to assess the strengths and weaknesses of those facts.

The Court may be faced with reports from a number of experts, and must choose which to accept in coming to a judgement. In the UK, most medico-legal issues are decided under an adversarial system, notwithstanding the so-called 'Wolff reforms'. These reforms, guided by the Civil Procedure Rules (CPR), are intended to facilitate access to civil justice by giving the Court the power to limit expert evidence to that which it sees as being both pertinent and necessary. What this means in practice is a reduction in the use of experts, often with the appointment of a 'single joint expert' to help the Court decide some lower value claims. In essence, the Court is looking for an unbiased opinion that can be substantiated by good scientific evidence, rather than an opinion potentially biased in favour of the party paying the bill. It follows that the Court will increasingly favour the evidence from experts who display impartiality and are able to offer a scientific basis for their evidence. In addition, experts are required, where there is a range of opinion, to summarise that range of opinion and give reasons for their own opinion.

This chapter offers a synthesis of the scientific evidence relevant to the questions posed above. It attempts to place the problem of low back 'disorders' into a scientific perspective that might help experts to comply with their duty to the Court, and may help the lawyers to interpret the reports they receive from experts.

There are two fundamental issues in personal injury claims: causation and liability. A claimant must persuade the Court on both counts to succeed in being awarded damages. The matter of liability for the injury is largely outside the scope of this chapter, which concerns only the medical and biological aspects of back disorders without attempting to interpret relevant legislation. However, one fundamental question relating to liability arises naturally from the evidence in this chapter, and that is: who is liable for genetic predisposition to disease? Is it the patient, the employer, or the state? If this wider issue is eventually laid at the door of the state, then medico-legal disputes concerning back injuries could lead to payments by the state to the injured party, because genetic predisposition is arguably the largest underlying cause of back pain and disability (p. 86).

BACKGROUND ISSUES

A simple mechanistic model of injury suggests that if an exposure is to be implicated in causation, there must be a cogent temporal and biomechanical relationship between exposure and injury. Furthermore, for the injury to be said to have occurred there should be some objective evidence that something has been damaged. This is readily seen in the case of a fractured hip resulting from a fall: there is an exposure to a biomechanical force that conceivably could break bone; it occurred at an identifiable point in time; and the resulting damage can be revealed radiographically. Whilst some alleged back injuries do fit such a model, many do not.

For example, take the case of a 35-year-old male book packer who has worked for a printer packing books (in 7 kg packs) for some years. He gradually becomes aware of mild back pain over a period of weeks, which seems to be aggravated at work and gradually deteriorates, culminating in an inability to continue the job because of pain. Here there is a lack of a clear temporal or biomechanical relationship between the exposure and development of symptoms, and there is unlikely to be radiographic evidence of mechanical damage. Instead, we have a report of symptoms that are clearly made worse by work, but there is no obvious triggering event and no detectable lesion. The man is convinced that repeatedly taking books from the production line and putting them on a pallet was the cause of his back pain – but is he really injured? Does the fact that he had been absent from work due to back pain 2 years previously make a difference? What if he regularly worked out at the gym? Would it make a difference if he was aged 55 and had radiographic evidence of lumbar disc degeneration, or magnetic resonance imaging (MRI) evidence of a disc prolapse? Was he likely to develop back pain anyway and, if so, when? Is he at greater risk of future back pain and, if so, when, how frequently, and how severe? Would he be prevented from returning to a manual job? Would the presence of leg pain make a difference? Suppose that the weights being handled were of the order of 25 kg – would that have an influence?

Alternatively, suppose that he had been transferred to the packing job only a few days previously, and his pain came on quite suddenly – are those significant factors? What if he had complained of pain some time prior to the onset of symptoms – would that be relevant?

These are typical scenarios and questions on which the Court must endeavour to make a fair and reasoned judgement. There are no simple answers, and this chapter does not purport to provide them, for that is rightly the responsibility of the Court.

EPIDEMIOLOGY

Before bringing biomechanics to bear on the matter, it is worth reiterating some of the information from Chapter 6. It is imperative that the issue of causation is viewed against the background of the epidemiology of back pain.

Back pain is a symptom that afflicts most people at some point in their lives, usually in the absence of a relevant, clinically detectable source. For many it is a recurrent complaint, and for a few it results in chronic disability. This pattern does not have a close statistical correlation with exposure to obvious physical stressors (including work); it has been observed in schoolchildren, sedentary workers and non-workers; it is the same in males and females, the physically fit and the unfit; and training in working practices (such as manual handling) has not been shown substantially to influence the pattern. Work loss is certainly related to physical exposures, but it is also related to psychosocial factors. Age-related degenerative changes, detected by imaging techniques, are related to physical exposures, but the strength of that association is swamped by the influence of genetic factors. Extreme physical demands have been related to reduced intervertebral disc height, which may or may not have been symptomatic.[118] More moderate physical demands (lifting and driving) have been related to symptomatic disc prolapse,[419,571] but psychosocial factors are also related to symptomatology.[101]

Epidemiology, by the nature of its methods, paints a broad picture – it cannot, nor does it attempt to, explain what actually happens to an individual. Yet its messages cannot be ignored, and it offers an important background to the legal question (in the UK) – 'on *the balance of probabilities* was this injury caused by the alleged event/circumstances?' It is appropriate to bear in mind the distinction between the presence of symptoms, the reporting of back pain, attributing symptoms to work, reporting an 'injury', seeking health care, loss of time from work, and long term damage (see Ch. 6). These matters have different determinants that are important from a medico-legal (as well as clinical) perspective, so they cannot simply be lumped together. It would be irrational to suggest that back injuries do not occur, but what is at issue is whether the particular circumstances of the case are conducive with the alleged injury. Largely leaving aside the difficult matters of diagnostic veracity and consequent disability, the following sections discuss the biomechanical issues pertinent to expert evidence offered to the Court.

'UNDERLYING' AND 'PRECIPITATING' CAUSES OF BACK DISORDERS

Most back disorders do not have a single cause. 'Underlying' factors may render certain tissues vulnerable to mechanical loading, so that injury or fatigue failure is then 'precipitated' during a particular activity or incident. Sometimes tissue vulnerability plays the dominant role, so that a back disorder follows normal everyday loading. On other occasions, a back disorder is precipitated by a loading event which is severe enough to injure all but the strongest backs. Generally, however, it is useful to consider both underlying and precipitating causes of the problem.

ALL BACKS ARE MORE OR LESS 'VULNERABLE'

Epidemiological studies suggest that 60% of back pain[540] and 70% of disc degeneration[72,698] is 'associated with' genetic inheritance. This statistical jargon just means that two features (e.g. back pain, and a specific genetic inheritance) are often found together in the same person. An association does not necessarily mean that one feature causes the other.

Although the genetic influence on back disorders is large, it is poorly understood. In rare cases, a particular gene mutation can be held responsible for a medical problem, such as when a specific mutation of the collagen type II gene leads inexorably to failure of articular cartilage, and severe joint disease.[667] Usually, however, various mutations of various genes contribute to a greater or lesser extent to a person's predisposition to 'disease'. For example, intervertebral disc degeneration is known to be influenced by variants of the genes for collagen type IX, for proteoglycans, and for vitamin D metabolism (p. 86). Another known risk factor for back pain that has some genetic basis is a long stiff back.[24] Other genetic risk factors could possibly include physical characteristics such as small discs, a heavy body, or small internal lever arms (which would lead to increased muscle forces, as described in Fig. 7.2). Intervertebral discs with a small ratio of area to height are likely to be subjected to particularly high stresses during complex loading.[588] Genetically determined risk factors could even involve inadequate proprioception or neuromuscular control (p. 172), which would increase the risk of accidents, and psychosocial factors, which could increase the risk of them being reported as 'injuries'.

Genetic predisposition to back disorders is important, but rarely decisive. The environment must still play a role, because defective genes are present from the moment of conception, whereas tissue degeneration and failure does not normally occur for a long time after birth (in the case of disc failure, 30 to 50 years after). Even then it is generally those tissues which are subjected to most mechanical loading that tend to be severely affected, such as the lower lumbar discs. Evidently, environmental influences such as mechanical loading do contribute to tissue failure in addition to genetic predisposition.

Genetic vulnerability is modified by age, which leads to progressive reductions in the strength and stiffness of skeletal tissues (Ch. 4). Age-related vulnerability to spinal disorders may be attributable to the accumulation of fatigue 'wear and tear' damage, and to the slow biochemical process of non-enzymatic glycation which leaves cartilaginous tissues more 'brittle' (p. 61). Also, of course, an older person has had more opportunity to become involved in an 'accident', and more time to express their genetic vulnerability. In the case of the intervertebral discs, tissue vulnerability does not increase relentlessly with age: it appears to peak between 35–50 years, and then decreases.[753] This could be due to the fact that certain disc injuries are less likely to occur when the nucleus pulposus becomes dehydrated (p. 149), as it generally does in old age.

A closely related cause of tissue vulnerability is fatigue loading, which can propagate micro-damage throughout the tissue so that failure occurs at only 30–45% of the normal failure load (p. 136). Fatigue damage may partly explain age-related weakening, but the two processes should not be equated. An abrupt increase in the level of physical activity over a period of just a few days or longer could give rise to fatigue damage, even though the age-related changes are negligible in such a time span. A more gradual change to hard physical work could have the opposite effect: it could lead to hypertrophy and strengthening of spinal tissues ('work hardening') so that the spine becomes less vulnerable to mechanical damage (p. 70).

A fourth cause of tissue vulnerability is prior injury. Poorly-vascularised tissues such as large tendons and intervertebral discs have only a limited capacity to heal (see Ch. 4) so that some degree of weakness can remain for several years, if not for life. Links between tissue failure and pain are complicated (p. 201) so it is conceivable that a painful injury could be largely attributable to a previous injury that produced only mild symptoms. This is not very likely, however, if that previous injury involved tissues such as muscle or bone which are capable of rapid and full healing. We know that a previous history of back pain is highly predictive of future pain (p. 83), but it cannot always be assumed that a previous injury predisposes to future injury: it depends very much on the tissue involved, and on the age and health of the individual patient. And it must be borne in mind that back pain is frequently a recurrent phenomenon unrelated to physical exposures.

Prior injury and fatigue damage are both capable of instigating cell-mediated degenerative changes in affected tissues, leading to inferior biochemical composition, and reduced strength (Ch 4). It is also possible that some primary 'disease' process (other than the ones considered above) could leave a tissue vulnerable to subsequent mechanical damage. However, the balance of evidence indicates that cell-mediated degenerative changes usually follow tissue damage rather than precede it (p. 199).

Because there are so many causes of tissue vulnerability, it is inappropriate to label any individual as having either a 'vulnerable' or a 'normal' back. Vulnerability should be assessed on a continuous scale, with a person's position on that scale depending on all of the factors mentioned above. To insist that a back is either 'vulnerable' or 'normal' can lead to circular definitions, such as when a medico-legal report asserts that: 'this tissue failed because it was vulnerable (or diseased)', while at the same time maintaining that 'this tissue must have been vulnerable/diseased because it failed in response to mechanical loading'. In the medico-legal context, it is desirable to attempt to identify the nature and extent of any tissue vulnerability. Medical reports presented to the Court frequently refer to a condition as being 'constitutional' which broadly can be defined as 'something that is inherent in the nature of a person', and is thus not the result of some outside force for which compensation should be awarded. Science is now showing that this seemingly simple concept is far from simple. The concept of vulnerability can impact on issues of liability: for example, should a worker be held responsible for his own genes? Should his present employer be held responsible for fatigue damage sustained in a previous occupation? These difficult problems will not be considered further here.

MECHANISMS OF INJURY AND FATIGUE FAILURE

Descriptions of injury mechanisms to spinal tissues, and the forces required to cause them, are given in Chapter 9. The site and nature of injury depend on variable factors including the following:

- the time of day (p. 170),
- the speed of loading (p. 135 and p. 146)
- the curvature (posture) of the lumbar spine at the time of maximal loading (p. 161)
- the age of the subject, and the degenerative state of the tissues (p. 149).

CAN MECHANICAL LOADING CAUSE A HEALTHY DISC TO PROLAPSE?

This particular question is often raised in medico-legal cases, even though it has been answered long ago (in the affirmative!) by mechanical experiments, albeit on cadaveric specimens (see p. 148). The relevance of these experiments to living spines has been justified at length (p. 113), and the mechanism of prolapse has been explained in detail by mathematical models (p. 149). There is, then, a challenge to the previously held view (the stuff of science!), and personal dislike, or ignorance, of new evidence should not be confused with scientific debate. The new evidence indicates that:

- 'Normal' intervertebral discs can prolapse in-vitro if loaded severely in bending and compression, yet the magnitude of the forces required cannot reliably be quantified.
- A component of lateral bending and/or torsion facilitates prolapse.
- Most L4–5 and L5–S1 discs aged 40–50 years can be made to prolapse in-vitro, so it is not necessary to assume that any degenerative condition (other than normal ageing) must precede prolapse in-vivo.

- Either the bending moment or the compressive force must exceed normal limits if prolapse is to occur in-vitro in a single loading cycle. (Note, all injuries involve supra-physiological loading.)
- Neither bending nor compression need exceed normal limits if prolapse is to occur in-vitro during repetitive loading.
- Prolapse is easier to obtain in-vitro when discs are swollen with fluid, as they are at the start of the day in-vivo.
- Animal experiments show that disc tissue degenerates after mechanical disruption. (It remains possible that disc degeneration could precede mechanical disruption in humans.)
- Displaced disc tissue swells markedly during the 2–3 hours following prolapse, so any symptoms arising from prolapse in-vivo could intensify during this period (p. 151).

RETROSPECTIVE ANALYSES OF SPINAL LOADING

Because of limited in-vivo data, it may be necessary to compare the maximum forces generated at the material time with those required to injure spinal tissues in-vitro. Spinal loading is discussed at length in Chapter 7, but the following details are particularly relevant to medico-legal cases:

- Most compressive loading of the spine comes from muscle tension (p. 95) rather than gravity.
- Trunk muscle forces can rise to very high levels during alarming incidents (p. 101), especially when the spine is flexed and the muscles are contracting eccentrically. (Trunk muscle forces can crush vertebrae during epileptic fits.[822])
- Traditional static analyses of peak spinal loading (see Figure. 7.2) ignore inertial forces associated with accelerations of the spine, which can increase the peak compressive force by up to 60%.[217] Static analyses often ignore antagonistic muscle action, which can

account for up to 45% of spinal compression in upright postures (p. 171).
- Back muscles usually prevent the bending moment on the spine from exceeding physiological limits, but muscle protection is reduced following fatigue, or creep, in sustained flexed posture (p. 172).
- The bending moment acting on the spine in the sagittal plane in-vivo can be quantified in the laboratory (p. 102), but it is currently impossible to quantify the bending moment in the frontal plane, or the axial torque acting on the spine.
- Fatigue loading can cause injury at levels as low as 30–45% of the normal failure load (p. 136).

HOW STRONG IS THE BACK?

The 'strength' of a skeletal structure is the force required to break it. Average values for the strength of the lumbar spine are given in Table 9.1, and the weakening effects of fatigue are shown in Table 9.2. Unfortunately, spinal strength varies so widely between individuals (for reasons explained above under 'Vulnerability') that it is difficult to relate averaged values to any particular individual. In short, it is impossible to say how strong a person's back is: there is just a wide range of likely strengths depending on factors such as age, gender, genetic inheritance, and work history. Each case must be assessed on the basis of the available facts, though these may, of course, be limited.

RELATING SPINAL LOADING TO PATHOLOGY AND PAIN

Except in cases involving an obvious traumatic incident, it is rarely possible to state dogmatically that the forces exerted on the spine during a particular incident were sufficient to damage a particular tissue. This is partly because of the complications inherent in retrospective analyses of spinal loading in-vivo (see above) and partly because of the large inter-individual variability in the strength of spinal tissues. Similarly, it is unsafe to infer that spinal pathology is responsible for pain and disability; the relationship is complex and at the mercy of factors such as pain-sensitisation, stress-shielding, and the human personality (p. 201).

Fortunately, medico-legal reports can usually call upon two additional pieces of evidence when attempting to relate mechanical loading to pathology, and pathology to pain, in a particular person. Firstly, there may be evidence from MRI scans to indicate what pathological changes are present. Whilst spinal pathology is a particularly common finding on X-rays and MRI scans, even in pain-free people, certain features are more common in those with severe back pain and can not be considered normal, even though they are not necessarily associated with pain. Such features include disc prolapse, and a radial fissure in the posterior anulus (p. 84). Therefore, the medical report does not need to state (for example) whether or not a given loading incident would cause most discs to prolapse; rather, it need only state whether or not the loading is consistent with this particular disc prolapse. Secondly, the report does not need to declare whether or not the pathology is painful (the patient can do that!). The report need only state if the alleged pain and disability is consistent with the demonstrated pathology.

If the injured worker is untruthful or exaggerating about his pain, then the report may attribute pain to pathology which is in fact painless. However, it is important that a report from an expert witness should be confined to matters in which the writer is expert, and this should not include judging the truthfulness of a claimant's evidence; that is the responsibility of the Court.

SUMMARY

It is clear that the expert advising the Court on matters of causation faces a significant challenge for which there is no simple formula. We have attempted here to introduce some of the issues the Court may find helpful in reaching a decision – it is for the expert to provide advice and guidance to facilitate that process, by way of presenting a rational opinion based on the available scientific evidence. The summary below highlights the major issues that may be pertinent to an expert opinion.

- Back pain is common and likely to recur: sick leave and chronic disability are not inevitable consequences, and are not closely related to work.
- It is not appropriate to deny employment on the basis of a previous history of LBP, (though care should be taken if the job is heavy) and an injured worker need not be symptom free before returning to work after back pain.[152,841]
- The relationship between back pain and spinal pathology is complex, and either one can exist without the other. Certain pathological entities such as disc extrusions are associated with an increased risk of symptoms, but in the individual case the symptoms need to be clinically consistent with the pathology for a causative link to be made.
- Symptoms and/or pathology may be precipitated or aggravated by work activities even though there are other important causes contributing to the problem, such as genetics, age or work history.
- Mechanical overload damage to vertebrae and intervertebral discs can occur with especially heavy work, either by injury or by 'fatigue failure'.
- In laboratory experiments, normal intervertebral discs can be made to prolapse by the application of severe or repetitive mechanical loading, and animal experiments suggest that disc degeneration follows mechanical failure, rather than precedes it.
- Most spinal compressive loading comes from back muscles, and forces are likely to rise to high levels during sudden and alarming incidents. These forces are

difficult to quantify in retrospective analyses.

- Bending stresses acting on the spine are a potential contributor to 'injury', particularly to the intervertebral discs. Bending stresses are highest in the early morning, and following sustained or repetitive bending.

- Most back 'injuries' should, and generally do, recover (in a clinical sense if not necessarily in a physiological sense). Persisting disability is best explained by psychosocial influences (see Chs 6 and 9).

13

Summary: spinal ageing, degeneration and pain

INTRODUCTION

The focus of this book is embodied in its title. It explores the scientific evidence concerning the biomechanics of low back pain (LBP), and attempts to present it in a comprehensive and rational fashion. Whilst the subject has been approached from a biomechanical perspective, mechanical, biological and psychological influences have been fully integrated in order to provide a mechanistic account of back pain. This final chapter draws together the main evidence into a concise summary of the natural history of spinal ageing, degeneration and pain.

GENETIC INHERITANCE PREDISPOSES TO TISSUE DAMAGE

In a statistical sense, genetic inheritance 'accounts for' approximately 70% of intervertebral disc degeneration, and 60% of back pain (p. 86). The most plausible interpretation of these data is that inherited characteristics make us more vulnerable to environmental influences which then precipitate tissue damage and pain. For example, we may inherit genes which produce inferior collagen or proteoglycans in our intervertebral discs, so that mechanical disc failure can then occur at lower load levels than in a person with a more fortunate inheritance.

Genetic predisposition need not involve biochemical composition. It could involve inefficient

197

metabolic pathways; or innate clumsiness (inadequate proprioceptive/neuromuscular control) leading to more accidents; or physical factors such as small discs, a heavy body, or short internal lever arms which would lead to higher muscle forces (Fig. 7.2).

It is important to realize that genetic predisposition to musculo-skeletal disorders is rarely simple, and rarely decisive. Usually, many genes contribute to a person's predisposition to 'disease', and the environment must still play an important role (p. 192). It follows that an individual should not be considered to have a 'vulnerable' or 'normal' back. Rather, each person lies on a continuous scale of vulnerability depending on the environment in which they have lived and worked, as well as on their age and genetic inheritance. The problem of genetic predisposition to disease looks likely to become one of the major health issues of our times.

AGEING CONTRIBUTES TO TISSUE VULNERABILITY

Ageing causes progressive biochemical changes in spinal tissues, and altered chemical composition can lead to impaired function. The biochemical process of non-enzymatic glycation of collagen (p. 61) causes an inexorable age-related stiffening in tissues such as cartilage and tendon which have a high collagen content and a low metabolic rate. Stiffened tissues may be unable to absorb much strain energy (p. 7), so that they are vulnerable to mechanical failure. Close links between tissue ageing and structural disruption are probably attributable to this biochemical vulnerability, and also to the fact that old tissues have been subjected to more wear and tear loading, and have had more time to sustain an injury. However, old tissues do not necessarily show structural changes, so ageing and degeneration are not the same thing (p. 67). Ageing is not closely linked to back pain (p. 82).

EXCESSIVE OR ABNORMAL LOADING PRECIPITATES TISSUE DAMAGE

Many environmental factors, including diet and smoking, could precipitate problems in vulnerable spinal tissues, but mechanical loading is the most important factor, the best understood, and probably the most easily controlled. Generally speaking, mechanical loading is good for the back, because all spinal tissues are strengthened by exercise, and weakened by inactivity (see Ch. 4). However, under certain circumstances, mechanical loading can be harmful.

Certain postures concentrate spinal loading in specific tissues, especially if the posture is maintained for a long period of time (Ch. 10). Stress concentrations in innervated tissues can probably explain temporary backache in the absence of pathological changes, and can certainly explain why some postures may be painful/uncomfortable, particularly during an episode of back pain. The concept of 'functional pathology' (see Ch. 10), which includes abnormal posture and muscle activation patterns, may possibly explain some persistent or episodic backache, especially if the dysfunction is associated with psychosocial pressures as well.

Severe and chronic back pain, however, is often related to structural changes in spinal tissues. High forces are generated by vigorous contraction of the back muscles, and these are most likely to rise to damaging levels during activities such as heavy lifting, or when movements are fast, or when the lifter is alarmed or falls (p. 138). Mechanisms of injury have been investigated in cadaveric tissues and animal models, as described in Chapter 9. Briefly, back muscles can sustain injury during vigorous eccentric contractions; ligaments of the neural arch by forward bending movements; the zygapophysial joint surfaces by torsion and backwards bending; the vertebral body by compression; and the intervertebral discs by asymmetrical bending and compression, or following compressive damage to the vertebral body. Sacroiliac joint injury mechanisms have not been investigated to the same extent, but probably involve high asymmetrical loading of the pelvis. In most cases, damage can occur during a single loading event, or by the process of accumulating 'fatigue failure' in which the peak forces can be as low as 30–40% of those required for sudden failure (see Table 9.2).

The concept of 'fatigue' (p. 8) was developed originally to explain the failure of engineering materials, and the concept must be modified when applied to living tissues. Connective tissue cells respond to repetitive loading by producing more extra-cellular matrix, making the tissue stiffer and stronger (Fig. 4.9), and this 'adaptive remodelling' opposes the accumulation of micro-damage which leads to fatigue failure. Essentially, repetitive loading of connective tissues sets up a 'race' between damage accumulation and adaptive remodelling, and the outcome can be either mechanical fatigue failure, or a strengthened tissue, depending on circumstances. The rate of damage accumulation increases with the severity of loading, whereas the rate of adaptive remodelling increases with the health and youth of the individual, and with the metabolic rate of the tissue in question. Therefore, fatigue failure is most likely to 'win the race' in large poorly vascularised tissues (such as intervertebral discs, tendons and ligaments), of unhealthy individuals, who are no longer young, but who engage in hard physical work or exercise. If fatigue failure does not occur, then adaptive remodelling will eventually increase tissue strength to match the mechanical demands placed upon it. This suggests that fatigue failure of poorly vascularised tissues is more likely to be associated with an abrupt increase in the level of physical activity, rather than with a consistently high level of such activity, and there is some evidence in support of this hypothesis.[17]

The risk of fatigue failure to spinal connective tissues is compounded by the tendency of muscles to strengthen rapidly in response to physical activity. Thus a novice weight-trainer might double his 'poundage' during repetitive lifts in just 1 year, and although some of this increase is due to increased skill and neurological 'facilitation', it nevertheless implies that his skeleton will be subjected to increased peak muscle forces (possibly 50% greater) at the end of the year. It seems unlikely that bone would strengthen as quickly as this (p. 58), and intervertebral discs and ligaments certainly would not. Therefore, a miss-match in strength between muscle, bone, ligaments and discs could persist for months or years until a new balance is reached or injury occurs.

'DEGENERATION' REPRESENTS A CELL-MEDIATED RESPONSE TO TISSUE DAMAGE

Damage is an acquired defect that leads to an impaired resistance to applied load (p. 131). Micro-damage can stimulate the adaptive remodelling response described above, especially in muscle and bone, but gross structural failure induces very different responses from the tissue's cells. Injured muscles are able to regenerate damaged muscle fibres, although the extra-cellular matrix may become more fibrous after healing (p. 54). Ruptured ligaments and tendon do not fully regain their original collagen architecture, and cysts and fat can appear in the matrix (p. 64). Damaged vertebrae do heal, but the original shape is not usually regained,[232] presumably because the spine is not relieved of all compressive force during the healing process. Minor damage to the cancellous bone of the vertebral body results in 'micro-calluses' forming on individual trabeculae[824] and their reduced support allows the vertebral endplates to bulge into the body. Osteophytes can appear around the margin of a vertebral body (Plate 4D), possibly in an attempt to increase its cross-sectional area and hence reduce compressive stress. Damaged zygapophysial joints can become osteoarthritic, with characteristic marginal osteophytes, cartilage fibrillation, and sclerosis of the subchondral bone. Injured intervertebral discs degenerate progressively, with little sign of true healing (p. 66). Scar tissue in the outer anulus can effectively seal old radial fissures so that nucleus pulposus material does not escape easily, but the disrupted collagen fibre bundles are not completely remodelled.

We propose that 'degeneration' within a musculoskeletal tissue represents an attempt by its cells to respond to paradoxical stimuli created by structural disruption. For example, habitually increased tension in a ligament would normally strengthen it, but if the tension were sufficient to cause damage, then disrupted regions of the ligament would cease to transmit a substantial tensile force, and the cells would respond to their local mechanical environment as if the overall peak loading of the ligament were reduced, rather than increased. The injured part of the ligament would become weaker still. This would constitute an inappropriate 'degenerative' response by the cells to a (local) paradoxical stimulus, with the trigger for the response being the loss of structural integrity by the ligament.

Similarly, intervertebral disc degeneration could represent a progressive response to structural damage to the anulus fibrosus or vertebral endplate. Damage to either structure causes the hydrostatic pressure within the nucleus to fall, and high concentrations of compressive stress to appear in the inner anulus (p. 137). Cells within the nucleus could conceivably restore normal disc function by producing more proteoglycans to increase nuclear volume and pressure. However, the reduced pressure in the nucleus provides a paradoxical stimulus to these cells, encouraging them to respond as if the overall loading of the disc has been reduced, even though loading of the disc, and the anulus in particular, has actually increased. In this way, nucleus cells would reduce their synthesis of proteoglycans, and further reduce nucleus volume and pressure, intensifying stress concentrations in the anulus (p. 137). Cells in the anulus would respond to greatly increased mechanical stress by producing more matrix-degrading enzymes.[329] Hence, the initial damage to the anulus or endplate would precipitate a progressive degenerative process in the disc, rather than a reversible remodelling one. A recent study on adolescents has provided powerful evidence that previous injury to a vertebral body often leads on to degenerative changes in the adjacent disc, although that degeneration is not often painful.[421]

Little is known about the transduction mechanisms which allow connective tissue cells to respond to their mechanical environment. However, cells will be most influenced by their local environment, and may be insensitive to events occurring just a few millimetres away. Structural disruption has such a harmful effect on connective tissue metabolism precisely because it uncouples the local tissue environment from the overall loading of the structure.

Inappropriate cell-mediated responses to limited structural disruption could serve to weaken the tissue and leave it vulnerable to further mechanical damage, so that a 'vicious circle' of tissue weakening and re-injury occurs. Such a process may underlie the episodic nature of some musculo-skeletal disorders, including back pain and osteoarthrosis.

Structural damage could possibly lead to disc degeneration by other means. Endplate fracture and subsequent healing could reduce the number of marrow cavities in contact with the cartilage endplate, and hence reduce metabolite transport into the nucleus (p. 166). Alternatively, a fractured endplate could allow contact between nucleus pulposus tissue and vertebral marrow, leading to an inflammatory or autoimmune response (p. 138). A radial fissure in the anulus fibrosus would allow nucleus pulposus to make contact with the innervated outer anulus. If the rupture is complete, extruded nucleus pulposus would reach adjacent nerve tissue. The biochemical and biological consequences of such contact are just beginning to be understood (p. 151), and it seems clear that displaced nucleus pulposus can do more than simply apply mechanical pressure to adjacent tissues.

It could be argued that tissue degeneration causes structural disruption, rather than the other way round. For example, inherited defects or prolonged high loading could adversely affect cell metabolism, leading to a weakened extracellular matrix which is then vulnerable to injury under normal loading. This is the traditional concept of some primary connective tissue 'disease' leading on to subsequent mechanical failure. However, there is comparatively little evidence to suggest that degeneration does cause structural failure. Indeed, cadaveric experiments suggest that, as far as intervertebral disc prolapse is concerned, structural failure does not follow severe degenerative changes (p. 149). On the other hand, many animal models have shown that primary structural damage to connective tissues leads quickly to cell-mediated degenerative changes similar to those seen in living people (see Ch. 4).

DEGENERATION IS NOT ALWAYS PAINFUL

Structural failure prevents a tissue from resisting mechanical loading in an even manner, so that regions of high and low stress appear within it, and become progressively worse as the cells respond inappropriately. It is easy to imagine that high stress concentrations can provoke pain from innervated tissues (think of a stone in your shoe!), and a direct association between stress concentrations and discogenic pain,[547] suggests one mechanism by which disc degeneration can cause pain.

Fortunately, things are not that simple! Intervertebral disc degeneration, vertebral body osteoporosis, and zygapophysial joint osteoarthritis are very common in middle-aged and elderly people, but they are not closely correlated with back pain. Certain structural abnormalities, such as a disc prolapse, do carry an increased risk of pain, but similar abnormalities in another person can be entirely unrelated to symptoms. Why then is spinal degeneration in general, and disc degeneration in particular, not always painful?

There is an obvious mechanical reason: damaged or degenerated structures are mechanically incompetent and tend to be protected by adjacent healthy tissue. For example, a narrowed and severely degenerated intervertebral disc can be 'stress-shielded' by the neural arch to such an extent that only 30% of the compressive force on the spine actually passes through the disc (p. 117). Similarly, pain-sensitive regions of an osteoarthritic synovial joint could be protected by adjacent healthy tissue, or by osteophytes. This logic suggests that, under certain circumstances, moderate degenerative changes in a tissue should be more painful than advanced changes, because they do not relieve that tissue from its primary mechanical function. There is little evidence to support this speculation, other than the fact that the prevalence of back pain is lower after middle age, whereas degenerative changes in the spine get progressively worse. On the other hand, there is no reason to suppose the contrary: that pain increases in proportion to the severity of degeneration.

Another possible reason why spinal degeneration is not always painful is that severe and chronic pain could arise only when the tissue has become sensitised to mechanical stimulation. Biochemical changes in the vicinity of nerve endings can amplify the pain sensation, and this is well demonstrated by pain-provocation experiments in which a full symptomatic pain response is induced from patients with severe back pain by relatively innocuous probing of specific tissues (Ch. 5). Pain sensitisation in degenerating tissues could be initiated by the breaking down of physical barriers, for example, allowing displaced nucleus pulposus to irritate the innervated outer anulus, or bony endplate, or nerve root. Experiments in small animals have shown that transplanted nucleus pulposus causes morphological and functional changes in a nerve root, and also causes the animal to behave in a manner which suggests pain (p. 70). If pain-sensitisation is a normal feature of discogenic pain, then small differences in the length of a radial fissure, or in the mechanical and biochemical properties of the migrating nucleus, could have a large influence on the resulting symptoms.

A third complicating factor in the relationship between spinal degeneration and pain is muscle action. 'Protective' antagonistic muscle activity increases the overall force acting on the spine, and small postural adjustments can have a relatively large effect on how this force is distributed between, and within, specific tissues (see Ch. 10). Excessive muscle 'splinting' of a painful or unstable segment could exacerbate small injuries, and lead to more or prolonged pain. Pain-induced reflex-inhibition can also occur, and lead to muscle atrophy, leaving the muscle weakened and less able to protect underlying structures from excessive deformation.

Evidently, the links between spinal degeneration and pain are complex, and require further investigation. It would be unfortunate if spinal degeneration, and the pathological processes which underlie it, were dismissed as clinically irrelevant simply because their association with pain is more complicated than was originally anticipated.

PSYCHOSOCIAL FACTORS INFLUENCE PAIN BEHAVIOUR

Psychosocial factors do not predict more than a few percent of first-time back pain, and the back pain they do predict tends to be relatively trivial.[24] However, psychosocial factors do exert a large influence on what people actually do about their back pain. Back pain behaviour includes the initial recognition of a discomfort as back pain; the decision to report it as such; to seek and respond to treatment; to become disabled; and to seek financial compensation. This behaviour is itself influenced by interactions with other people, including work colleagues and medical practitioners. Not surprisingly, epidemiological studies of back pain find that psychosocial risk factors feature prominently in their predictive models of who reports back pain and disability. Recognition of the importance of these factors has quite rightly been termed a 'back pain revolution'[840] and there is now little doubt that studies of any aspect of back pain behaviour (such as response to treatment) must consider psychosocial factors if they are to be of much value.

This is especially true of chronic back pain and disability, which are influenced by psychosocial influences to such an extent that some sufferers are treated solely by cognitive behavioural and other psychosocial approaches (p. 184). Chronic back pain involves complex interactions between mind and body, with altered muscle function

perhaps playing an intermediary role. Rehabilitation programmes which involve active exercise are able to reduce the severity of pain in many chronic sufferers, and get others back to normal activity and work. These programmes work directly on the body by increasing factors such as mobility, muscle strength, muscle endurance, and cardiovascular fitness. Indirectly, they may influence posture and manual handling technique. In addition, they doubtless affect the mind, by increasing motivation, reducing fear, and fostering self-belief.

WHY DO WE CURRENTLY HAVE AN 'EPIDEMIC' OF BACK PAIN?

Back pain-related disability has increased greatly during the last 20 years, despite the enormous investment in labour-saving devices, and the introduction of more stringent manual handling regulations. Whilst prevalence rates have remained stable, there may be an increased tendency for some populations to report symptoms. It could be that people are becoming less prepared to tolerate pain, and are encouraged to seek treatment and time off work by generous social welfare provision, and thus are over-reacting to symptoms that were previously accepted as a normal life experience. But is this the whole answer, or is there something else about our modern lifestyle that is causing real harm to our backs?

Perhaps the disability related to mechanical back pain is not decreasing in line with the decreasing physical demands of work because it is not high loading which is bad for the back, but *excessive* loading (for that spine). Reducing physical demands on the back weakens both the spine and its supporting musculature, resulting in what could be referred to as an 'eggshell' back. This in turn increases the risk of injury during falls and other direct impacts. Furthermore, any abrupt increase in the level of physical activity, whether at work or at play, will strengthen muscles faster than poorly vascularised tissues such as intervertebral ligaments and discs. In this way, cultural innovations such as labour-saving devices, habitual inactivity, changing occupations, and recreational fads, may all conspire against these poorly vascularised spinal tissues. Other cultural inventions, such as car seats, high-heeled shoes, and vibrating environments, could also contribute to the back pain problem by affecting posture and spinal creep, and thereby increasing stress concentrations within spinal tissues.

CONCLUDING REMARKS

A typical natural history of spinal ageing, degeneration and pain is summarised in Figure 13.1.

For many patients, a blend of physical and psychological strengthening (perhaps accompanied by appropriate therapy) may be sufficient to bring their history of back pain to a natural conclusion. For others, however, the organic problems underlying severe back pain will require more specific interventions, including manual therapy and surgery. There is no reason to believe that back pain is fundamentally different from other joint pain, or that it can not be treated successfully by physical means, but the limited success currently enjoyed by available treatments reflects the complicated origins of back pain, and the practical problems inherent in treating such a deep structure as the spine.

Accurate diagnostic criteria and effective treatments for back pain are unlikely to be developed by considering just one aspect of the problem. Rather we need to integrate the evidence from genetics, biomechanics, biochemistry, cell biology and psychology to construct a comprehensive model of the natural history of spinal ageing, degeneration and pain, and then apply the model to the problems of prevention, diagnosis and cure. The 'history' presented in the present chapter has gaps in it, and probably some mistakes as well, but at least it has a beginning and an end, and incorporates all aspects of the scientific evidence in between. We hope it will encourage others to adopt an integrative approach, and to believe that spinal degeneration and pain can be explained in rigorous scientific terms.

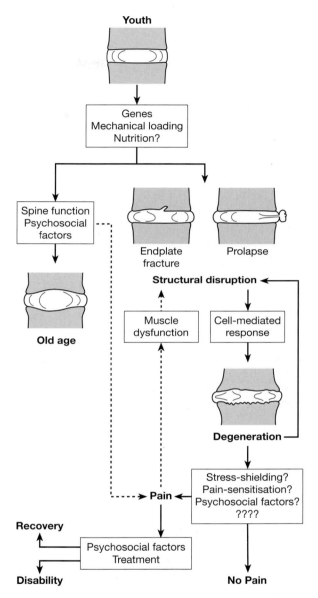

Figure 13.1 Spinal tissues can age biochemically without becoming degenerated or painful (left). However, genetic predisposition, combined with mechanical loading which is excessive for that spine, can disrupt spinal tissues (in this example, an intervertebral disc). Degeneration follows as the tissue's cells respond to their altered mechanical environment in an inappropriate way. This can lead to further tissue weakness and disruption. Degeneration can lead to pain, but this depends on variable factors such as stress-shielding and chemical sensitisation of damaged tissues. The patient's responses to pain and treatment are influenced greatly by psychosocial factors, and pain-induced alterations in muscle function may possibly lead to re-injury.

References

1. Acaroglu E R, Iatridis J C, Setton L A et al. 1995 Degeneration and aging affect the tensile behavior of human lumbar anulus fibrosus. Spine 20: 2690–2701
2. Adams M 1989 'Masonry arch' model of the spine [letter] [see comments]. Spine 14: 1272
3. Adams M A 1980 The mechanical properties of lumbar intervertebral joints with special reference to the causes of low back pain. PhD thesis. Polytechnic of Central London, London, UK
4. Adams M A 1995 Mechanical testing of the spine. An appraisal of methodology, results, and conclusions. Spine 20: 2151–2156
5. Adams M A 1995 Letter to the Editor. Proc Instn Mech Egrs: 135
6. Adams M A, Hutton W C 1980 The effect of posture on the role of the apophysial joints in resisting intervertebral compressive forces. J Bone Joint Surg [Br] 62: 358–362
7. Adams M A, Hutton W C 1981 The relevance of torsion to the mechanical derangement of the lumbar spine. Spine 6: 241–248
8. Adams M A, Hutton W C 1982 Prolapsed intervertebral disc. A hyperflexion injury. Spine 7: 184–191
9. Adams M A, Hutton W C 1983 The effect of posture on the fluid content of lumbar intervertebral discs. Spine 8: 665–671
10. Adams M A, Hutton W C 1983 The mechanical function of the lumbar apophyseal joints. Spine 8: 327–330
11. Adams M A, Hutton W C 1985 Gradual disc prolapse. Spine 10: 524–531
12. Adams M A, Hutton W C 1986 The effect of posture on diffusion into lumbar intervertebral discs. J Anat 147: 121–134
13. Adams M A, Hutton W C 1986 Has the lumbar spine a margin of safety in forward bending? Clin Biomech 1: 3–6
14. Adams M A, Dolan P 1991 A technique for quantifying the bending moment acting on the lumbar spine in vivo. J Biomech 24: 117–126
15. Adams M A, Green T P 1993 Tensile properties of the annulus fibrosus. Part I The contribution of fibre–matrix interactions to tensile stiffness and strength. Eur Spine J 2: 203–208
16. Adams M A, Dolan P 1996 Time-dependent changes in the lumbar spine's resistance to bending. Clin Biomech 11: 194–200
17. Adams M A, Dolan P 1997 Could sudden increases in physical activity cause degeneration of intervertebral discs? Lancet 350: 734–735
18. Adams M A, Hutton W C, Stott J R 1980 The resistance to flexion of the lumbar intervertebral joint. Spine 5: 245–253
19. Adams M A, Dolan P, Hutton W C 1986 The stages of disc degeneration as revealed by discograms. J Bone Joint Surg [Br] 68: 36–41
20. Adams M A, Dolan P, Hutton W C 1987 Diurnal variations in the stresses on the lumbar spine. Spine 12: 130–137
21. Adams M A, Dolan P, Hutton W C 1988 The lumbar spine in backward bending. Spine 13: 1019–1026
22. Adams M A, Green T P, Dolan P 1994 The strength in anterior bending of lumbar intervertebral discs. Spine 19: 2197–2203
23. Adams M A, McNally D S, Dolan P 1996 Stress distributions inside intervertebral discs. The effects of age and degeneration. J Bone Joint Surg Br 78: 965–972
24. Adams M A, Mannion A F, Dolan P 1999 Personal risk factors for first-time low back pain. Spine 24: 2497–2505
25. Adams M A, Dolan P, Marx C et al. 1986 An electronic inclinometer technique for measuring lumbar curvature. Clin Biomech 1: 130–134
26. Adams M A, McNally D S, Wagstaff J et al. 1993 Abnormal stress concentrations in lumbar intervertebral discs following damage to the vertebral body: a cause of disc failure. Eur Spine J 1: 214–221
27. Adams M A, McNally D S, Chinn H et al. 1994 Posture and the compressive strength of the lumbar spine. Clin Biomech 9: 5–14
28. Adams M A, McMillan D W, Green T P et al. 1996 Sustained loading generates stress concentrations in lumbar intervertebral discs. Spine 21: 434–438
29. Adams M A, May S, Freeman B J et al. 2000 Effects of backward bending on lumbar intervertebral discs. Relevance to physical therapy treatments for low back pain. Spine 25: 431–437; discussion 438

30. Adams M A, Freeman B J, Morrison H P et al. 2000 Mechanical initiation of intervertebral disc degeneration. Spine 25: 1625–1636

31. Ahern D K, Follick M J, Council J R et al. 1988 Comparison of lumbar paravertebral EMG patterns in chronic low back pain patients and non-patient controls. Pain 34: 153–160

32. Ahern D K, Hannon D J, Goreczny A J et al. 1990 Correlation of chronic low-back pain behavior and muscle function examination of the flexion-relaxation response. Spine 15: 92–95

33. Ahlgren B D, Vasavada A, Brower R S et al. 1994 Anular incision technique on the strength and multidirectional flexibility of the healing intervertebral disc. Spine 19: 948–954

34. Ahmed A M, Duncan N A, Burke D L 1990 The effect of facet geometry on the axial torque-rotation response of lumbar motion segments. Spine 15: 391–401

35. Aigner T, Gresk-Otter K R, Fairbank J C et al. 1998 Variation with age in the pattern of type X collagen expression in normal and scoliotic human intervertebral discs. Calcif Tissue Int 63: 263–268

36. Akerblom B 1948 Standing and sitting posture. With special reference to the construction of chairs. Nordiska Bokhandeln, Stockholm

37. Alexander R M 1988 Elastic mechanisms in animal movement. Cambridge University Press, Cambridge

38. Alexander R M 1997 Elasticity in human and animal backs. In: Vleeming A, Mooney V, Dorman T et al. (eds) Movement, stability and low back pain. Churchill Livingstone, Edinburgh, p. 227

39. Althoff I, Brinckmann P, Frobin W et al. 1992 An improved method of stature measurement for quantitative determination of spinal loading. Application to sitting postures and whole body vibration. Spine 17: 682–693

40. Anderson C K, Chaffin D B, Herrin G D et al. 1985 A biomechanical model of the lumbosacral joint during lifting activities. J Biomech 18: 571–584

41. Andersson B J, Ortengren R, Nachemson A L et al. 1975 The sitting posture: an electromyographic and discometric study. Orthop Clin North Am 6: 105–120

42. Andersson G, Bogduk N et al. 1989 Muscle: clinical perspectives. In: Frymoyer J W, Gordon S L (eds) New perspectives on low back pain. American Academy of Orthopaedic Surgeons, Park Ridge, Illinois, 293–334

43. Andersson G B 1998 Epidemiology of low back pain. Acta Orthop Scand Suppl 281: 28–31

44. Andersson G B, Schultz A B 1979 Effects of fluid injection on mechanical properties of intervertebral discs. J Biomech 12: 453–458

45. Andersson G B, Ortengren R, Nachemson A 1977 Intradiskal pressure, intra-abdominal pressure and myoelectric back muscle activity related to posture and loading. Clin Orthop: 156–164

46. Andersson G B, Murphy R W, Ortengren R et al. 1979 The influence of backrest inclination and lumbar support on lumbar lordosis. Spine 4: 52–58

47. Andersson G B, Lucente T, Davis A M et al. 1999 A comparison of osteopathic spinal manipulation with standard care for patients with low back pain. N Engl J Med 341: 1426–1431

48. Andersson G B J 1997 The epidemiology of spinal disorders. In: Frymoyer J W (ed) The adult spine: principles and practice. Lippincott-Raven, Philadelphia 93–141

49. Andersson G B J, Deyo R 1997 Sensitivity, specificity and predictive value. In: Frymoyer J W (ed) The adult spine: principles and practice. Lippincott-Raven, 2nd edn, Philadelphia, 308–310

50. Anon 1994 Acute low-back problems in adults. Clinical practice guideline number 14. Agency for Health Care Policy and Research, US Government Printing Office, Washington DC

51. Anon 1997 New Zealand acute low back pain guide. ACC and the National Health Committee, Ministry of Health, Wellington, NZ

52. Anon 1997 Handlungsleitlinie – ruckenschmerzen. Empfehlungen zur therapie von ruckenschmerzen. Artzneimittelkommission der Deutschen Arzteschaft. [Treatment guidelines – backache. Drug committee of the German Medical Society.] Zeitschr Artzliche Fortbild Qualitatssich 91: 457–460

53. Anon 1999 Clinical guidelines for the management of acute low back pain. Royal College of General Practitioners, London

54. Anon 2000 Back pain and neck pain. An evidence based review. The Swedish Council on Technology Assessment in Health Care

55. Aprill C, Bogduk N 1992 High-intensity zone: a diagnostic sign of painful lumbar disc on magnetic resonance imaging. Br J Radiol 65: 361–369

56. Argoubi M, Shirazi-Adl A 1996 Poroelastic creep response analysis of a lumbar motion segment in compression. J Biomech 29: 1331–1339

57. Armstrong R B, Ogilvie R W, Schwane J A 1983 Eccentric exercise-induced injury to rat skeletal muscle. J Appl Physiol 54: 80–93

58. Arokoski J P, Jurvelin J S, Vaatainen U et al. 2000 Normal and pathological adaptations of articular cartilage to joint loading [In Process Citation]. Scand J Med Sci Sports 10: 186–198

59. Aspden R M 1989 The spine as an arch. A new mathematical model [see comments]. Spine 14: 266–274

60. Baker R 2001 Is it time to review the idea of compliance with guidelines (Editorial). Br J Gen Pract 51: 7

61. Baldwin M L, Johnson W G, Butler R J 1996 The error of using returns-to-work to measure the outcomes of health care. Am J Ind Med 29: 632–641

62. Bank R A, Bayliss M T, Lafeber F P et al. 1998 Ageing and zonal variation in post-translational modification of collagen in normal human articular cartilage. The age-related increase in non-enzymatic glycation affects biomechanical properties of cartilage. Biochem J 330: 345–351

63. Bank R A, Soudry M, Maroudas A et al. 2000 The increased swelling and instantaneous deformation of osteoarthritic cartilage is highly correlated with collagen degradation. Arthritis Rheum 43: 2202–2210

64. Barnsley L, Lord S M, Wallis B J et al. 1995 The prevalence of chronic cervical zygapophysial joint pain after whiplash. Spine 20: 20–25; discussion 26

65. Bartelink D L 1957 The role of abdominal pressure in relieving the pressure on the lumbar intervertebral discs. J Bone Joint Surg [Br] 39: 718–725

66. Basmajian J V 1989 Acute back pain and spasm. A controlled multicenter trial of combined analgesic and antispasm agents. Spine 14: 438–439

67. Bass E C, Duncan N A, Hariharan J S et al. 1997 Frozen storage affects the compressive creep behavior of the porcine intervertebral disc. Spine 22: 2867–2876

68. Bassey E J 1995 Exercise in primary prevention of osteoporosis in women. Ann Rheum Dis 54: 861–862

69. Bassey E J, Ramsdale S J 1994 Increase in femoral bone density in young women following high-impact exercise. Osteoporos Int 4: 72–75

70. Battie M C, Bigos S J, Sheehy A et al. 1987 Spinal flexibility and individual factors that influence it. Physical Therapy 67: 653–658

71. Battie M C, Haynor D R, Fisher L D et al. 1995 Similarities in degenerative findings on magnetic resonance images of the lumbar spines of identical twins. J Bone Joint Surg Am 77: 1662–1670

72. Battie M C, Videman T, Gibbons L E et al. 1995 1995 Volvo Award in clinical sciences. Determinants of lumbar disc degeneration. A study relating lifetime exposures and magnetic resonance imaging findings in identical twins. Spine 20: 2601–2612

73. Battie M C, Bigos S J, Fisher L D et al. 1990 The role of spinal flexibility in back pain complaints within industry. A prospective study. Spine 15: 768–773

74. Battie M C, Videman T, Gill K et al. 1991 1991 Volvo Award in clinical sciences. Smoking and lumbar intervertebral disc degeneration: an MRI study of identical twins. Spine 16: 1015–1021

75. Baumgartner W, Grob D, Kramers de Quervain I et al. 2001 Position of instantaneous axis of rotation during standardised movements. Paper presented at the International Society for the Study of the Lumbar Spine. Edinburgh, UK, 2001

76. Bayliss M T, Johnstone B, O'Brien J P 1988 Proteoglycan synthesis in the human intervertebral disc. Variation with age, region and pathology. Spine 13: 972–981

77. Bearn J G 1961 The significance of the activity of the abdominal muscles in weight lifting. Acta Anat 45: 83–89

78. Becker C K, Savelberg H H, Barneveld A 1994 In vitro mechanical properties of the accessory ligament of the deep digital flexor tendon in horses in relation to age. Equine Vet J 26: 454–459

79. Beighton P, Solomon L, Soskolne C L 1973 Articular mobility in an African population. Ann Rheum Dis 32: 413–418

80. Belcastro A N, Shewchuk L D, Raj D A 1998 Exercise-induced muscle injury: a calpain hypothesis. Mol Cell Biochem 179: 135–145

81. Belkoff S M, Mathis J M, Fenton D C et al. 2001 An ex vivo biomechanical evaluation of an inflatable bone tamp used in the treatment of compression fracture. Spine 26: 151–156

82. Bernick S, Walker J M, Paule W J 1991 Age changes to the anulus fibrosus in human intervertebral discs. Spine 16: 520–524

83. Biering-Sorensen F 1984 Physical measurements as risk indicators for low-back trouble over a one-year period. Spine 9: 106–119

84. Bigland B, Lippold O C 1954 The relationship between force, velocity and integrated electrical activity in human muscles. J Physiol 123: 214–220

85. Bigos S J, Battie M C, Fisher L D et al. 1992 A prospective evaluation of preemployment screening methods for acute industrial back pain. Spine 17: 922–926

86. Birch H L, Wilson A M, Goodship A E 1997 The effect of exercise-induced localised hyperthermia on tendon cell survival. J Exp Biol 200: 1703–1708

87. Bishop J B, Szpalski M, Ananthraman S K et al. 1997 Classification of low back pain from dynamic motion characteristics using an artificial neural network. Spine 22: 2991–2998

88. Bishop P B, Pearce R H 1993 The proteoglycans of the cartilaginous end-plate of the human intervertebral disc change after maturity. J Orthop Res 11: 324–331

89. Bleasel J F, Poole A R, Heinegard D et al. 1999 Changes in serum cartilage marker levels indicate altered cartilage metabolism in families with the osteoarthritis-related type II collagen gene COL2A1 mutation. Arthritis Rheum 42: 39–45

90. Boden S D, Davis D O, Dina T S et al. 1990 Abnormal magnetic-resonance scans of the lumbar spine in asymptomatic subjects. A prospective investigation. J Bone Joint Surg [Am] 72: 403–408

91. Boden S D, Riew K D, Yamaguchi K et al. 1996 Orientation of the lumbar facet joints: association with degenerative disc disease. J Bone Joint Surg Am 78: 403–411

92. Bogduk N 1991 The lumbar disc and low back pain. Neurosurg Clin N Am 2: 791–806

93. Bogduk N 1997 Clinical anatomy of the lumbar spine, 3rd edn. Churchill Livingstone, Edinburgh

94. Bogduk N 1998 Point of View on Ito et al. Spine 23: 1259–1260

95. Bogduk N 2000 What's in a name? The labelling of back pain. Med J Aust 173: 400–401

96. Bogduk N 2000 Draft evidence-based clinical guidelines for the management of acute low back pain. National Health and Medical Research Council of Australia

97. Bogduk N, Macintosh J E 1984 The applied anatomy of the thoracolumbar fascia. Spine 9: 164–170

98. Bogduk N, Macintosh J E, Pearcy M J 1992 A universal model of the lumbar back muscles in the upright position. Spine 17: 897–913

99. Bogduk N, Lord, S M 1997 Commentary on: Donelson R, Aprill C, Medcalf R, Grant W. (1997). A prospective study of centralization of lumbar and referred pain. Pain Med Journal Club J 3: 246–248

100. Bongers P M, de Winter C R, Kompier M A et al. 1993 Psychosocial factors at work and musculoskeletal disease. Scand J Work Environ Health 19: 297–312

101. Boos N, Rieder R, Schade V et al. 1995 The diagnostic accuracy of magnetic resonance imaging, work perception, and psychosocial factors in identifying symptomatic disc herniations. Spine 20: 2613–2625

102. Boos N, Semmer N, Elfering A et al. 2000 Natural history of individuals with asymptomatic disc abnormalities in magnetic resonance imaging: predictors of low back pain-related medical consultation and work incapacity. Spine 25: 1484–1492

103. Borkan J, Reis S, Werner S et al. 1996 Guidelines for treating low back pain in primary care. The Israeli

Low Back Pain Guideline Group. Harefuah 130: 145–151; 224

104. Botsford D J, Esses S I, Ogilvie-Harris D J 1994 In vivo diurnal variation in intervertebral disc volume and morphology. Spine 19: 935–940

105. Bovenzi M, Hulshof C T 1999 An updated review of epidemiologic studies on the relationship between exposure to whole-body vibration and low back pain (1986–1997). Int Arch Occup Environ Health 72: 351–365

106. Bradbury N, Wilson L F, Mulholland R C 1996 Adolescent disc protrusions. A long-term follow-up of surgery compared to chymopapain. Spine 21: 372–377

107. Bradford D S, Cooper K M, Oegema T R, Jr. 1983 Chymopapain, chemonucleolysis, and nucleus pulposus regeneration. J Bone Joint Surg [Am] 65: 1220–1231

108. Bressler H B, Keyes W J, Rochon P A et al. 1999 The prevalence of low back pain in the elderly. A systematic review of the literature. Spine 24: 1813–1819

109. Brinckmann P 1986 Injury of the annulus fibrosus and disc protrusions. An in vitro investigation on human lumbar discs. Spine 11: 149–153

110. Brinckmann P, Horst M 1985 The influence of vertebral body fracture, intradiscal injection, and partial discectomy on the radial bulge and height of human lumbar discs. Spine 10: 138–145

111. Brinckmann P, Grootenboer H 1991 Change of disc height, radial disc bulge, and intradiscal pressure from discectomy. An in vitro investigation on human lumbar discs. Spine 16: 641–646

112. Brinckmann P, Porter R W 1994 A laboratory model of lumbar disc protrusion. Fissure and fragment [see comments]. Spine 19: 228–235

113. Brinckmann P, Biggemann M, Hilweg D 1988 Fatigue fracture of human lumbar vertebrae. Clin Biomech 3 (Suppl 1)

114. Brinckmann P, Biggemann M, Hilweg D 1989 Prediction of the compressive strength of human lumbar vertebrae. Spine 14: 606–610

115. Brinckmann P, Biggemann M, Hilweg D 1989 Prediction of the compressive strength of human lumbar vertebrae. Clin Biomech 4 (Suppl 2)

116. Brinckmann P, Frobin W, Hierholzer E et al. 1983 Deformation of the vertebral end-plate under axial loading of the spine. Spine 8: 851–856

117. Brinckmann P, Frobin W, Biggemann M et al. 1998 Quantification of overload injuries to thoracolumbar vertebrae and discs in persons exposed to heavy physical exertions or vibration at the workplace: Part II Occurrence and magnitude of overload injury in exposed cohorts. Clin Biomech 13: S1–S36

118. Brinckmann P, Frobin W, Biggemann M et al. 1998 Quantification of overload injuries to the thoracolumbar spine in persons exposed to heavy physical exertions or vibration at the workplace: Part 2 – Occurrence and magnitude of overload injury in exposed cohorts. Clin Biomech 13: s(2)1–s(2)36

119. Brisby H, Byrod G, Olmarker K et al. 2000 Nitric oxide as a mediator of nucleus pulposus-induced effects on spinal nerve roots. J Orthop Res 18: 815–820

120. Broberg K B 1993 Slow deformation of intervertebral discs. J Biomech 26: 501–512

121. Brock M, Patt S, Mayer H M 1992 The form and structure of the extruded disc. Spine 17: 1457–1461

122. Broom N D, Silyn-Roberts H 1989 The three-dimensional 'knit' of collagen fibrils in articular cartilage. Conn Tissue Res 23: 261–277

123. Broom N D, Silyn-Roberts H 1990 Collagen–collagen versus collagen–proteoglycan interactions in the determination of cartilage strength. Arthritis Rheum 33: 1512–1517

124. Brown M F, Hukkanen M V, McCarthy I D et al. 1997 Sensory and sympathetic innervation of the vertebral endplate in patients with degenerative disc disease. J Bone Joint Surg Br 79: 147–153

125. Buchbinder R, Jolley D, Wyatt M 2001 Population based intervention to change back pain beliefs and disability: three part evaluation. BMJ 322: 1516–1520

126. Buckwalter J A 1995 Aging and degeneration of the human intervertebral disc. Spine 20: 1307–1314

127. Burdorf A, Sorock G 1997 Positive and negative evidence of risk factors for back disorders. Scand J Work Environ Health 23: 243–256

128. Burton A K, Tillotson K M 1988 Reference values for 'normal' regional lumbar sagittal mobility. Clin Biomech 3: 106–113

129. Burton A K, Erg E 1997 Back injury and work loss. Biomechanical and psychosocial influences. Spine 22: 2575–2580

130. Burton A K, Waddell G 1998 Clinical guidelines in the management of low back pain. Bailliere's Clinical Rheumatology 12: 17–35

131. Burton A K, Leivseth G 1998 Manipulative therapy. In: Szpalski M, Gunzburg R, Pope M H (eds) Lumbar segmental instability. Lippincott Williams and Wilkins, Philadelphia, 153–158

132. Burton A K, Main C J 2000 Relevance of biomechanics in occupational musculoskeletal disorders. In: Mayer T G, Gatchel R J, Polatin P B (eds) Occupational musculoskeletal disorders: function, outcomes and evidence. Lipincott-Raven, Philadelphia, 157–166

133. Burton A K, Main C J 2000 Obstacles to recovery from work-related musculoskeletal disorders. In: Karwowski W (ed) International encyclopedia of ergonomics and human factors. Taylor and Francis, London, 1542–1544

134. Burton A K, Tillotson K M, Troup J D 1989 Variation in lumbar sagittal mobility with low-back trouble. Spine 14: 584–590

135. Burton A K, Tillotson K M, Boocock M G 1994 Estimation of spinal loads in overhead work. Ergonomics 37: 1311–1321

136. Burton A K, Tillotson K M, Cleary J 2000 Single-blind randomised controlled trial of chemonucleolysis and manipulation in the treatment of symptomatic lumbar disc herniation. Eur Spine J 9: 202–207

137. Burton A K, Clarke R D, McClune T D et al. 1996 The natural history of low back pain in adolescents. Spine 21: 2323–2328

138. Burton A K, Waddell G, Tillotson K M et al. 1999 Information and advice to patients with back pain can have a positive effect. A randomized controlled

trial of a novel educational booklet in primary care. Spine 24: 2484–2491

139. Burton A K, Tillotson K M, Symonds T L et al. 1996 Occupational risk factors for the first-onset and subsequent course of low back trouble. A study of serving police officers. Spine 21: 2612–2620

140. Burton A K, Tillotson K M, Main C J et al. 2001 Four-year follow-up of patients with low back pain – outcomes and predictors. Spine (submitted)

141. Buseck M, Schipplein O D, Andersson G B et al. 1988 Influence of dynamic factors and external loads on the moment at the lumbar spine in lifting. Spine 13: 918–921

142. Bush-Joseph C, Schipplein O, Andersson G B et al. 1988 Influence of dynamic factors on the lumbar spine moment in lifting. Ergonomics 31: 211–216

143. Butler D, Trafimow J H, Andersson G B et al. 1990 Discs degenerate before facets. Spine 15: 111–113

144. Byrod G, Rydevik B, Nordborg C et al. 1998 Early effects of nucleus pulposus application on spinal nerve root morphology and function. Eur Spine J 7: 445–449

145. Cady L D, Bischoff D P, O'Connell E R et al. 1979 Strength and fitness and subsequent back injuries in firefighters. J Occup Med 21: 269–272

146. Callaghan J P, McGill S M 1995 Frozen storage increases the ultimate compressive load of porcine vertebrae. J Orthop Res 13: 809–812

147. Cannon J G, St Pierre B A 1998 Cytokines in exertion-induced skeletal muscle injury. Mol Cell Biochem 179: 159–167

148. Cannon J G, Meydani S N, Fielding R A et al. 1991 Acute phase response in exercise. II. Associations between vitamin E, cytokines, and muscle proteolysis. Am J Physiol 260: R1235–1240

149. Cao K D, Grimm M J, Yang K H 2001 Load sharing within a human lumbar vertebral body using the finite element method. Spine 26: E253–E260

150. Carey T S, Garrett J M, Jackman A et al. 1999 Recurrence and care seeking after acute back pain: results of a long-term follow-up study. North Carolina Back Pain Project. Med Care 37: 157–164

151. Carosella A M, Lackner J M, Feuerstein M 1994 Factors associated with early discharge from a multidisciplinary work rehabilitation program for chronic low back pain. Pain 57: 69–76

152. Carter J T, Birrell L N 2000 Occupational health guidelines for the management of low back pain at work – principal recommendations. Faculty of Occupational Medicine, London

153. Cassidy J D, Young-Hing K, Kirkaldy-Willis W H et al. 1988 A study of the effects of bipedism and upright posture on the lumbosacral spine and paravertebral muscles of the Wistar rat. Spine 13: 301–308

154. Cassidy J J, Hiltner A, Baer E 1989 Hierarchical structure of the intervertebral disc. Connect Tissue Res 23: 75–88

155. Cassisi J E, Robinson M E, O'Conner P et al. 1993 Trunk strength and lumbar paraspinal muscle activity during isometric exercise in chronic low-back pain patients and controls. Spine 18: 245–251

156. Cavanaugh J M, Ozaktay A C, Yamashita H T et al. 1996 Lumbar facet pain: biomechanics, neuroanatomy and neurophysiology. J Biomech 29: 1117–1129

157. Chaffin D 1969 Computerised biomechanical models – development and use in studying gross body actions. J Biomech 2: 429–441

158. Chatterjee S, Foy P M, Findlay G F 1995 Report of a controlled clinical trial comparing automated percutaneous lumbar discectomy and microdiscectomy in the treatment of contained lumbar disc herniation. Spine 20: 734–738

159. Cheadle A, Franklin G, Wolfhagen C et al. 1994 Factors influencing the duration of work-related disability: a population-based study of Washington State workers' compensation. Am J Public Health 84: 190–196

160. Cherkin D C, Deyo R A, Battie M et al. 1998 A comparison of physical therapy, chiropractic manipulation, and provision of an educational booklet for the treatment of patients with low back pain. N Engl J Med 339: 1021–1029

161. Cholewicki J, McGill S M 1992 Lumbar posterior ligament involvement during extremely heavy lifts estimated from fluoroscopic measurements. J Biomech 25: 17–28

162. Cholewicki J, McGills S M, Norman R W 1995 Comparison of muscle forces and joint load from an optimization and EMG assisted lumbar spine model: towards development of a hybrid approach. J Biomech 28: 321–331

163. Cholewicki J, Crisco J J, 3rd, Oxland T R et al. 1996 Effects of posture and structure on three-dimensional coupled rotations in the lumbar spine. A biomechanical analysis. Spine 21: 2421–2428

164. Chow D H, Luk K D, Leong J C et al. 1989 Torsional stability of the lumbosacral junction. Significance of the iliolumbar ligament. Spine 14: 611–615

165. Clarke J M 1985 The organisation of collagen in cryofractured rabbit articular cartilage: a scanning electron microscopic study. J Orthop Res 3: 17–29

166. Clarkson P M, Kroll W, McBride T C 1980 Maximal isometric strength and fiber type composition in power and endurance athletes. Eur J Appl Physiol Occup Physiol 44: 35–42

167. Coggan D, Rose G, Barker D J P 1997 Epidemiology for the uninitiated. BMJ Publishing Group, London

168. Cohen R E, Hooley C J, McCrum N G 1976 Viscoelastic creep of collagenous tissue. J Biomech 9: 175–184

169. Collee G, Dijkmans B A, Vandenbroucke J P et al. 1991 Iliac crest pain syndrome in low back pain: frequency and features. J Rheumatol 18: 1064–1067

170. Colombini D, Occhipinti E, Grieco A et al. 1989 Estimation of lumbar disc areas by means of anthropometric parameters [published erratum appears in Spine 1989 May; 14(5):533]. Spine 14: 51–55

171. Conley K E, Jubrias S A, Esselman P C 2000 Oxidative capacity and ageing in human muscle. J Physiol 526 Pt 1: 203–210

172. Conley K E, Esselman P C, Jubrias S A et al. 2000 Ageing, muscle properties and maximal O(2) uptake rate in humans. J Physiol 526 Pt 1: 211–217

173. Cooper C, McAlindon T, Coggon D et al. 1994 Occupational activity and osteoarthritis of the knee. Ann Rheum Dis 53: 90–93

174. Coppes M H, Marani E, Thomeer R T et al. 1997 Innervation of 'painful' lumbar discs. Spine 22: 2342–2349; discussion 2349–2350

175. Corlett E N, Eklund J A E, Reilly T et al. 1989 Assessment of workload from measurements of stature. Applied Ergonomics 18: 65–71

176. Cossette J W, Farfan H F, Robertson G H et al. 1971 The instantaneous center of rotation of the third lumbar intervertebral joint. J Biomech 4: 149–153

177. Cox V M, Williams P E, Wright H et al. 2000 Growth induced by incremental static stretch in adult rabbit latissimus dorsi muscle. Exp Physiol 85: 193–202

178. Crock H V 1986 Internal disc disruption. A challenge to disc prolapse fifty years on. Spine 11: 650–653

179. Croft P, Papageorgiou A C, McNally R 1997 Low back pain. In: Stevens A, Rafferty J (eds) Health care needs assessment, 2nd series. Radcliffe Medical Press, Oxford, 129–182

180. Croft P R, Macfarlane G J, Papageorgiou A C et al. 1998 Outcome of low back pain in general practice: a prospective study. BMJ 316: 1356–1359

181. Croft P R, Papageorgiou A C, Thomas E et al. 1999 Short-term physical risk factors for new episodes of low back pain. Prospective evidence from the South Manchester Back Pain Study. Spine 24: 1556–1561

182. Croft P R, Papageorgiou A C, Ferry S et al. 1995 Psychologic distress and low back pain. Evidence from a prospective study in the general population. Spine 20: 2731–2737

183. Curtis P, Carey T S, Evans P et al. 2000 Training primary care physicians to give limited manual therapy for low back pain: patient outcomes. Spine 25: 2954–2961

184. Cyron B M, Hutton W C 1978 The fatigue strength of the lumbar neural arch in spondylolysis. J Bone Joint Surg [Br] 60-B: 234–238

185. Cyron B M, Hutton W C 1979 Variations in the amount and distribution of cortical bone across the partes interarticulares of L5. A predisposing factor in spondylolysis? Spine 4: 163–167

186. Cyron B M, Hutton W C 1980 Articular tropism and stability of the lumbar spine. Spine 5: 168–172

187. Cyron B M, Hutton W C 1981 The behaviour of the lumbar intervertebral disc under repetitive forces. Int Orthop 5: 203–207

188. Cyron B M, Hutton W C 1981 The tensile strength of the capsular ligaments of the apophyseal joints. J Anat 132: 145–150

189. Cyron B M, Hutton W C, Troup J D 1976 Spondylolytic fractures. J Bone Joint Surg [Br] 58-B: 462–466

190. Daltroy L H, Iversen M D, Larson M G et al. 1997 A controlled trial of an educational program to prevent low back injuries. N Engl J Med 337: 322–328

191. Davis K G, Heaney C A 2000 The relationship between psychosocial work characteristics and low back pain: underlying methodological issues. Clin Biomech 15: 389–406

192. Davis P R, Troup J D G, Burnard J H 1965 Movements of the thoracic and lumbar spine when lifting: a chrono-cyclophotographic study. J Anat 99: 13–26

193. Day R, Puustjarvi K, Adams M A 1999 Can physical exercise strengthen intervertebral discs? Proceedings of the Society for Back Pain Research. Cardiff, UK

194. DePukey P 1935 The physiological oscillation of the length of the body. Acta Orthop Scand 6: 338

195. DeGroot J, Verzijl N, Bank R A et al. 1999 Age-related decrease in proteoglycan synthesis of human articular chondrocytes: the role of nonenzymatic glycation. Arthritis Rheum 42: 1003–1009

196. DeGroot J, Verzijl N, Wenting-van Wijk M et al. 2001 Nonenzymatic glycation increases the severity of osteoarthritis in the canine ACLT model: a biochemical basis for age as a risk factor of OA. Proceedings of the Orthopaedic Research Society. San Francisco, USA

197. Denis F 1983 The three column spine and its significance in the classification of acute thoracolumbar spinal injuries. Spine 8: 817–831

198. Devereux J J, Buckle P W, Vlachonikolis I G 1999 Interactions between physical and psychosocial risk factors at work increase the risk of back disorders: an epidemiological approach. Occup Environ Med 56: 343–353

199. Devor S T, Faulkner J A 1999 Regeneration of new fibers in muscles of old rats reduces contraction-induced injury. J Appl Physiol 87: 750–756

200. Deyo R A 1993 Practice variations, treatment fads, rising disability. Do we need a new clinical research paradigm? Spine 18: 2153–2162

201. Deyo R A, Diehl A K 1988 Cancer as a cause of back pain: frequency, clinical presentation, and diagnostic strategies. J Gen Intern Med 3: 230–238

202. Deyo R A, Rainville J, Kent D L 1992 What can the history and physical examination tell us about low back pain? JAMA 268: 760–765

203. Dhillon N, Bass E C, Lotz J C 2001 Effect of frozen storage on the creep behavior of human intervertebral discs. Spine 26: 883–888

204. van Dieen J H, Toussaint H M 1993 Spinal shrinkage as a parameter of functional load. Spine 18: 1504–1514

205. van Dieen J H, Creemers M, Draisma I et al. 1994 Repetitive lifting and spinal shrinkage, effects of age and lifting technique. Clin Biomech 9: 367–374

206. van Dieen J H, van der Burg P, Raaijmakers T A J et al. 1998 Effects of repetitive lifting on kinematics: inadequate anticipatory control or adaptive changes? J Motor Behaviour 30: 20–32

207. Dionne C E 1999 Low back pain. In: Crombie I K (ed) Epidemiology of pain. IASP Press, Seattle 283–297

208. Dishman R K, Oldenburg B, O'Neal H et al. 1998 Worksite physical activity interventions. Am J Prev Med 15: 344–361

209. Dolan P, Adams M A 1993 The relationship between EMG activity and extensor moment generation in the erector spinae muscles during bending and lifting activities. J Biomech 26: 513–522

210. Dolan P, Adams M A 1993 Influence of lumbar and hip mobility on the bending stresses acting on the lumbar spine. Clin Biomech 8: 185–192

211. Dolan P, Adams M A 1998 Repetitive lifting tasks fatigue the back muscles and increase the bending moment acting on the lumbar spine. J Biomech 31: 713–721

212. Dolan P, Adams M A 2001 Recent advances in lumbar spinal mechanics and their significance for modelling. Clin Biomech 16: S8–S16

213. Dolan P, Adams M A, Hutton W C 1987 The short-term effects of chymopapain on intervertebral discs. J Bone Joint Surg [Br] 69: 422–428

214. Dolan P, Adams M A, Hutton W C 1988 Commonly adopted postures and their effect on the lumbar spine. Spine 13: 197–201

215. Dolan P, Adams M A 2001 Recent advances in lumbar spinal mechanics and their significance for modelling. Clin Biomech 16 (Suppl. 1): S8–S16

216. Dolan P, Mannion A F, Adams M A 1994 Passive tissues help the back muscles to generate extensor moments during lifting. J Biomech 27: 1077–1085

217. Dolan P, Earley M, Adams M A 1994 Bending and compressive stresses acting on the lumbar spine during lifting activities. J Biomech 27: 1237–1248

218. Dolan P, Mannion A F, Adams M A 1995 'Schober test' measurements do not correlate well with angular movements of the lumbar spine. Proceedings of the International Society for the Study of the Lumbar Spine, Helsinki, Finland

219. Dolan P, Greenfield K, Nelson R J et al. 2000 Can exercise therapy improve the outcome of microdiscectomy? Spine 25: 1523–1532

220. Dolan P, Kingma I, van Dieen J et al. 1999 Dynamic forces acting on the lumbar spine during manual handling. Can they be estimated using electromyographic techniques alone? Spine 24: 698–703

221. Dolan P, Kingma I, De Looze M P et al. 2001 An EMG technique for measuring spinal loading during asymmetric lifting. Clin Biomech 16: S17–S24

222. Donceel P, Du Bois M 1998 Fitness for work after surgery for lumbar disc herniation: a retrospective study. Eur Spine J 7: 29–35

223. Donelson R, Aprill C, Medcalf R et al. 1997 A prospective study of centralization of lumbar and referred pain. A predictor of symptomatic discs and anular competence. Spine 22: 1115–1122

224. Dreyfuss P, Michaelsen M, Pauza K et al. 1996 The value of medical history and physical examination in diagnosing sacroiliac joint pain [see comments]. Spine 21: 2594–2602

225. Duance V C, Crean J K, Sims T J et al. 1998 Changes in collagen cross-linking in degenerative disc disease and scoliosis. Spine 23: 2545–2551

226. Dumas G A, Beaudoin L, Drouin G 1987 In situ mechanical behavior of posterior spinal ligaments in the lumbar region. An in vitro study. J Biomech 20: 301–310

227. Dumas G A, Reid J G, Wolfe L A et al. 1995 Exercise, posture, and back pain during pregnancy. Clin Biomech 10: 104–109

228. Duncan N A, Ahmed A M 1991 The role of axial rotation in the etiology of unilateral disc prolapse. An experimental and finite-element analysis. Spine 16: 1089–1098

229. Dunlop R B, Adams M A, Hutton W C 1984 Disc space narrowing and the lumbar facet joints. J Bone Joint Surg [Br] 66: 706–710

230. Dvorak J, Vajda E G, Grob D et al. 1995 Normal motion of the lumbar spine as related to age and gender. Eur Spine J 4: 18–23

231. Dvorak J, Panjabi M M, Chang D G et al. 1991 Functional radiographic diagnosis of the lumbar spine. Flexion–extension and lateral bending. Spine 16: 562–571

232. Eastell R, Cedel S L, Wahner H W et al. 1991 Classification of vertebral fractures. J Bone Miner Res 6: 207–215

233. Ebara S, Iatridis J C, Setton L A et al. 1996 Tensile properties of nondegenerate human lumbar anulus fibrosus. Spine 21: 452–461

234. Egund N, Olsson T H, Schmid H et al. 1978 Movements in the sacroiliac joints demonstrated with roentgen stereophotogrammetry. Acta Radiol [Diagn] 19: 833–846

235. Eie N 1966 Load capacity of the low back. J Oslo City Hosp 16: 73–98

236. Eie N 1973 Recent measurements of the intra-abdominal pressure. In: Kenedi R M (ed) Perspectives in biomedical engineering. Macmillan Press, London, p. 121

237. Eisenstein S 1978 Spondylolysis. A skeletal investigation of two population groups. J Bone Joint Surg [Br] 60-B: 488–494

238. El Mahdi M A, Latif F Y A, Janko M 1981 The spinal nerve root innervation, and a new concept of the clinicopathological interrelations in back pain and sciatica. Neurochirurgia 24: 137–141

239. Ensink F B, Saur P M, Frese K et al. 1996 Lumbar range of motion: influence of time of day and individual factors on measurements. Spine 21: 1339–1343

240. Esola M A, McClure P W, Fitzgerald G K et al. 1996 Analysis of lumbar spine and hip motion during forward bending in subjects with and without a history of low back pain. Spine 21: 71–78

241. Eyre D R, Muir H 1977 Quantitative analysis of types I and II collagens in human intervertebral discs at various ages. Biochim Biophys Acta 492: 29–42

242. Faas A, Chavannes A W, Koes B W et al. 1996 NHG-standaard lage-rugpijn. Huisarts Wet 39: 18–31

243. Fahrni W H 1975 Conservative treatment of lumbar disc degeneration: our primary responsibility. Orthop Clin North Am 6: 93–103

244. Fahrni W H, Trueman G E 1965 Comparative radiological study of the spines of a primitive population with North Americans and North Europeans. J Bone Joint Surg [Br] 47: 552–555

245. Farfan H F, Sullivan J D 1967 The relation of facet orientation to intervertebral disc failure. Can J Surg 10: 179–185

246. Farfan H F, Huberdeau R M, Dubow H I 1972 Lumbar intervertebral disc degeneration: the influence of geometrical features on the pattern of disc degeneration – a post mortem study. J Bone Joint Surg [Am] 54: 492–510

247. Farfan H F, Cossette J W, Robertson G H et al. 1970 The effects of torsion on the lumbar intervertebral joints: the role of torsion in the production of disc degeneration. J Bone Joint Surg [Am] 52: 468–497

248. Fathallah F A, Marras W S, Parnianpour M 1998 The role of complex, simultaneous trunk motions in the risk of occupation-related low back disorders. Spine 23: 1035–1042

249. Fathallah F A, Marras W S, Parnianpour M 1998 An assessment of complex spinal loads during dynamic lifting tasks. Spine 23: 706–716

250. Feinstein B, Langton J N K, Jameson R M, Schiller F 1954 Experiments on pain referred from deep somatic tissues. J Bone Joint Surg 35 A: 981–987

251. Ferguson S A, Marras W S 1997 A literature review of low back disorder surveillance measures and risk factors. Clin Biomech 12: 211–226

252. Ferguson S A, Marras W S, Waters T R 1992 Quantification of back motion during asymmetric lifting. Ergonomics 35: 845–859

253. Findlay G F, Hall B I, Musa B S et al. 1998 A 10-year follow-up of the outcome of lumbar microdiscectomy. Spine 23: 1168–1171

254. Fishbain D A, Cutler R B, Rosomoff H L et al. 1997 Impact of chronic pain patients' job perception variables on actual return to work. Clin J Pain 13: 197–206

255. Floyd W F, Silver P H S 1955 The function of the erectores spinae muscles in certain movements and postures in man. J Physiol 129: 184–203

256. Fordyce W E 1995 Back pain in the workplace: management of disability in non-specific conditions. IASP Press, Seattle

257. Foreman T K, Troup J D G 1987 Diurnal variations in spinal loading and the effects on stature: a preliminary study of nursing activities. Clin Biomech 2: 48–54

258. Fortin J D, Dwyer A P, West S et al. 1994 Sacroiliac joint: pain referral maps upon applying a new injection/arthrography technique. Part I: Asymptomatic volunteers. Spine 19: 1475–1482

259. Frank J W, Kerr M S, Brooker A S et al. 1996 Disability resulting from occupational low back pain. Part I: What do we know about primary prevention? A review of the scientific evidence on prevention before disability begins. Spine 21: 2908–2917

260. Frankel B S, Moffett J K, Keen S et al. 1999 Guidelines for low back pain: changes in GP management. Fam Pract 16: 216–222

261. Fredrickson B E, Edwards W T, Rauschning W et al. 1992 Vertebral burst fractures: an experimental, morphologic, and radiographic study. Spine 17: 1012–1021

262. Friden J, Sjostrom M, Ekblom B 1983 Myofibrillar damage following intense eccentric exercise in man. Int J Sports Med 4: 170–176

263. Fritzell P, Hagg O, Wessberg P et al. 2001 Lumbar fusion for chronic low back pain. A multicentre RCT comparing fusion with non-surgical treatment. A report from the Swedish Lumbar Spine Study. Proceedings of the International Society for the Study of the Lumbar Spine, Edinburgh, UK

264. Fritzell P, Hagg O, Wessberg P et al. 2001 Chronic low back pain and fusion – a comparison of three surgical techniques. A report from the Swedish Lumbar Spine Study Group. Proceedings of the International Society for the Study of the Lumbar Spine, Edinburgh, UK

265. Frobin W, Brinckmann P, Biggemann M et al. 1997 Precision measurement of disc height, vertebral height and sagittal plane displacement from lateral radiographic views of the lumbar spine. Clin Biomech 12: S1–S64

266. Frost H, Klaber Moffett J A, Moser J S et al. 1995 Randomised controlled trial for evaluation of fitness programme for patients with chronic low back pain [see comments]. BMJ 310: 151–154

267. Frost H M 1987 Bone 'mass' and the 'mechanostat': a proposal. Anat Rec 219: 1–9

268. Fujita Y, Duncan N A, Lotz J C 1997 Radial tensile properties of the lumbar annulus fibrosus are site and degeneration dependent. J Orthop Res 15: 814–819

269. Fujiwara A, Tamai K, An H S et al. 2000 The interspinous ligament of the lumbar spine. Magnetic resonance images and their clinical significance. Spine 25: 358–363

270. Fukui S, Ohseto K, Shiotani M et al. 1997 Distribution of referred pain from the lumbar zygapophyseal joints and dorsal rami. Clin J Pain 13: 303–307

271. Furlan A D, Clarke J, Esmail R et al. 2001 A critical review of reviews on the treatment of chronic low back pain. Spine 26: E155–E162

272. Gagnon D, Gagnon M 1992 The influence of dynamic factors on triaxial net muscular moments at the L5/S1 joint during asymmetrical lifting and lowering. J Biomech 25: 891–901

273. Galante J O 1967 Tensile properties of the human lumbar annulus fibrosus. Acta Orthop Scand Suppl: 1–91

274. Gallagher D, Ruts E, Visser M et al. 2000 Weight stability masks sarcopenia in elderly men and women. Am J Physiol Endocrinol Metab 279: E366–E375

275. Gardner-Morse M G, Stokes I A 1998 The effects of abdominal muscle coactivation on lumbar spine stability. Spine 23: 86–91; discussion 91–82

276. Garg A, Moore J S 1992 Epidemiology of low-back pain in industry. Occup Med 7: 593–608

277. Garg A, Moore J S 1992 Prevention strategies and the low back in industry. Occup Med 7: 629–640

278. Garrett W E, Jr., Seaber A V, Boswick J et al. 1984 Recovery of skeletal muscle after laceration and repair. J Hand Surg [Am] 9: 683–692

279. Gatton M L, Pearcy M J 1999 Kinematics and movement sequencing during flexion of the lumbar spine. Clin Biomech 14: 376–383

280. Gebhardt W A 1994 Effectiveness of training to prevent job-related back pain: a meta-analysis. Br J Clin Psychol 33: 571–574

281. Gedalia U, Solomonow M, Zhou B H et al. 1999 Biomechanics of increased exposure to lumbar injury caused by cyclic loading. Part 2. Recovery of reflexive muscular stability with rest. Spine 24: 2461–2467

282. Gelb D E, Lenke L G, Bridwell K H et al. 1995 An analysis of sagittal spinal alignment in 100 asymptomatic middle and older aged volunteers. Spine 20: 1351–1358

283. Gertzbein S D, Seligman J, Holtby R et al. 1985 Centrode patterns and segmental instability in degenerative disc disease. Spine 10: 257–261

284. Gibala M J, MacDougall J D, Tarnopolsky M A et al. 1995 Changes in human skeletal muscle ultrastructure and force production after acute resistance exercise. J Appl Physiol 78: 702–708

285. Gibson J N, Smith K, Rennie M J 1988 Prevention of disuse muscle atrophy by means of electrical stimulation: maintenance of protein synthesis. Lancet 2: 767–770

286. Gibson J N, Grant I C, Waddell G 1999 The Cochrane review of surgery for lumbar disc prolapse and degenerative lumbar spondylosis. Spine 24: 1820–1832

287. Gibson J N, Halliday D, Morrison W L et al. 1987 Decrease in human quadriceps muscle protein turnover consequent upon leg immobilization. Clin Sci (Colch) 72: 503–509

288. Gill K, Videman T, Shimizu T et al. 1987 The effect of repeated extensions on the discographic dye patterns in cadaveric lumbar motion segments. Clin Biomech 2: 205–210

289. Giori N J, Beaupre G S, Carter D R 1993 Cellular shape and pressure may mediate mechanical control of tissue composition in tendons. J Orthop Res 11: 581–591

290. Goel V K, Gilbertson L G 1995 Applications of the finite element method to thoracolumbar spinal research – past, present, and future. Spine 20: 1719–1727

291. Goel V K, Monroe B T, Gilbertson L G et al. 1995 Interlaminar shear stresses and laminae separation in a disc. Finite element analysis of the L3–L4 motion segment subjected to axial compressive loads. Spine 20: 689–698

292. Goel V K, Kong W, Han J S et al. 1993 A combined finite element and optimization investigation of lumbar spine mechanics with and without muscles. Spine 18: 1531–1541

293. Goldspink G 1992 Cellular and molecular aspects of adaptation in skeletal muscle. In: Komi P V (ed) The encyclopaedia of sports medicine III: strength and power in sport. Blackwell Science, Oxford, 211–229

294. Goldspink G, Waterson S E 1971 The effect of growth and inanition on the total amount of nitroblue tetrazolium deposited in individual muscle fibres of fast and slow rat skeletal muscle. Acta Histochem 40: 16–22

295. Goldspink G, Ward P S 1979 Changes in rodent muscle fibre types during post-natal growth, undernutrition and exercise. J Physiol 296: 453–469

296. Goldspink G, Williams P E 1979 The nature of the increased passive resistance in muscle following immobilization of the mouse soleus muscle [proceedings]. J Physiol 289: 55P

297. Goodship A E, Lanyon L E, McFie H 1979 Functional adaptation of bone to increased stress. An experimental study. J Bone Joint Surg [Am] 61: 539–546

298. Goodship A E, Birch H L, Wilson A M 1994 The pathobiology and repair of tendon and ligament injury. Vet Clin North Am Equine Pract 10: 323–349

299. Gordon S J, Yang K H, Mayer P J et al. 1991 Mechanism of disc rupture. A preliminary report. Spine 16: 450–456

300. Gracovetsky S, Farfan H 1986 The optimum spine. Spine 11: 543–573

301. Gracovetsky S, Farfan H F, Lamy C 1977 A mathematical model of the lumbar spine using an optimized system to control muscles and ligaments. Orthop Clin North Am 8: 135–153

302. Gracovetsky S, Farfan H F, Lamy C 1981 The mechanism of the lumbar spine. Spine 6: 249–262

303. Gracovetsky S, Farfan H, Helleur C 1985 The abdominal mechanism. Spine 10: 317–324

304. Granata K P, Marras W S 1993 An EMG-assisted model of loads on the lumbar spine during asymmetric trunk extensions. J Biomech 26: 1429–1438

305. Granata K P, Marras W S 1995 The influence of trunk muscle coactivity on dynamic spinal loads. Spine 20: 913–919

306. Granata K P, Marras W S 2000 Cost-benefit of muscle cocontraction in protecting against spinal instability. Spine 25: 1398–1404

307. Granata K P, Marras W S, Davis K G 1997 Biomechanical assessment of lifting dynamics, muscle activity and spinal loads while using three different styles of lifting belt. Clin Biomech 12: 107–115

308. Granata K P, Marras W S, Davis K G 1999 Variation in spinal load and trunk dynamics during repeated lifting exertions. Clin Biomech 14: 367–375

309. Granhed H, Jonson R, Hansson T 1987 The loads on the lumbar spine during extreme weight lifting. Spine 12: 146–149

310. Granhed H, Jonson R, Hansson T 1989 Mineral content and strength of lumbar vertebrae. A cadaver study. Acta Orthop Scand 60: 105–109

311. Green H J, Thomson J A, Daub W D et al. 1979 Fiber composition, fiber size and enzyme activities in vastus lateralis of elite athletes involved in high intensity exercise. Eur J Appl Physiol Occup Physiol 41: 109–117

312. Green T P, Adams M A, Dolan P 1993 Tensile properties of the annulus fibrosus. Part II Ultimate tensile strength and fatigue life. Eur Spine J 2: 209–214

313. Green T P, Allvey J C, Adams M A 1994 Spondylolysis. Bending of the inferior articular processes of lumbar vertebrae during simulated spinal movements. Spine 19: 2683–2691

314. Gregersen G G, Lucas D B 1967 An in vivo study of the axial rotation of the human thoracolumbar spine. J Bone Joint Surg [Am] 49: 247–262

315. Grimby G, Saltin B 1983 The ageing muscle. Clin Physiol 3: 209–218

316. Groen G J, Baljet B, Drukker J 1990 Nerves and nerve plexuses of the human vertebral column. Am J Anat 188: 282–296

317. Guilak F 1995 Compression-induced changes in the shape and volume of the chondrocyte nucleus. J Biomech 28: 1529–1541

318. Guilak F, Ting-Beall H P, Baer A E et al. 1999 Viscoelastic properties of intervertebral disc cells. Identification of two biomechanically distinct cell populations. Spine 24: 2475–2483

319. Gundewall B, Liljeqvist M, Hansson T 1993 Primary prevention of back symptoms and absence from work. A prospective randomized study among hospital employees. Spine 18: 587–594

320. Gunzburg R, Hutton W, Fraser R 1991 Axial rotation of the lumbar spine and the effect of flexion. An in vitro and in vivo biomechanical study. Spine 16: 22–28

321. Gunzburg R, Parkinson R, Moore R et al. 1992 A cadaveric study comparing discography, magnetic resonance imaging, histology, and mechanical behavior of the human lumbar disc. Spine 17: 417–426

322. Gupta A 2001 Analyses of myo-electrical silence of erectors spinae. J Biomech 34: 491–496

323. Hadler N M 1997 Back pain in the workplace. What you lift or how you lift matters far less than whether you lift or when. Spine 22: 935–940

324. Hadler N M 1999 Backache: predicament at home, nemesis at work. In: Hadler N M (ed) Occupational musculoskeletal disorders, 2nd edn. Lippincott, Williams and Wilkins, Philadelphia, 7–17

325. Haldorsen E M, Indahl A, Ursin H 1998 Patients with low back pain not returning to work. A 12-month follow-up study. Spine 23: 1202–1207; discussion 1208

326. Hall A C, Urban J P, Gehl K A 1991 The effects of hydrostatic pressure on matrix synthesis in articular cartilage. J Orthop Res 9: 1–10

327. Hamanishi C, Kawabata T, Yosii T et al. 1994 Schmorl's nodes on magnetic resonance imaging. Their incidence and clinical relevance. Spine 19: 450–453

328. Hampton D, Laros G, McCarron R et al. 1989 Healing potential of the anulus fibrosus. Spine 14: 398–401

329. Handa T, Ishihara H, Ohshima H et al. 1997 Effects of hydrostatic pressure on matrix synthesis and matrix metalloproteinase production in the human lumbar intervertebral disc. Spine 22: 1085–1091

330. Hansen F R, Bendix T, Skov P et al. 1993 Intensive, dynamic back-muscle exercises, conventional physiotherapy, or placebo-control treatment of low-back pain. A randomized, observer-blind trial. Spine 18: 98–108

331. Hansson T, Roos B 1983 The amount of bone mineral and Schmorl's nodes in lumbar vertebrae. Spine 8: 266–271

332. Hansson T, Roos B, Nachemson A 1980 The bone mineral content and ultimate compressive strength of lumbar vertebrae. Spine 5: 46–55

333. Hansson T H, Hansson E K 2000 The effects of common medical interventions on pain, back function, and work resumption in patients with chronic low back pain: A prospective 2-year cohort study in six countries. Spine 25: 3055–3064

334. Hansson T H, Keller T S, Spengler D M 1987 Mechanical behavior of the human lumbar spine. II. Fatigue strength during dynamic compressive loading [published erratum appears in J Orthop Res 1988; 6(3): 465]. J Orthop Res 5: 479–487

335. Harada Y, Nakahara S 1989 A pathologic study of lumbar disc herniation in the elderly. Spine 14: 1020–1024

336. Hardcastle P, Annear P, Foster D H et al. 1992 Spinal abnormalities in young fast bowlers. J Bone Joint Surg [Br] 74: 421–425

337. Harreby M, Neergaard K, Hesselsoe G et al. 1995 Are radiologic changes in the thoracic and lumbar spine of adolescents risk factors for low back pain in adults? A 25-year prospective cohort study of 640 school children. Spine 20: 2298–2302

338. Hartigan C, Miller L, Liewehr S C 1996 Rehabilitation of acute and subacute low back and neck pain in the work-injured patient. Orthop Clin North Am 27: 841–860

339. Hartvigsen J, Leboeuf-Yde C, Lings S et al. 2000 Is sitting-while-at-work associated with low back pain? A systematic, critical literature review. Scand J Public Health 28: 230–239

340. Hasberry S, Pearcy M J 1986 Temperature dependence of the tensile properties of interspinous ligaments of sheep. J Biomed Eng 8: 62–66

341. Hazard R G, Reid S, Haugh L D et al. 2000 A controlled trial of an educational pamphlet to prevent disability after occupational low back injury. Spine 25: 1419–1423

342. Hazard R G, Haugh L D, Reid S et al. 1997 Early physician notification of patient disability risk and clinical guidelines after low back injury: a randomized, controlled trial. Spine 22: 2951–2958

343. Hedtmann A, Steffen R, Methfessel J et al. 1989 Measurement of human lumbar spine ligaments during loaded and unloaded motion. Spine 14: 175–185

344. Heliovaara M 1987 Body height, obesity, and risk of herniated lumbar intervertebral disc. Spine 12: 469–472

345. Hemingway H, Shipley M J, Stansfeld S et al. 1997 Sickness absence from back pain, psychosocial work characteristics and employment grade among office workers. Scand J Work Environ Health 23: 121–129

346. Herring S W, Grimm A F, Grimm B R 1984 Regulation of sarcomere number in skeletal muscle: a comparison of hypotheses. Muscle Nerve 7: 161–173

347. Heylings D J 1978 Supraspinous and interspinous ligaments of the human lumbar spine. J Anat 125: 127–131

348. Hides J A, Stokes M J, Saide M et al. 1994 Evidence of lumbar multifidus muscle wasting ipsilateral to symptoms in patients with acute/subacute low back pain. Spine 19: 165–172

349. Hilton R C, Ball J 1984 Vertebral rim lesions in the dorsolumbar spine. Ann Rheum Dis 43: 302–307

350. Hilton R C, Ball J, Benn R T 1976 Vertebral end-plate lesions (Schmorl's nodes) in the dorsolumbar spine. Ann Rheum Dis 35: 127–132

351. Hilton R C, Ball J, Benn R T 1979 In-vitro mobility of the lumbar spine. Ann Rheum Dis 38: 378–383

352. Hindle R J, Pearcy M J, Cross A 1990 Mechanical function of the human lumbar interspinous and supraspinous ligaments. J Biomed Eng 12: 340–344

353. Hindle R J, Pearcy M J, Cross A T et al. 1990 Three-dimensional kinematics of the human back. Clin Biomech 5: 218–228

354. Hirabayashi S, Kumano K, Ogawa Y et al. 1993 Microdiscectomy and second operation for lumbar disc herniation. Spine 18: 2206–2211

355. Hirsch C, Schajowicz F 1953 Studies on structural changes in the lumbar annulus fibrosus. Acta Orthop Scand 22: 184–231

356. Hirsch C, Nachemson A 1961 Clinical observations on the spine in ejected pilots. Acta Orthop Scand 31: 135–145

357. Hirsch C, Inglemark B, Miller M 1963 The anatomical basis for low back pain. Acta Orthop Scand 33: 1–17

358. Hodgson D R, Rose R J 1994 The athletic horse. W.B. Saunders, Philadelphia

359. Holdsworth F W 1963 Fractures, dislocations and fracture-dislocations of the spine. J Bone Joint Surg [Br] 45: 6–20

360. Holm S, Nachemson A 1982 Nutritional changes in the canine intervertebral disc after spinal fusion. Clin Orthop: 243–258

361. Holmes A D, Hukins D W, Freemont A J 1993 End-plate displacement during compression of lumbar vertebra–disc vertebra segments and the mechanisms of failure. Spine 18: 128–135

362. Honeyman P T, Jacobs E A 1996 Effects of culture on back pain in Australian aboriginals. Spine 21: 841–843

363. Hoppeler H, Lindstedt S L 1985 Malleability of skeletal muscle in overcoming limitations: structural elements. J Exp Biol 115: 355–364

364. Horner H, Urban J P G 2001 The effect of nutrient supply on viability of cells from the nucleus pulposus of the intervertebral disc. Proceedings of the International Society for the Study of the Lumbar Spine, Edinburgh, UK

365. Hukins D W, Aspden R M, Yarker Y E 1984 Fibre reinforcement and mechanical stability in articular cartilage. Eng Med 13: 153–156

366. Hukins D W, Kirby M C, Sikoryn T A et al. 1990 Comparison of structure, mechanical properties, and functions of lumbar spinal ligaments. Spine 15: 787–795

367. Hukins D W L 1988 Disc structure and function. In: Ghosh P (ed) The biology of the intervertebral disc. CRC Press, Boca Raton, Florida, 24–27

368. Hukins D W L, Aspden R M 1985 Composition and properties of connective tissue. TIBS 10: 260–264

369. Hunt A, Habeck R 1993. The Michigan disability prevention study. W.E. Upjohn Institute for Employment Research, Kalamazoo, Michigan

370. Hunter S K, Thompson M W, Adams R D 2000 Relationships among age-associated strength changes and physical activity level, limb dominance, and muscle group in women. J Gerontol A Biol Sci Med Sci 55: B264–273

371. Hutton W C, Adams M A 1982 Can the lumbar spine be crushed in heavy lifting? Spine 7: 586–590

372. Hutton W C, Stott J R R, Cyron B M 1977 Is spondylolysis a fatigue fracture? Spine 2: 202–209

373. Hutton W C, Cyron B M, Stott J R 1979 The compressive strength of lumbar vertebrae. J Anat 129: 753–758

374. Hutton W C, Toribatake Y, Elmer W A et al. 1998 The effect of compressive force applied to the intervertebral disc in vivo. A study of proteoglycans and collagen. Spine 23: 2524–2537

375. Huxley A F 1957 Muscle structure and theories of contraction. Progr Biophys 7: 255–318

376. Huxley H E 1965 The mechanism of muscular contraction. Sci Am 213: 18–27

377. Iatridis J C, Weidenbaum M, Setton L A et al. 1996 Is the nucleus pulposus a solid or a fluid? Mechanical behaviors of the nucleus pulposus of the human intervertebral disc. Spine 21: 1174–1184

378. Iatridis J C, Mente P L, Stokes I A et al. 1999 Compression-induced changes in intervertebral disc properties in a rat tail model. Spine 24: 996–1002

379. Igarashi T, Kikuchi S, Shubayev V et al. 2000 Exogenous tumor necrosis factor-alpha mimics nucleus pulposus-induced neuropathology. Molecular,

380. Infante-Rivarde C, Lortie M 1997 Relapse and short sickness absence for back pain in the six months after returning to work. Occup Environ Med 54: 328–334

381. Inufusa A, An H S, Lim T H et al. 1996 Anatomic changes of the spinal canal and intervertebral foramen associated with flexion-extension movement. Spine 21: 2412–2420

382. Ishihara H, McNally D S, Urban J P et al. 1996 Effects of hydrostatic pressure on matrix synthesis in different regions of the intervertebral disk. J Appl Physiol 80: 839–846

383. Ito M, Incorvaia K M, Yu S F et al. 1998 Predictive signs of discogenic lumbar pain on magnetic resonance imaging with discography correlation. Spine 23: 1252–1258; discussion 1259–1260

384. Jackson D W, Wiltse L L, Cirincoine R J 1976 Spondylolysis in the female gymnast. Clin Orthop: 68–73

385. Jackson R P, McManus A C 1994 Radiographic analysis of sagittal plane alignment and balance in standing volunteers and patients with low back pain matched for age, sex, and size. A prospective controlled clinical study. Spine 19: 1611–1618

386. Janevic J, Ashton-Miller J A, Schultz A B 1991 Large compressive preloads decrease lumbar motion segment flexibility. J Orthop Res 9: 228–236

387. Jarvik J G, Deyo R A 2000 Imaging of lumbar intervertebral disk degeneration and aging, excluding disk herniations. Radiol Clin North Am 38: 1255–1266, vi

388. Jeffery A K, Blunn G W, Archer C W et al. 1991 Three-dimensional collagen architecture in bovine articular cartilage. J Bone Joint Surg [Br] 73: 795–801

389. Jensen M C, Brant-Zawadzki M N, Obuchowski N et al. 1994 Magnetic resonance imaging of the lumbar spine in people without back pain. N Engl J Med 331: 69–73

390. Jiang H, Raso J V, Moreau M J et al. 1994 Quantitative morphology of the lateral ligaments of the spine. Assessment of their importance in maintaining lateral stability. Spine 19: 2676–2682

391. Johnstone B, Urban J P, Roberts S et al. 1992 The fluid content of the human intervertebral disc. Comparison between fluid content and swelling pressure profiles of discs removed at surgery and those taken postmortem. Spine 17: 412–416

392. Jonck L M, Van Niekerk J M 1961 A roentgenological study of the motion of the lumbar spine of the Bantu. S A J Lab Clin Med 7: 67–71

393. Jones D A, Newham D J, Round J M et al. 1986 Experimental human muscle damage: morphological changes in relation to other indices of damage. J Physiol 375: 435–448

394. Jones H H, Priest J D, Hayes W C et al. 1977 Humeral hypertrophy in response to exercise. J Bone Joint Surg [Am] 59: 204–208

395. Jones J R, Hodgson J T, Clegg T A et al. 1998 Self-reported work-related illness in 1995. Results from a household survey. Her Majesty's Stationery Office, Norwich

396. Kaapa E, Han X, Holm S et al. 1995 Collagen synthesis and types I, III, IV, and VI collagens in

an animal model of disc degeneration. Spine 20: 59–66; discussion 66–57

397. Kanayama M, Abumi K, Kaneda K et al. 1996 Phase lag of the intersegmental motion in flexion-extension of the lumbar and lumbosacral spine. An in vivo study. Spine 21: 1416–1422

398. Kanayama M, Tadano S, Kaneda K et al. 1995 A cineradiographic study on the lumbar disc deformation during flexion and extension of the trunk. Clin Biomech 10: 193–199

399. Kaneoka K, Ono K, Inami S et al. 1999 Motion analysis of cervical vertebrae during whiplash loading. Spine 24: 763–769; discussion 770

400. Kanerva A, Kommonen B, Gronblad M et al. 1997 Inflammatory cells in experimental intervertebral disc injury. Spine 22: 2711–2715

401. Kang J D, Georgescu H I, McIntyre-Larkin L et al. 1996 Herniated lumbar intervertebral discs spontaneously produce matrix metalloproteinases, nitric oxide, interleukin-6, and prostaglandin E2. Spine 21: 271–277

402. Kankaanpaa M, Taimela S, Airaksinen O et al. 1999 The efficacy of active rehabilitation in chronic low back pain. Effect on pain intensity, self-experienced disability, and lumbar fatigability. Spine 24: 1034–1042

403. Kaplansky B D, Wei F Y, Reecer M V 1998 Prevention strategies for occupational low back pain. Occup Med 13: 33–45

404. Karjalainen K, Malmivaara A, van Tulder M et al. 2000 Multidisciplinary biopsychosocial rehabilitation for neck and shoulder pain among working age adults. Cochrane Database Syst Rev 3

405. Kaser L, Mannion A F, Rhyner A et al. 2001 Active therapy for chronic low back pain: Part 2. effects on paraspinal muscle cross-sectional area, fiber type size, and distribution. Spine 26: 909–919

406. Kastelic J, Galeski A, Baer E 1978 The multicomposite structure of tendon. Connect Tissue Res 6: 11–23

407. Katake K 1961 Studies on the strength of human skeletal muscles. J Kyoto Pref Med Univ 69: 463–483

408. Kawaguchi Y, Osada R, Kanamori M et al. 1999 Association between an aggrecan gene polymorphism and lumbar disc degeneration. Spine 24: 2456–2460

409. Kawakami M, Tamaki T, Hayashi N et al. 2000 Mechanical compression of the lumbar nerve root alters pain-related behaviors induced by the nucleus pulposus in the rat. J Orthop Res 18: 257–264

410. Kayama S, Konno S, Olmarker K et al. 1996 Incision of the annulus fibrosus induces nerve root morphologic, vascular, and functional changes. An experimental study. Spine 21: 2539–2543

411. Kazimirski J C 1997 CMA Policy Summary: The physician's role in helping patients return to work after an illness or injury. Can Med Assoc J 156: 680A–680C

412. Keel P, Weber M, Roux E 1998 Kreuzschmerzen: Hintergrunde, pravention, behandlung. Basisdokumentation Verbindung der Schweizer Arzte, Bern

413. Keller T S, Holm S H, Hansson T H et al. 1990 The dependence of intervertebral disc mechanical properties on physiologic conditions. Spine 15: 751–761

414. Keller T S, Hansson T H, Holm S H et al. 1989 In vivo creep behaviour of the normal and degenerated porcine intervertebral disc: a preliminary report. J Spinal Disord 1: 267–278

415. Kellgren J H 1938 Observations on referred pain arising from muscle. Clin Sci 3: 175–190

416. Kellgren J H 1939 On the distribution of pain arising from deep somatic structures with charts of segmental pain areas. Clin Sci 4: 35–46

417. Kelsey J L, Hardy R J 1975 Driving of motor vehicles as a risk factor for acute herniated lumbar intervertebral disc. Am J Epidemiol 102: 63–73

418. Kelsey J L, Githens P B, O'Conner T et al. 1984 Acute prolapsed lumbar intervertebral disc. An epidemiologic study with special reference to driving automobiles and cigarette smoking. Spine 9: 608–613

419. Kelsey J L, Githens P B, White III A A et al. 1984 An epidemiologic study of lifting and twisting on the job and risk for acute prolapsed lumbar intervertebral disc. J Orthop Res 2: 61–66

420. Kempson G E 1991 Age-related changes in the tensile properties of human articular cartilage: a comparative study between the femoral head of the hip joint and the talus of the ankle joint. Biochim Biophys Acta 1075: 223–230

421. Kerttula L I, Serlo W S, Tervonen O A et al. 2000 Post-traumatic findings of the spine after earlier vertebral fracture in young patients: clinical and MRI study. Spine 25: 1104–1108

422. Khan K M, Cook J L, Bonar F et al. 1999 Histopathology of common tendinopathies. Update and implications for clinical management. Sports Med 27: 393–408

423. Kimura T, Nakata K, Tsumaki N et al. 1996 Progressive degeneration of articular cartilage and intervertebral discs. An experimental study in transgenic mice bearing a type IX collagen mutation. Int Orthop 20: 177–181

424. Kingma I, de Looze M P, Toussaint H M et al. 1996 Validation of a full body 3-D dynamic linked segment model. Hum Move Sci 15: 833–860

425. Kingma I, van Dieen J H, de Looze M et al. 1998 Asymmetric low back loading in asymmetric lifting movements is not prevented by pelvic twist [see comments]. J Biomech 31: 527–534

426. Kingma I, Baten C T M, Dolan P et al. 2001 Lumbar loading during lifting: a comparative study of three measurement techniques. J Electromyogr Kinesiol 11: 337–345

427. Kippers V, Parker A W 1984 Posture related to myoelectric silence of erectores spinae during trunk flexion. Spine 9: 740–745

428. Kissling R O, Jacob H A C 1997 The mobility of sacroiliac joints in healthy subjects. In: Vleeming A et al. (ed) Movement, stability and low back pain. Churchill Livingstone, Edinburgh

429. Kjellby-Wendt G, Styf J 1998 Early active training after lumbar discectomy. A prospective, randomized, and controlled study. Spine 23: 2345–2351

430. Klaber Moffett J A, Hughes G I, Griffiths P 1993 A longitudinal study of low back pain in student nurses. Int J Nurs Stud 30: 197–212

431. Klein J A, Hukins D W 1982 Collagen fibre orientation in the annulus fibrosus of intervertebral disc during bending and torsion measured by x-ray diffraction. Biochim Biophys Acta 719: 98–101

432. Koeller W, Funke F, Hartmann F 1984 Biomechanical behavior of human intervertebral discs subjected to long lasting axial loading. Biorheology 21: 675–686

433. Koeller W, Muehlhaus S, Meier W et al. 1986 Biomechanical properties of human intervertebral discs subjected to axial dynamic compression – influence of age and degeneration. J Biomech 19: 807–816

434. Koes B W, van Tulder M W, Ostelo R et al. 2001 Clinical guidelines for the management of low back pain in primary care: an international comparison. Spine 26: 2504–2512

435. Komori H, Shinomiya K, Nakai O et al. 1996 The natural history of herniated nucleus pulposus with radiculopathy. Spine 21: 225–229

436. Kopsidas G, Kovalenko S A, Heffernan D R et al. 2000 Tissue mitochondrial DNA changes. A stochastic system. Ann N Y Acad Sci 908: 226–243

437. Korkala O, Gronblad M, Liesi P et al. 1985 Immunohistochemical demonstration of nociceptors in the ligamentous structures of the lumbar spine. Spine 10: 156–157

438. Kotani Y, Cunningham B W, Cappuccino A et al. 1998 The effects of spinal fixation and destabilization on the biomechanical and histologic properties of spinal ligaments. An in vivo study. Spine 23: 672–682; discussion 682–673

439. Kotilainen E 1994 Microinvasive lumbar disc surgery. A study on patients treated with microdiscectomy or percutaneous nucleotomy for disc herniation. Ann Chir Gynaecol Suppl 209: 1–50

440. Kraemer J, Kolditz D, Gowin R 1985 Water and electrolyte content of human intervertebral discs under variable load. Spine 10: 69–71

441. Krag M H, Cohen M C, Haugh L D et al. 1990 Body height change during upright and recumbent posture. Spine 15: 202–207

442. Krajcarski S R, Potvin J R, Chiang J 1999 The in vivo dynamic response of the spine to perturbations causing rapid flexion: effects of pre-load and step input magnitude. Clin Biomech 14: 54–62

443. Krismer M, Haid C, Rabl W 1996 The contribution of anulus fibers to torque resistance. Spine 21: 2551–2557

444. Kujala U M, Oksanen A, Taimela S et al. 1997 Training does not increase maximal lumbar extension in healthy adolescents. Clin Biomech 12: 181–184

445. Kumar S 1984 The physiological cost of three different methods of lifting in sagittal and lateral planes. Ergonomics 27: 425–433

446. Kuslich S D, Ulstrom C L, Michael C J 1991 The tissue origin of low back pain and sciatica: a report of pain response to tissue stimulation during operations on the lumbar spine using local anesthesia. Orthop Clin North Am 22: 181–187

447. Lahad A, Malter A D, Berg A O et al. 1994 The effectiveness of four interventions for the prevention of low back pain. JAMA 272: 1286–1291

448. Laible J P, Pflaster D S, Krag M H et al. 1993 A poroelastic-swelling finite element model with application to the intervertebral disc. Spine 18: 659–670

449. Lamy C, Bazergui A, Kraus H et al. 1975 The strength of the neural arch and the etiology of spondylolysis. Orthop Clin North Am 6: 215–231

450. Lancourt J, Kettelhut M 1992 Predicting return to work for lower back pain patients receiving worker's compensation. Spine 17: 629–640

451. Lane R J M 1996 Handbook of muscle disease. Marcel Dekker, New York

452. Lanyon L E, Rubin C T 1984 Static vs dynamic loads as an influence on bone remodelling. J Biomech 17: 897–905

453. Lark M W, Gordy J T, Weidner J R et al. 1995 Cell-mediated catabolism of aggrecan. Evidence that cleavage at the 'aggrecanase' site (Glu373-Ala374) is a primary event in proteolysis of the interglobular domain. J Biol Chem 270: 2550–2556

454. Larsson L 1982 Physical training effects on muscle morphology in sedentary males at different ages. Med Sci Sports Exerc 14: 203–206

455. Lavender S A, Shakeel K, Andersson G B et al. 2000 Effects of a lifting belt on spine moments and muscle recruitments after unexpected sudden loading. Spine 25: 1569–1578

456. Lavender S A, Tsuang Y H, Hafezi A et al. 1992 Coactivation of the trunk muscles during asymmetric loading of the torso. Hum Factors 34: 239–247

457. Leboeuf-Yde C 1999 Smoking and low back pain. A systematic literature review of 41 journal articles reporting 47 epidemiologic studies. Spine 24: 1463–1470

458. Lehman G J, McGill S M 2001 Spinal manipulation causes variable spine kinematic and trunk muscle electromyographic responses. Clin Biomech 16: 293–299

459. Leivseth G, Drerup B 1997 Spinal shrinkage during work in a sitting posture compared to work in a standing posture. Clin Biomech 12: 409–418

460. Leivseth G, Salvesen R, Hemminghytt S et al. 1999 Do human lumbar discs reconstitute after chemonucleolysis? A 7-year follow-up study. Spine 24: 342–347; discussion 348

461. Lemaire J P, Skalli W, Lavaste F et al. 1997 Intervertebral disc prosthesis. Results and prospects for the year 2000. Clin Orthop: 64–76

462. Leong J C, Luk K D, Chow D H et al. 1987 The biomechanical functions of the iliolumbar ligament in maintaining stability of the lumbosacral junction. Spine 12: 669–674

463. Leppilahti J, Puranen J, Orava S 1996 Incidence of Achilles tendon rupture. Acta Orthop Scand 67: 277–279

464. Lewin T 1964 Osteoarthritis in lumbar synovial joints. A morphologic study. Acta Orthop Scand, supplement 73

465. Lieber R L, Friden J 1999 Mechanisms of muscle injury after eccentric contraction. J Sci Med Sport 2: 253–265

466. Lindblom K 1952 Experimental ruptures of intervertebral discs in rats' tails. J Bone Joint Surg [Am] 34: 123–128

467. Lindblom K 1957 Intervertebral disc degeneration considered as a pressure atrophy. J Bone Joint Surg [Am] 39: 933–945

468. Linton S J 2000 A review of psychological risk factors in back and neck pain. Spine 25: 1148–1156

469. Linton S J, van Tulder M W 2001 Preventive interventions for back and neck pain problems: what is the evidence? Spine 26: 778–787

470. Little C B, Flannery C R, Hughes C E et al. 1999 Aggrecanase versus matric metalloproteinases in the catabolism of the interglobular domain of aggrecan in vitro. Biochem J 344 Pt 1: 61–68

471. Liu Y K, Nijus G, Buckwater J et al. 1983 Fatigue response of lumbar intervertebral joints under axial cyclic loading. Spine 8: 857–865

472. Liu Y K, Goel V K, Dejong A et al. 1985 Torsional fatigue of the lumbar intervertebral joints. Spine 10: 894–900

473. Liyang D, Yinkan X, Wenming Z et al. 1989 The effect of flexion-extension motion of the lumbar spine on the capacity of the spinal canal. An experimental study. Spine 14: 523–525

474. de Looze M P, Visser B, Houting I et al. 1996 Weight and frequency effect on spinal loading in a bricklaying task. J Biomech 29: 1425–1433

475. Lord M J, Small J M, Dinsay J M et al. 1997 Lumbar lordosis. Effects of sitting and standing. Spine 22: 2571–2574

476. Lotz J C 1999 The biomechanics of prevention and treatment for low back pain: 2nd international workshop. Clin Biomech 14: 220–223

477. Lotz J C, Colliou O K, Chin J R et al. 1998 Compression-induced degeneration of the intervertebral disc: an in vivo mouse model and finite-element study. Spine 23: 2493–2506

478. Lu Y M, Hutton W C, Gharpuray V M 1996 Do bending, twisting, and diurnal fluid changes in the disc affect the propensity to prolapse? A viscoelastic finite element model. Spine 21: 2570–2579

479. Lu Y M, Hutton W C, Gharpuray V M 1996 Can variations in intervertebral disc height affect the mechanical function of the disc? Spine 21: 2208–2216; discussion 2217

480. Lumsden R M D, Morris J M 1968 An in vivo study of axial rotation and immoblization at the lumbosacral joint. J Bone Joint Surg [Am] 50: 1591–1602

481. Lundin O, Ekstrom L, Hellstrom M et al. 1998 Injuries in the adolescent porcine spine exposed to mechanical compression. Spine 23: 2574–2579

482. Macfarlane G J, Thomas E, Papageorgiou A C et al. 1997 Employment and physical work activities as predictors of future low back pain. Spine 22: 1143–1149

483. Macintosh J E, Bogduk N 1986 The biomechanics of the lumbar multifidus. Clin Biomech 1: 205–213

484. Macintosh J E, Bogduk N 1991 The attachments of the lumbar erector spinae. Spine 16: 783–792

485. Macintosh J E, Bogduk N, Gracovetsky S 1987 The biomechanics of the thoracolumbar fascia. Clin Biomech 2: 78–83

486. Macintosh J E, Pearcy M J, Bogduk N 1993 The axial torque of the lumbar back muscles: torsion strength of the back muscles. Aust N Z J Surg 63: 205–212

487. Macintosh J E, Bogduk N, Pearcy M J 1993 The effects of flexion on the geometry and actions of the lumbar erector spinae. Spine 18: 884–893

488. Mackay C, Burton K, Boocock M et al. 1998 Musculoskeletal disorders in supermarket cashiers. HMSO, Norwich

489. Macrae I F, Wright V 1969 Measurement of back movement. Ann Rheum Dis 28: 584–589

490. Maeda S, Kokubun S 2000 Changes with age in proteoglycan synthesis in cells cultured in vitro from the inner and outer rabbit annulus fibrosus. Responses to interleukin-1 and interleukin-1 receptor antagonist protein. Spine 25: 166–169

491. Magnusson M L, Aleksiev A R, Spratt K F et al. 1996 Hyperextension and spine height changes. Spine 21: 2670–2675

492. Magnusson M L, Bishop J B, Hasselquist L et al. 1998 Range of motion and motion patterns in patients with low back pain before and after rehabilitation. Spine 23: 2631–2639

493. Magnusson M L, Aleksiev A, Wilder D G et al. 1996 Unexpected load and asymmetric posture as etiologic factors in low back pain. Eur Spine J 5: 23–35

494. Magnusson M L, Pope M H, Hasselquist L et al. 1999 Cervical electromyographic activity during low-speed rear impact. Eur Spine J 8: 118–125

495. Magora A 1973 Investigation of the relation between low back pain and occupation. IV. Physical requirements: bending, rotation, reaching and sudden maximal effort. Scand J Rehabil Med 5: 186–190

496. Maigne J Y, Aivaliklis A, Pfefer F 1996 Results of sacroiliac joint double block and value of sacroiliac pain provocation tests in 54 patients with low back pain. Spine 21: 1889–1892

497. Main C J, Spanswick C C 2000 Pain management. An interdisciplinary approach. Churchill Livingstone, Edinburgh

498. Malinsky J 1959 The ontogenetic development of nerve terminations in the intervertebral discs of man. Acta Anat 38: 96–113

499. Malko J A, Hutton W C, Fajman W A 1999 An in vivo magnetic resonance imaging study of changes in the volume (and fluid content) of the lumbar intervertebral discs during a simulated diurnal load cycle. Spine 24: 1015–1022

500. Malmivaara A, Kotilainen E, Laasonen E et al. 1999 Clinical practice guidelines of the Finnish Medical Association Duodecim. In: Diseases of the low back. Finnish Medical Association

501. Manniche C 1999 Low back pain; frequency, management and prevention from HTA perspective. Danish Institute for Health Technology Assessment

502. Manniche C, Lundberg E, Christensen I et al. 1991 Intensive dynamic back exercises for chronic low back pain: a clinical trial. Pain 47: 53–63

503. Mannion A F, Dolan P 1996 Relationship between myoelectric and mechanical manifestations of fatigue in the quadriceps femoris muscle group. Eur J Appl Physiol 74: 411–419

504. Mannion A F, Dolan P 1996 The effects of muscle length and force output on the EMG power spectrum of the erector spinae. J Electromyogr Kinesiol 6: 159–168

505. Mannion A F, Dolan P, Adams M A 1996 Psychological questionnaires: do 'abnormal' scores precede or follow first-time low back pain? Spine 21: 2603–2611

506. Mannion A F, Adams M A, Dolan P 2000 People who load their spines heavily during standard lifting tasks are more likely to develop low back pain. Proceedings of the International Society for the Study of the Lumbar Spine, Singapore

507. Mannion A F, Adams M A, Dolan P 2000 Sudden and unexpected loading generates high forces on the lumbar spine. Spine 25: 842–852

508. Mannion A F, Connolly B, Wood K et al. 1997 The use of surface EMG power spectral analysis in the evaluation of back muscle function. J Rehabil Res Dev 34: 427–439

509. Mannion A F, Muntener M, Taimela S et al. 1999 A randomized clinical trial of three active therapies for chronic low back pain. Spine 24: 2435–2448

510. Mannion A F, Taimela S, Muntener M et al. 2001 Active therapy for chronic low back pain. Part 1: effects on back muscle activation, fatigability, and strength. Spine 26: 897–908

511. Mannion A F, Weber B R, Dvorak J et al. 1997 Fibre type characteristics of the lumbar paraspinal muscles in normal healthy subjects and in patients with low back pain. J Orthop Res 15: 881–887

512. Marchand F, Ahmed A M 1989 Mechanical properties and failure mechanisms: constituent components of the annulus fibrosus. Proceedings of the 10th Annual Conference of the Canadian Biomaterials Society, 74–77

513. Marchand F, Ahmed A M 1990 Investigation of the laminate structure of lumbar disc anulus fibrosus. Spine 15: 402–410

514. Markolf K L, Morris J M 1974 The structural components of the intervertebral disc. A study of their contributions to the ability of the disc to withstand compressive forces. J Bone Joint Surg Am 56: 675–687

515. Maroudas A, Rigler D, Schneiderman R 1999 Young and aged cartilage differ in their response to dynamic compression as far as the rate of glycosaminoglycan synthesis is concerned. Proceedings of the Orthopaedic Research Society, Anaheim, California

516. Maroudas A, Stockwell R A, Nachemson A et al. 1975 Factors involved in the nutrition of the human lumbar intervertebral disc: cellularity and diffusion of glucose in vitro. J Anat 120: 113–130

517. Marras W S, Mirka G A 1990 Muscle activities during asymmetric trunk angular accelerations. J Orthop Res 8: 824–832

518. Marras W S, Sommerich C M 1991 A three-dimensional motion model of loads on the lumbar spine: I. Model structure. Hum Factors 33: 123–137

519. Marras W S, Granata K P 1995 A biomechanical assessment and model of axial twisting in the thoracolumbar spine. Spine 20: 1440–1451

520. Marras W S, Mirka G A 1996 Intra-abdominal pressure during trunk extension motions. Clin Biomech 11: 267–274

521. Marras W S, Jorgensen M J, Granata K P et al. 2001 Female and male trunk geometry: size and prediction of the spine loading trunk muscles derived from MRI. Clin Biomech 16: 38–46

522. Marras W S, Davies K G, Heaney C A et al. 2000 The influence of psychosocial stress, gender, and personality on mechanical loading of the lumbar spine. Spine 25: 3045–3054

523. Marras W S, Lavender S A, Leurgans S E et al. 1993 The role of dynamic three-dimensional trunk motion in occupationally-related low back disorders. The effects of workplace factors, trunk position, and trunk motion characteristics on risk of injury. Spine 18: 617–628

524. Matsumoto T, Kawakami M, Kuribayashi K et al. 1999 Cyclic mechanical stretch stress increases the growth rate and collagen synthesis of nucleus pulposus cells in vitro. Spine 24: 315–319

525. Mayer T, Tabor J, Bovasso E et al. 1994 Physical progress and residual impairment quantification after functional restoration. Part I: Lumbar mobility. Spine 19: 389–394

526. McBroom R J, Hayes W C, Edwards W T et al. 1985 Prediction of vertebral body compressive fracture using quantitative computed tomography. J Bone Joint Surg [Am] 67: 1206–1214

527. McCall I W, Park W M, O'Brien J P 1979 Induced pain referral from posterior lumbar elements in normal subjects. Spine 4: 441–446

528. McGill S, Seguin J, Bennett G 1994 Passive stiffness of the lumbar torso in flexion, extension, lateral bending, and axial rotation. Effect of belt wearing and breath holding. Spine 19: 696–704

529. McGill S, Juker D, Kropf P 1996 Appropriately placed surface EMG electrodes reflect deep muscle activity (psoas, quadratus lumborum, abdominal wall) in the lumbar spine. J Biomech 29: 1503–1507

530. McGill S M 1991 Electromyographic activity of the abdominal and low back musculature during the generation of isometric and dynamic axial trunk torque: implications for lumbar mechanics. J Orthop Res 9: 91–103

531. McGill S M 1992 A myoelectrically based dynamic three-dimensional model to predict loads on lumbar spine tissues during lateral bending. J Biomech 25: 395–414

532. McGill S M 1992 The influence of lordosis on axial trunk torque and trunk muscle myoelectric activity. Spine 17: 1187–1193

533. McGill S M, Norman R W 1985 Dynamically and statically determined low back moments during lifting. J Biomech 18: 877–885

534. McGill S M, Norman R W 1987 Effects of an anatomically detailed erector spinae model on L4/L5 disc compression and shear. J Biomech 20: 591–600

535. McGill S M, Brown S 1992 Creep response of the lumbar spine to prolonged full flexion. Clin Biomech 7: 43–46

536. McGill S M, Kippers V 1994 Transfer of loads between lumbar tissues during the flexion–relaxation phenomenon. Spine 19: 2190–2196

537. McGill S M, Norman R W, Sharratt M T 1990 The effect of an abdominal belt on trunk muscle activity and intra-abdominal pressure during squat lifts. Ergonomics 33: 147–160

538. McGill S M, Yingling V R, Peach J P 1999 Three-dimensional kinematics and trunk muscle myoelectric activity in the elderly spine – a database compared to young people. Clin Biomech 14: 389–395

539. McGorry R W, Hsiang S M, Fathallah F A et al. 2001 Timing of activation of the erector spinae and

hamstrings during a trunk flexion and extension task. Spine 26: 418–425

540. McGregor A H 1999 Genetic basis of low back pain. Proceedings of the Society for Back Pain Research, Cardiff, UK

541. McGregor A H, McCarthy I D, Dore C J et al. 1997 Quantitative assessment of the motion of the lumbar spine in the low back pain population and the effect of different spinal pathologies of this motion. Eur Spine J 6: 308–315

542. McMillan D W, Garbutt G, Adams M A 1996 Effect of sustained loading on the water content of intervertebral discs: implications for disc metabolism. Ann Rheum Dis 55: 880–887

543. McMillan D W, McNally D S, Garbutt G et al. 1996 Stress distributions inside intervertebral discs: the validity of experimental 'stress profilometry'. Proc Inst Mech Eng [H] 210: 81–87

544. McNally D S, Adams M A 1992 Internal intervertebral disc mechanics as revealed by stress profilometry. Spine 17: 66–73

545. McNally D S, Adams M A, Goodship A E 1992 Development and validation of a new transducer for intradiscal pressure measurement. J Biomed Eng 14: 495–498

546. McNally D S, Adams M A, Goodship A E 1993 Can intervertebral disc prolapse be predicted by disc mechanics? Spine 18: 1525–1530

547. McNally D S, Shackleford I M, Goodship A E et al. 1996 In vivo stress measurement can predict pain on discography. Spine 21: 2580–2587

548. McNeil P L, Khakee R 1992 Disruptions of muscle fiber plasma membranes. Role in exercise-induced damage. Am J Pathol 140: 1097–1109

549. McNeill T, Warwick D, Andersson G et al. 1980 Trunk strengths in attempted flexion, extension, and lateral bending in healthy subjects and patients with low-back disorders. Spine 5: 529–538

550. Mellin G P 1989 Comparison between tape measurements of forward and lateral flexion of the spine. Clin Biomech 4: 121–123

551. Melrose J, Ghosh P, Taylor T K et al. 1992 A longitudinal study of the matrix changes induced in the intervertebral disc by surgical damage to the annulus fibrosus. J Orthop Res 10: 665–676

552. Mercer S, Bogduk N 1999 The ligaments and anulus fibrosus of human adult cervical intervertebral discs. Spine 24: 619–626; discussion 627–628

553. Merskey H, Bogduk N 1994 Classification of chronic pain: descriptions of chronic pain syndromes and definitions of pain terms, 2nd edn. IASP Press, Seattle

554. Miller J A, Schultz A B, Andersson G B 1987 Load-displacement behavior of sacroiliac joints. J Orthop Res 5: 92–101

555. Miller J A, Schmatz C, Schultz A B 1988 Lumbar disc degeneration: correlation with age, sex, and spine level in 600 autopsy specimens. Spine 13: 173–178

556. Miller J A, Schultz A B, Warwick D N et al. 1986 Mechanical properties of lumbar spine motion segments under large loads. J Biomech 19: 79–84

557. Miller S A, Mayer T, Cox R et al. 1992 Reliability problems associated with the modified Schober technique for true lumbar flexion measurement. Spine 17: 345–348

558. Mimura M, Panjabi M M, Oxland T R et al. 1994 Disc degeneration affects the multidirectional flexibility of the lumbar spine. Spine 19: 1371–1380

559. Miyamoto K, Iinuma N, Maeda M et al. 1999 Effects of abdominal belts on intra-abdominal pressure, intra-muscular pressure in the erector spinae muscles and myoelectrical activities of trunk muscles. Clin Biomech 14: 79–87

560. Monemi M, Kadi F, Liu J X et al. 1999 Adverse changes in fibre type and myosin heavy chain compositions of human jaw muscle vs. limb muscle during ageing. Acta Physiol Scand 167: 339–345

561. Monemi M, Eriksson P O, Kadi F et al. 1999 Opposite changes in myosin heavy chain composition of human masseter and biceps brachii muscles during aging. J Muscle Res Cell Motil 20: 351–361

562. Moneta G B, Videman T, Kaivanto K et al. 1994 Reported pain during lumbar discography as a function of anular ruptures and disc degeneration. A re-analysis of 833 discograms. Spine 19: 1968–1974

563. Moon S H, Gilbertson L G, Nishida K et al. 2000 Human intervertebral disc cells are genetically modifiable by adenovirus-mediated gene transfer: implications for the clinical management of intervertebral disc disorders. Spine 25: 2573–2579

564. Mooney V, Robertson J 1976 The facet syndrome. Clin Orthop 115: 149–156

565. Moore J E, Von Korff M, Cherkin D, Saunders K, Lorig K 2000 A randomized clinical trial of a cognitive-behavioral program for enhancing back pain care in a primary care setting. Pain 88: 145–154

566. Moore R J 2000 The vertebral end-plate: what do we know? Eur Spine J 9: 92–96

567. Moore R J, Osti O L, Vernon-Roberts B et al. 1992 Changes in endplate vascularity after an outer anulus tear in the sheep. Spine 17: 874–878

568. Moore R J, Vernon-Roberts B, Osti O L et al. 1996 Remodeling of vertebral bone after outer anular injury in sheep. Spine 21: 936–940

569. Moore R J, Vernon-Roberts B, Fraser R D et al. 1996 The origin and fate of herniated lumbar intervertebral disc tissue. Spine 21: 2149–2155

570. Moreton R D 1966 Spondylolysis. JAMA 195: 671–674

571. Mundt D J, Kelsey J L, Golden A L et al. 1993 An epidemiologic study of non-occupational lifting as a risk factor for herniated lumbar intervertebral disc. The Northeast Collaborative Group on Low Back Pain. Spine 18: 595–602

572. Murray R C, Zhu C F, Goodship A E et al. 1999 Exercise affects the mechanical properties and histological appearance of equine articular cartilage. J Orthop Res 17: 725–731

573. Myers E R, Wilson S E 1997 Biomechanics of osteoporosis and vertebral fracture. Spine 22: 25S–31S

574. Myklebust J B, Pintar F, Yoganandan N et al. 1988 Tensile strength of spinal ligaments. Spine 13: 526–531

575. Nachemson A 1966 The load on lumbar disks in different positions of the body. Clin Orthop 45: 107–122

576. Nachemson A, Morris J M 1964 In-vivo measurements of intradiscal pressure. J Bone Joint Surg [Am] 46: 1077–1092

577. Nachemson A, Vingard E 2000 Influences of individual factors and smoking on neck and low back pain. In: Nachemson A L, Jonsson E (eds) Neck and back pain: the scientific evidence of causes, diagnosis and treatment. Lippincott, Williams and Wilkins, Philadelphia, 79–96

578. Nachemson A, Jonsson E 2001 Evidence based treatment for back pain. Swedish Council on Technology Assessment in Health Care. Lippincott, Stockholm/Philadelphia (English translation in press)

579. Nachemson A, Lewin T, Maroudas A et al. 1970 In vitro diffusion of dye through the end-plates and the annulus fibrosus of human lumbar inter-vertebral discs. Acta Orthop Scand 41: 589–607

580. Nachemson A L 1960 Lumbar intradiscal pressure. Acta Orthop Scand, supplement 73

581. Nachemson A L 1963 The influence of spinal movements on the lumbar intradiscal pressure and on the tensile stresses in the annulus fibrosus. Acta Orthop Scand 33: 183–207

582. Nachemson A L 1981 Disc pressure measurements. Spine 6: 93–97

583. Nachemson A L 2000 Introduction to treatment of neck and back pain. In: Nachemson A L, Jonsson E (eds) Neck and back pain: the scientific evidence of causes, diagnosis and treatment. Lippincott, Williams and Wilkins, Philadelphia, 237–240

584. Nachemson A L, Evans J H 1968 Some mechanical properties of the third human lumbar interlaminar ligament (ligamentum flavum). J Biomech 1: 211–220

585. Nachemson A L, Wadell G, Norlund A I 2000 Epidemiology of neck and low back pain. In: Nachemson A L, Jonsson E (eds) Neck and back pain: the scientific evidence of causes, diagnosis and treatment. Lippincott, Williams and Wilkins, Philadelphia, 165–188

586. Nahit E S, Macfarlane G J, Pritchard C M et al. 2001 Short term influence of mechanical factors on regional musculoskeletal pain: a study of new workers from 12 occupational groups. Occup Environ Med 58: 374–381

587. Nakamura N, Hart D A, Boorman R S et al. 2000 Decorin antisense gene therapy improves functional healing of early rabbit ligament scar with enhanced collagen fibrillogenesis in vivo. J Orthop Res 18: 517–523

588. Natarajan R N, Andersson G B 1999 The influence of lumbar disc height and cross-sectional area on the mechanical response of the disc to physiologic loading. Spine 24: 1873–1881

589. Nelson J M, Walmsley R P, Stevenson J M 1995 Relative lumbar and pelvic motion during loaded spinal flexion/extension. Spine 20: 199–204

590. Nerlich A G, Schleicher E D, Boos N 1997 Immunohistologic markers for age-related changes of human lumbar intervertebral discs. Spine 22: 2781–2795

591. Neumann P, Nordwall A, Osvalder A L 1995 Traumatic instability of the lumbar spine. A dynamic in vitro study of flexion-distraction injury. Spine 20: 1111–1121

592. Neumann P, Keller T S, Ekstrom L et al. 1994 Effect of strain rate and bone mineral on the structural properties of the human anterior longitudinal ligament. Spine 19: 205–211

593. Neumann P, Osvalder A L, Nordwall A et al. 1992 The mechanism of initial flexion-distraction injury in the lumbar spine. Spine 17: 1083–1090

594. Neumann P, Keller T, Ekstrom L et al. 1993 Structural properties of the anterior longitudinal ligament. Correlation with lumbar bone mineral content. Spine 18: 637–645

595. Newham D J, Jones D A, Clarkson P M 1987 Repeated high-force eccentric exercise: effects on muscle pain and damage. J Appl Physiol 63: 1381–1386

596. Newham D J, McPhail G, Mills K R et al. 1983 Ultrastructural changes after concentric and eccentric contractions of human muscle. J Neurol Sci 61: 109–122

597. Newman P H 1952 Sprung back. J Bone Joint Surg [Br] 34: 30–37

598. Newton M, Waddell G 1993 Trunk strength testing with iso-machines. Part 1: Review of a decade of scientific evidence [see comments]. Spine 18: 801–811

599. Newton M, Thow M, Somerville D et al. 1993 Trunk strength testing with iso-machines. Part 2: Experimental evaluation of the Cybex II Back Testing System in normal subjects and patients with chronic low back pain. Spine 18: 812–824

600. Nice D A, Riddle D L, Lamb R L et al. 1992 Intertester reliability of judgments of the presence of trigger points in patients with low back pain. Arch Phys Med Rehabil 73: 893–898

601. NIOSH 1997 Low back musculoskeletal disorders: evidence for work-relatedness. Musculoskeletal disorders and workplace factors. National Institute of Occupational Safety and Health, Cincinatti, USA

602. Njoo K H, van der Does E 1994 The occurrence and inter-rater reliability of myofascial trigger points in the quadratus lumborum and gluteus medius: a prospective study in non-specific low back pain patients and controls in general practice. Pain 58: 317–323

603. Njoo K H, van der Does E, Stam H J 1995 Interobserver agreement on iliac crest pain syndrome in general practice. J Rheumatol 22: 1532–1535

604. Nordin M et al. 1997 Early predictors of delayed return to work in patients with low back pain. J Musculoskel Pain 5: 5–27

605. Noren R, Trafimow J, Andersson G B et al. 1991 The role of facet joint tropism and facet angle in disc degeneration. Spine 16: 530–532

606. Norman R et al. 1998 A comparison of peak vs cumulative physical work exposure risk factors for the reporting of low back pain in the automotive industry. Clin Biomech 13: 561–573

607. Oda K, Shibayama Y, Abe M et al. 1998 Morphogenesis of vertebral deformities in involutional osteoporosis. Age-related, three-dimensional trabecular structure. Spine 23: 1050–1055; discussion 1056

608. Oegema T R, Jr., Johnson S L, Aguiar D J et al. 2000 Fibronectin and its fragments increase with degeneration in the human intervertebral disc. Spine 25: 2742–2747

609. Ogata K, Whiteside L A 1981 Nutritional pathways of the intervertebral disc. An experimental study using hydrogen washout technique. Spine 6: 211–216

610. Ogon M, Bender B R, Hooper D M et al. 1997 A dynamic approach to spinal instability. Part II: Hesitation and giving-way during interspinal motion. Spine 22: 2859–2866

611. O'Hara B P, Urban J P, Maroudas A 1990 Influence of cyclic loading on the nutrition of articular cartilage. Ann Rheum Dis 49: 536–539

612. Okawa A, Shinomiya K, Komori H et al. 1998 Dynamic motion study of the whole lumbar spine by videofluoroscopy. Spine 23: 1743–1749

613. Oleinick A, Gluck J V, Guire K 1996 Factors affecting first return to work following a compensable occupational back injury. Am J Ind Med 30: 540–555

614. Oliver M J, Twomey L T 1995 Extension creep in the lumbar spine. Clin Biomech 10: 363–368

615. Olmarker K, Rydevik B, Nordborg C 1993 Autologous nucleus pulposus induces neurophysiologic and histologic changes in porcine cauda equina nerve roots [see comments]. Spine 18: 1425–1432

616. Olmarker K, Blomquist J, Stromberg J et al. 1995 Inflammatogenic properties of nucleus pulposus. Spine 20: 665–669

617. Osti O L, Vernon-Roberts B, Fraser R D 1990 Anulus tears and intervertebral disc degeneration. An experimental study using an animal model. Spine 15: 762–767

618. Ostry A, Stringer B, Berkowitz J et al. 1999 Workplace organisation questionnaire. Proceedings of the 9th World Congress on Pain, Vienna

619. Osvalder A L, Neumann P, Lovsund P et al. 1990 Ultimate strength of the lumbar spine in flexion – an in vitro study. J Biomech 23: 453–460

620. Osvalder A L, Neumann P, Lovsund P et al. 1993 A method for studying the biomechanical load response of the (in vitro) lumbar spine under dynamic flexion-shear loads. J Biomech 26: 1227–1236

621. Otani K, Arai I, Mao G P et al. 1997 Experimental disc herniation: evaluation of the natural course. Spine 22: 2894–2899

622. Otterness I G, Eskra J D, Bliven M L et al. 1998 Exercise protects against articular cartilage degeneration in the hamster. Arthritis Rheum 41: 2068–2076

623. Oxland T R, Lund T, Jost B et al. 1996 The relative importance of vertebral bone density and disc degeneration in spinal flexibility and interbody implant performance. An in vitro study. Spine 21: 2558–2569

624. Paassilta P, Lohiniva J, Goring H H et al. 2001 Identification of a novel common genetic risk factor for lumbar disk disease. JAMA 285: 1843–1849

625. Panjabi M, Yamamoto I, Oxland T et al. 1989 How does posture affect coupling in the lumbar spine? Spine 14: 1002–1011

626. Panjabi M, Brown M, Lindahl S et al. 1988 Intrinsic disc pressure as a measure of integrity of the lumbar spine [see comments]. Spine 13: 913–917

627. Panjabi M M, Goel V K, Takata K 1982 Physiologic strains in the lumbar spinal ligaments. An in vitro biomechanical study. Spine 7: 192–203

628. Panjabi M M, Krag M H, Chung T Q 1984 Effects of disc injury on mechanical behavior of the human spine. Spine 9: 707–713

629. Panjabi M M, Krag M, Summers D et al. 1985 Biomechanical time-tolerance of fresh cadaveric human spine specimens. J Orthop Res 3: 292–300

630. Panjabi M M, Oxland T R, Lin R M et al. 1994 Thoracolumbar burst fracture. A biomechanical investigation of its multidirectional flexibility. Spine 19: 578–585

631. Panjabi M M, Andersson G B, Jorneus L et al. 1986 In vivo measurements of spinal column vibrations. J Bone Joint Surg [Am] 68: 695–702

632. Panjabi M M, Cholewicki J, Nibu K et al. 1998 Mechanism of whiplash injury. Clin Biomech 13: 239–249

633. Papageorgiou A C, Croft P R, Thomas E et al. 1996 Influence of previous pain experience on the episode incidence of low back pain: results from the South Manchester Back Pain Study. Pain 66: 181–185

634. Papageorgiou A C, Macfarlane G J, Thomas E et al. 1997 Psychosocial factors in the workplace – do they predict new episodes of low back pain? Evidence from the South Manchester Back Pain Study. Spine 22: 1137–1142

635. Patt S, Brock M, Mayer H M et al. 1993 Nucleus pulposus regeneration after chemonucleolysis with chymopapain? Spine 18: 227–231

636. Patwardhan A G, Havey R M, Meade K P et al. 1999 A follower load increases the load-carrying capacity of the lumbar spine in compression. Spine 24: 1003–1009

637. Pearcy M, Portek I, Shepherd J 1984 Three-dimensional x-ray analysis of normal movement in the lumbar spine. Spine 9: 294–297

638. Pearcy M, Portek I, Shepherd J 1985 The effect of low-back pain on lumbar spinal movements measured by three-dimensional X-ray analysis. Spine 10: 150–153

639. Pearcy M J 1993 Twisting mobility of the human back in flexed postures. Spine 18: 114–119

640. Pearcy M J, Tibrewal S B 1984 Axial rotation and lateral bending in the normal lumbar spine measured by three-dimensional radiography. Spine 9: 582–587

641. Pearcy M J, Tibrewal S B 1984 Lumbar intervertebral disc and ligament deformations measured in vivo. Clin Orthop: 281–286

642. Pearcy M J, Bogduk N 1988 Instantaneous axes of rotation of the lumbar intervertebral joints. Spine 13: 1033–1041

643. Pearcy M J, Hindle R J 1989 New method for the non-invasive three-dimensional measurement of human back movement. Clin Biomech 4: 73–79

644. Pearcy M J, Gill J M, Whittle M W et al. 1987 Dynamic back movement measured using a three-dimensional television system. J Biomech 20: 943–949

645. Perey O 1957 Fracture of the vertebral endplate. A biomechanical investigation. Acta Orthop Scand

646. Pflaster D S, Krag M H, Johnson C C et al. 1997 Effect of test environment on intervertebral disc hydration. Spine 22: 133–139

647. Pincus T, Burton A K, Vogel S et al. 2001 A systematic review of psychological factors as predictors of chronicity/disability in prospective cohorts of low back pain. Spine (in press)

648. Pintar F A, Yoganandan N, Myers T et al. 1992 Biomechanical properties of human lumbar spine ligaments. J Biomech 25: 1351–1356

649. Plamondon A, Gagnon M, Gravel D 1995 Moments at the L(5)/S(1) joint during asymmetrical lifting: effects of different load trajectories and initial load positions. Clin Biomech 10: 128–136

650. Pokharna H K, Phillips F M 1998 Collagen crosslinks in human lumbar intervertebral disc aging [see comments]. Spine 23: 1645–1648

651. Pollintine P, Dolan P, Tobias J H et al. 2001 Osteoporotic fractures and intervertebral disc degeneration. J Bone Min Res (submitted)

652. Polyani M F D, Eakin J, Frank J W et al. 1998 Creating healthier work environments: a critical review of the health impacts of workplace organisational change interventions. In: National forum on health, Canada Health Action: building on the legacy. Editions Multimondes, Quebec, Ste Foy

653. Pope M H, Broman H, Hansson T 1989 Impact response of the standing subject – a feasibility study. Clin Biomech 4: 195–200

654. Pope M H, Kaigle A M, Magnusson M et al. 1991 Intervertebral motion during vibration. Proc Inst Mech Eng [H] 205: 39–44

655. van Poppel M N, Koes B W, Smid T et al. 1997 A systematic review of controlled clinical trials on the prevention of back pain in industry. Occup Environ Med 54: 841–847

656. van Poppel M N, Koes B W, van der Ploeg T et al. 1998 Lumbar supports and education for the prevention of low back pain in industry: a randomized controlled trial. JAMA 279: 1789–1794

657. Portek I, Pearcy M J, Reader G P et al. 1983 Correlation between radiographic and clinical measurement of lumbar spine movement. Br J Rheumatol 22: 197–205

658. Porter J L, Wilkinson A 1997 Lumbar-hip flexion motion. A comparative study between asymptomatic and chronic low back pain in 18- to 36-year-old men. Spine 22: 1508–1513; discussion 1513–1504

659. Porter R W, Trailescu I F 1990 Diurnal changes in straight leg raising [see comments]. Spine 15: 103–106

660. Porter R W, Adams M A, Hutton W C 1989 Physical activity and the strength of the lumbar spine. Spine 14: 201–203

661. Postacchini F, Bellocci M, Massobrio M 1984 Morphologic changes in anulus fibrosus during aging. An ultrastructural study in rats. Spine 9: 596–603

662. Potvin J R, Norman R W 1993 Quantification of erector spinae muscle fatigue during prolonged, dynamic lifting tasks. Eur J Appl Physiol Occup Physiol 67: 554–562

663. Potvin J R, McGill S M, Norman R W 1991 Trunk muscle and lumbar ligament contributions to dynamic lifts with varying degrees of trunk flexion [see comments]. Spine 16: 1099–1107

664. Potvin J R, Norman R W, McGill S M 1991 Reduction in anterior shear forces on the L4/L5 disc by the lumbar musculature. Clin Biomech 6: 88–96

665. Potvin J R, Norman R W, McGill S M 1996 Mechanically corrected EMG for the continuous estimation of erector spinae muscle loading during repetitive lifting. Eur J Appl Physiol Occup Physiol 74: 119–132

666. Preuschoft H, Hayama S, Gunther M M 1988 Curvature of the lumbar spine as a consequence of mechanical necessities in Japanese macaques trained for bipedalism. Folia Primatol 50: 42–58

667. Pun Y L, Moskowitz R W, Lie S et al. 1994 Clinical correlations of osteoarthritis associated with a single-base mutation (arginine519 to cysteine) in type II procollagen gene. A newly defined pathogenesis. Arthritis Rheum 37: 264–269

668. Purslow P P 1989 Strain-induced reorientation of an intramuscular connective tissue network: implications for passive muscle elasticity. J Biomech 22: 21–31

669. Putto E, Tallroth K 1990 Extension-flexion radiographs for motion studies of the lumbar spine. A comparison of two methods. Spine 15: 107–110

670. Puustjarvi K 1994 Exercise-induced alterations in the metabolism of intervertebral disc matrix, vertebral mineral density and spinal muscle fibre types. In Kuopio, Finland: University of Kuopio

671. Puustjarvi K, Tammi M, Reinikainen M et al. 1994 Running training alters fiber type composition in spinal muscles. Eur Spine J 3: 17–21

672. Quinnell R C, Stockdale H R, Willis D S 1983 Observations of pressures within normal discs in the lumbar spine. Spine 8: 166–169

673. Rabischong P, Louis R, Vignaud J et al. 1978 The intervertebral disc. Anat Clin 1: 55–64

674. Radin E L, Rose R M 1986 Role of subchondral bone in the initiation and progression of cartilage damage. Clin Orthop: 34–40

675. Radin E L, Yang K H, Riegger C et al. 1991 Relationship between lower limb dynamics and knee joint pain [published erratum appears in J Orthop Res 1991 9(5): 776]. J Orthop Res 9: 398–405

676. Ranu H S 1993 Multipoint determination of pressure–volume curves in human intervertebral discs. Ann Rheum Dis 52: 142–146

677. Rauschning W, Jonsson H 1998 Injuries of the cervical spine in automobile accidents: pathoanatomic and clinical aspects. In: Gunzburg R, Szpalski M (eds) Whiplash injuries. Lippincott-Raven, Philadelphia, USA

678. Reigo T 2001 The nature of back pain in a general population: a longitudinal study. PhD thesis, Linkoping University

679. Reihsner R, Menzel E J 1998 Two-dimensional stress-relaxation behavior of human skin as influenced by non-enzymatic glycation and the inhibitory agent aminoguanidine. J Biomech 31: 985–993

680. Riihimaki H, Tola S, Videman T et al. 1989 Low-back pain and occupation. A cross-sectional questionnaire study of men in machine operating, dynamic physical work, and sedentary work. Spine 14: 204–209

681. Rissanen P M 1960 The surgical anatomy and pathology of the supraspinous and interspinous ligaments of the lumbar spine with special reference to ligament ruptures. Acta Orthop Scand, supplement 46

682. Roberts S, Menage J, Urban J P 1989 Biochemical and structural properties of the cartilage end-plate and its relation to the intervertebral disc. Spine 14: 166–174

683. Roberts S, Menage J, Eisenstein S M 1993 The cartilage end-plate and intervertebral disc in scoliosis: calcification and other sequelae. J Orthop Res 11: 747–757

684. Roberts S, Menage J, Duance V et al. 1991 Collagen types around the cells of the intervertebral disc and cartilage end plate: an immunolocalization study. Spine 16: 1030–1038

685. Roberts S, McCall I W, Menage J et al. 1997 Does the thickness of the vertebral subchondral bone reflect the composition of the intervertebral disc? Eur Spine J 6: 385–389

686. Roberts S, Caterson B, Menage J et al. 2000 Matrix metalloproteinases and aggrecanase: their role in disorders of the human intervertebral disc. Spine 25: 3005–3013

687. Robin S, Skalli W, Lavaste F 1994 Influence of geometrical factors on the behavior of lumbar spine segments: a finite element analysis. Eur Spine J 3: 84–90

688. Rockoff S D, Sweet E, Bleustein J 1969 The relative contribution of trabecular and cortical bone to the strength of human lumbar vertebrae. Calcif Tissue Res 3: 163–175

689. Roland M, Waddell G, Klaber-Moffett J et al. 1996 The back book. The Stationery Office, Norwich

690. Rolander S D 1966 Motion of the lumbar spine with special reference to the stabilizing effect of posterior fusion. An experimental study on autopsy specimens. Acta Orthop Scand Suppl: 1–144

691. Rothhaupt D, Laser T, Ziegler H et al. 1997 [Orthopedic hippotherapy in postoperative rehabilitation of lumbar intervertebral disk patients. A prospective, randomized therapy study]. Sportverletz Sportschaden 11: 63–69

692. Rubin C T, Lanyon L E 1984 Regulation of bone formation by applied dynamic loads. J Bone Joint Surg [Am] 66: 397–402

693. Rubin C T, Lanyon L E 1985 Regulation of bone mass by mechanical strain magnitude. Calcif Tissue Int 37: 411–417

694. Ruff S 1950 Brief acceleration: less than one second. In: German aviation medicine, World War II. Government Printing Office 1: Washington DC, USA, 584–597

695. Saal J A, Saal J S 2000 Intradiscal electrothermal treatment for chronic discogenic low back pain: a prospective outcome study with minimum 1-year follow-up. Spine 25: 2622–2627

696. Salminen J J, Erkintalo-Tertti M O, Paajanen H E 1993 Magnetic resonance imaging findings of lumbar spine in the young: correlation with leisure time physical activity, spinal mobility, and trunk muscle strength in 15-year-old pupils with or without low-back pain. J Spinal Disord 6: 386–391

697. Salminen J J, Erkintalo M O, Pentti J et al. 1999 Recurrent low back pain and early disc degeneration in the young. Spine 24: 1316–1321

698. Sambrook P N, MacGregor A J, Spector T D 1999 Genetic influences on cervical and lumbar disc degeneration: a magnetic resonance imaging study in twins. Arthritis Rheum 42: 366–372

699. Sandstrom J, Esbjornsson E 1986 Return to work after rehabilitation. The significance of the patient's own prediction. Scand J Rehabil Med 18: 29–33

700. Sargeant A J, Dolan P 1987 Human muscle function following prolonged eccentric exercise. Eur J Appl Physiol 56: 704–711

701. Sasaki N, Odajima S 1996 Elongation mechanism of collagen fibrils and force-strain relations of tendon at each level of structural hierarchy. J Biomech 29: 1131–1136

702. Sato K, Kikuchi S, Yonezawa T 1999 In vivo intradiscal pressure measurement in healthy individuals and in patients with ongoing back problems. Spine 24: 2468–2474

703. Saur P M, Ensink F B, Frese K et al. 1996 Lumbar range of motion: reliability and validity of the inclinometer technique in the clinical measurement of trunk flexibility. Spine 21: 1332–1338

704. Savage R A, Whitehouse G H, Roberts N 1997 The relationship between the magnetic resonance imaging appearance of the lumbar spine and low back pain, age and occupation in males. Eur Spine J 6: 106–114

705. Schechtman H, Bader D L 1997 In vitro fatigue of human tendons. J Biomech 30: 829–835

706. Schellhas K P, Pollei S R, Gundry C R et al. 1996 Lumbar disc high-intensity zone. Correlation of magnetic resonance imaging and discography. Spine 21: 79–86

707. Schendel M J, Wood K B, Buttermann G R et al. 1993 Experimental measurement of ligament force, facet force, and segment motion in the human lumbar spine. J Biomech 26: 427–438

708. Schipplein O D, Trafimow J H, Andersson G B et al. 1990 Relationship between moments at the L5/S1 level, hip and knee joint when lifting. J Biomech 23: 907–912

709. Schmidt M B, Mow V C, Chun L E et al. 1990 Effects of proteoglycan extraction on the tensile behavior of articular cartilage. J Orthop Res 8: 353–363

710. Schmidt T A, An H S, Lim T H et al. 1998 The stiffness of lumbar spinal motion segments with a high-intensity zone in the anulus fibrosus. Spine 23: 2167–2173

711. Schollmeier G, Lahr-Eigen R, Lewandrowski K U 2000 Observations on fiber-forming collagens in the anulus fibrosus. Spine 25: 2736–2741

712. Schonstrom N, Lindahl S, Willen J et al. 1989 Dynamic changes in the dimensions of the lumbar spinal canal: an experimental study in vitro. J Orthop Res 7: 115–121

713. Schrader P K, Grob D, Rahn B A et al. 1999 Histology of the ligamentum flavum in patients with degenerative lumbar spinal stenosis. Eur Spine J 8: 323–328

714. Schultz A B, Warwick D N, Berkson M H et al. 1979 Mechanical properties of human lumbar spine segments. Part 1. Response in flexion, extension, lateral bending and torsion. J Biomech Eng 101: 46–52

715. Schultz A B, Haderspeck-Grib K, Sinkora G et al. 1985 Quantitative studies of the flexion–relaxation phenomenon in the back muscles. J Orthop Res 3: 189–197

716. Schultz A B, Andersson G B, Haderspeck K et al. 1982 Analysis and measurement of lumbar trunk loads in tasks involving bends and twists. J Biomech 15: 669–675

717. Schwarzer A C, Aprill C N, Bogduk N 1995 The sacroiliac joint in chronic low back pain. Spine 20: 31–37

718. Schwarzer A C, Wang S C, Bogduk N et al. 1995 Prevalence and clinical features of lumbar zygapophysial joint pain: a study in an Australian population with chronic low back pain. Ann Rheum Dis 54: 100–106

719. Schwarzer A C, Aprill C N, Derby R et al. 1994 Clinical features of patients with pain stemming from the lumbar zygapophysial joints. Is the lumbar facet syndrome a clinical entity? Spine 19: 1132–1137

720. Schwarzer A C, Derby R, Aprill C N et al. 1994 Pain from the lumbar zygapophysial joints: a test of two models. J Spinal Disord 7: 331–336

721. Schwarzer A C, Aprill C N, Derby R et al. 1995 The prevalence and clinical features of internal disc disruption in patients with chronic low back pain [see comments]. Spine 20: 1878–1883

722. Schwarzer A C, Wang S C, O'Driscoll D et al. 1995 The ability of computed tomography to identify a painful zygapophysial joint in patients with chronic low back pain. Spine 20: 907–912

723. Sedlin E D, Hirsch C 1966 Factors affecting the determination of the physical properties of femoral cortical bone. Acta Orthop Scand 37: 29–48

724. Seroussi R E, Pope M H 1987 The relationship between trunk muscle electromyography and lifting moments in the sagittal and frontal planes. J Biomech 20: 135–146

725. Seroussi R E, Wilder D G, Pope M H 1989 Trunk muscle electromyography and whole body vibration. J Biomech 22: 219–229

726. Seroussi R E, Krag M H, Muller D L et al. 1989 Internal deformations of intact and denucleated human lumbar discs subjected to compression, flexion, and extension loads. J Orthop Res 7: 122–131

727. Setton L A, Zhu W, Mow V C 1993 The biphasic poroviscoelastic behavior of articular cartilage: role of the surface zone in governing the compressive behavior [see comments]. J Biomech 26: 581–592

728. Setton L A, Zhu W, Weidenbaum M et al. 1993 Compressive properties of the cartilaginous end-plate of the baboon lumbar spine. J Orthop Res 11: 228–239

729. Shah J S, Hampson W G, Jayson M I 1978 The distribution of surface strain in the cadaveric lumbar spine. J Bone Joint Surg [Br] 60-B: 246–251

730. Shannon H S, Walters V, Lewchuck W et al. 1996 Workplace organizational correlates of lost-time accident rates in manufacturing. Am J Ind Med 29: 258–268

731. Shapiro F, Koide S, Glimcher M J 1993 Cell origin and differentiation in the repair of full-thickness defects of articular cartilage. J Bone Joint Surg Am 75: 532–553

732. Shea M, Takeuchi T Y, Wittenberg R H et al. 1994 A comparison of the effects of automated percutaneous diskectomy and conventional diskectomy on intradiscal pressure, disk geometry, and stiffness. J Spinal Disord 7: 317–325

733. Shirado O, Kaneda K, Tadano S et al. 1992 Influence of disc degeneration on mechanism of thoracolumbar burst fractures. Spine 17: 286–292

734. Shirazi-Adl A 1989 Strain in fibers of a lumbar disc. Analysis of the role of lifting in producing disc prolapse. Spine 14: 96–103

735. Shirazi-Adl A 1991 Finite-element evaluation of contact loads on facets of an L2–L3 lumbar segment in complex loads. Spine 16: 533–541

736. Shirazi-Adl A 1992 Finite-element simulation of changes in the fluid content of human lumbar discs. Mechanical and clinical implications. Spine 17: 206–212

737. Shirazi-Adl A 1994 Biomechanics of the lumbar spine in sagittal/lateral moments. Spine 19: 2407–2414

738. Shirazi-Adl A 1994 Nonlinear stress analysis of the whole lumbar spine in torsion – mechanics of facet articulation. J Biomech 27: 289–299

739. Shirazi-Adl A, Drouin G 1987 Load-bearing role of facets in a lumbar segment under sagittal plane loadings. J Biomech 20: 601–613

740. Shirazi-Adl A, Parnianpour M 1999 Effect of changes in lordosis on mechanics of the lumbar spine-lumbar curvature in lifting. J Spinal Disord 12: 436–447

741. Silva M J, Keaveny T M, Hayes W C 1997 Load sharing between the shell and centrum in the lumbar vertebral body. Spine 22: 140–150

742. Simpson E K, Parkinson I H, Manthey B et al. 2001 Intervertebral disc disorganization is related to trabecular bone architecture in the lumbar spine. J Bone Miner Res 16: 681–687

743. Skaggs D L, Weidenbaum M, Iatridis J C et al. 1994 Regional variation in tensile properties and biochemical composition of the human lumbar annulus fibrosus [see comments]. Spine 19: 1310–1319

744. Smeathers J E 1984 Some time dependent properties of the intervertebral joint when under compression. Eng Med 13: 83–87

745. Smeathers J E, Joanes D N 1988 Dynamic compressive properties of human lumbar intervertebral joints: a comparison between fresh and thawed specimens. J Biomech 21: 425–433

746. Smidt G L, McQuade K, Wei S H et al. 1995 Sacroiliac kinematics for reciprocal straddle positions. Spine 20: 1047–1054

747. Smidt G L, Wei S H, McQuade K et al. 1997 Sacroiliac motion for extreme hip positions. A fresh cadaver study. Spine 22: 2073–2082

748. Smith G N, Jr., Brandt K D 1992 Hypothesis: can type IX collagen 'glue' together intersecting type II fibers in articular cartilage matrix? A proposed mechanism. J Rheumatol 19: 14–17

749. Smyth M J, Wright V 1959 Sciatica and the intervertebral disc. An experimental study. J Bone Joint Surg 40 A: 1401–1418

750. Snook S H, Webster B S, McGorry R W et al. 1998 The reduction of chronic nonspecific low back pain through the control of early morning lumbar flexion. A randomized controlled trial. Spine 23: 2601–2607

751. Solomonow M, Zhou B H, Baratta R V et al. 1999 Biomechanics of increased exposure to lumbar injury caused by cyclic loading: Part 1. Loss of reflexive muscular stabilization. Spine 24: 2426–2434

752. Solomonow M, He Zhou B, Baratta R V et al. 2000 Biexponential recovery model of lumbar viscoelastic laxity and reflexive muscular activity after prolonged cyclic loading. Clin Biomech 15: 167–175

753. Spangfort E V 1973 The lumbar disc herniation. Acta Orthop Scand, supplement 142

754. Spitzer W O, Skovron M L, Salmi L R et al. 1995 Scientific monograph of the Quebec Task Force on Whiplash-Associated Disorders: redefining 'whiplash' and its management. Spine 20: 8S–73S

755. Spratt K F, Weinstein J N, Lehmann T R et al. 1993 Efficacy of flexion and extension treatments incorporating braces for low-back pain patients with retrodisplacement, spondylolisthesis, or normal sagittal translation. Spine 18: 1839–1849

756. Stairmand J W, Holm S, Urban J P 1991 Factors influencing oxygen concentration gradients in the intervertebral disc. A theoretical analysis. Spine 16: 444–449

757. Steffen T, Baramki H G, Rubin R et al. 1998 Lumbar intradiscal pressure measured in the anterior and posterolateral annular regions during asymmetrical loading. Clin Biomech 13: 495–505

758. Steffen T, Rubin R K, Baramki H G et al. 1997 A new technique for measuring lumbar segmental motion in vivo. Method, accuracy, and preliminary results. Spine 22: 156–166

759. Steindler A, Luck J V 1938 Differential diagnosis of pain low in the back: allocation of the source of pain by procain hydrochloride method. JAMA 110: 106–112

760. Stewart T D 1953 The age incidence of neural arch defects in Alaskan natives – considered from the standpoint of aetiology. J Bone Joint Surg [Am] 35: 937–950

761. Stokes I A 1987 Surface strain on human intervertebral discs. J Orthop Res 5: 348–355

762. Stokes I A 1988 Bulging of lumbar intervertebral discs: non-contacting measurements of anatomical specimens. J Spinal Disord 1: 189–193

763. Stokes I A, Bevins T M, Lunn R A 1987 Back surface curvature and measurement of lumbar spinal motion. Spine 12: 355–361

764. Stokes I A, Wilder D G, Frymoyer J W et al. 1981 Assessment of patients with low- back pain by biplanar radiographic measurement of intervertebral motion. Spine 6: 233–240

765. Stokes I A, Gardner-Morse M, Henry S M et al. 2000 Decrease in trunk muscular response to perturbation with preactivation of lumbar spinal musculature. Spine 25: 1957–1964

766. Stokes M, Young A 1984 The contribution of reflex inhibition to arthrogenous muscle weakness. Clin Sci 67: 7–14

767. Stokes M J, Cooper R G, Morris G et al. 1992 Selective changes in multifidus dimensions in patients with chronic low back pain. Eur Spine J 1: 38–42

768. Stubbs M, Harris M, Solomonow M et al. 1998 Ligamento-muscular protective reflex in the lumbar spine of the feline. J Electromyogr Kinesiol 8: 197–204

769. Sturesson B 1997 Movement of the sacro-iliac joints: a fresh look. In: Vleeming A et al. (eds) Movement, stability and low back pain. Churchill Livingstone, Edinburgh

770. Sturesson B, Selvik G, Uden A 1989 Movements of the sacroiliac joints. A roentgen stereophotogrammetric analysis. Spine 14: 162–165

771. Sullivan A, McGill S M 1990 Changes in spine length during and after seated whole-body vibration. Spine 15: 1257–1260

772. Sullivan J D, Farfan H F 1975 The crumpled neural arch. Orthop Clin North Am 6: 199–214

773. Sullivan M S, Dickinson C E, Troup J D 1994 The influence of age and gender on lumbar spine sagittal plane range of motion. A study of 1126 healthy subjects. Spine 19: 682–686

774. Sumida K, Sato K, Aoki M et al. 1999 Serial changes in the rate of proteoglycan synthesis after chemo-nucleolysis of rabbit intervertebral discs. Spine 24: 1066–1070

775. Suwito W, Keller T S, Basu P K et al. 1992 Geometric and material property study of the human lumbar spine using the finite element method. J Spinal Disord 5: 50–59

776. Svensson M Y 1998 Injury biomechanics. In: Gunzburg R, Szpalski M (eds) Whiplash injuries. Lippincott-Raven, Philadelphia, USA

777. Swanepoel M W, Smeathers J E, Adams L M 1994 The stiffness of human apophyseal articular cartilage as an indicator of joint loading. Proc Inst Mech Eng 208: 33–43

778. Swanepoel M W, Adams L M, Smeathers J E 1995 Human lumbar apophyseal joint damage and intervertebral disc degeneration. Ann Rheum Dis 54: 182–188

779. Swanepoel M W, Adams L M, Smeathers J E 1997 Morphometry of human lumbar apophyseal joints. A novel technique. Spine 22: 2473–2483

780. Sward L, Hellstrom M, Jacobsson B et al. 1990 Back pain and radiologic changes in the thoraco-lumbar spine of athletes. Spine 15: 124–129

781. Sward L, Hellstrom M, Jacobsson B et al. 1991 Disc degeneration and associated abnormalities of the spine in elite gymnasts. A magnetic resonance imaging study. Spine 16: 437–443

782. Syczewska M, Oberg T, Karlsson D 1999 Segmental movements of the spine during treadmill walking with normal speed. Clin Biomech 14: 384–388

783. Symmons D P, van Hemert A M, Vandenbroucke J P et al. 1991 A longitudinal study of back pain and radiological changes in the lumbar spines of middle aged women. II. Radiographic findings. Ann Rheum Dis 50: 162–166

784. Symonds T L, Burton A K, Tillotson K M et al. 1995 Absence resulting from low back trouble can be reduced by psychosocial intervention at the work place. Spine 20: 2738–2745

785. Szpalski M, Michel F, Hayez J P 1996 Determination of trunk motion patterns associated with permanent or transient stenosis of the lumbar spine. Eur Spine J 5: 332–337

786. Tanaka M, Nakahara S, Inoue H 1993 A pathologic study of discs in the elderly. Separation between the cartilaginous endplate and the vertebral body. Spine 18: 1456–1462

787. Taylor J R, Twomey L T 1986 Age changes in lumbar zygapophyseal joints. Observations on structure and function. Spine 11: 739–745

788. Taylor J R, Twomey L T, Corker M 1990 Bone and soft tissue injuries in post-mortem lumbar spines. Paraplegia 28: 119–129

789. Teitz C C, Garrett W E, Miniachi A et al. 1997 Tendon problems in athletic individuals. J Bone Joint Surg [Am] 79: 138–152

790. Tesh K M, Dunn J S, Evans J H 1987 The abdominal muscles and vertebral stability. Spine 12: 501–508

791. Tew S R, Kwan A P, Hann A et al. 2000 The reactions of articular cartilage to experimental wounding: role of apoptosis. Arthritis Rheum 43: 215–225

792. Thompson J P, Pearce R H, Schechter M T et al. 1990 Preliminary evaluation of a scheme for grading the gross morphology of the human intervertebral disc. Spine 15: 411–415

793. Thorstensson A, Hulten B, von Dobeln W et al. 1976 Effect of strength training on enzyme activities and fibre characteristics in human skeletal muscle. Acta Physiol Scand 96: 392–398

794. Tkaczuk H 1968 Tensile properties of human lumbar longitudinal ligaments. Acta Orthop Scand, supplement

795. Tobias D, Ziv I, Maroudas A 1992 Human facet cartilage: swelling and some physico-chemical characteristics as a function of age. Part 1: Swelling of human facet joint cartilage. Spine 17: 694–700

796. Torstensen T A, Ljunggren A E, Meen H D et al. 1998 Efficiency and costs of medical exercise therapy, conventional physiotherapy, and self-exercise in patients with chronic low back pain. A pragmatic, randomized, single-blinded, controlled trial with 1-year follow-up. Spine 23: 2616–2624

797. Tracy M F, Gibson M J, Szypryt E P et al. 1989 The geometry of the muscles of the lumbar spine determined by magnetic resonance imaging. Spine 14: 186–193

798. Trafimow J H, Schipplein O D, Novak G J et al. 1993 The effects of quadriceps fatigue on the technique of lifting. Spine 18: 364–367

799. Trotter J A 1993 Functional morphology of force transmission in skeletal muscle. A brief review. Acta Anat 146: 205–222

800. Trotter J A, Purslow P P 1992 Functional morphology of the endomysium in series fibered muscles. J Morphol 212: 109–122

801. Truchon M, Fillion L 2000 Biopsychosocial determinants of chronic disability and low back pain: a review. J Occupat Rehab 10: 117–142

802. Tsuji H, Hirano N, Ohshima H et al. 1993 Structural variation of the anterior and posterior anulus fibrosus in the development of human lumbar intervertebral disc. A risk factor for intervertebral disc rupture. Spine 18: 204–210

803. van Tulder M W, Assendelft W J, Koes B W et al. 1997 Spinal radiographic findings and nonspecific low back pain. A systematic review of observational studies. Spine 22: 427–434

804. van Tulder M W, Goosens M, Waddell G et al. 2000 Conservative treatment of chronic low back pain. In: Nachemson A L, Jonsson E (eds) Neck and back pain: the scientific evidence of causation, diagnosis and treatment. Lippincott, Williams and Wilkins, Philadelphia 271–304

805. van Tulder M W, Cherkin D C, Berman B et al. 1999 The effectiveness of acupuncture in the management of acute and chronic low back pain. A systematic review within the framework of the Cochrane Collaboration Back Review Group. Spine 24: 1113–1123

806. van Tulder M W, Ostelo R W, Vlaeyen J W et al. 2000 Behavioural treatment for chronic low back pain. Cochrane Database Syst Rev 2

807. van Tulder M W, Ostelo R, Vlaeyen J W et al. 2000 Behavioral treatment for chronic low back pain: a systematic review within the framework of the Cochrane Back Review Group. Spine 25: 2688–2699

808. Tullberg T, Blomberg S, Branth B et al. 1998 Manipulation does not alter the position of the sacroiliac joint. A roentgen stereophotogrammetric analysis. Spine 23: 1124–1128; discussion 1129

809. Tveit P, Daggfeldt K, Hetland S et al. 1994 Erector spinae lever arm length variations with changes in spinal curvature. Spine 19: 199–204

810. Twomey L, Taylor J 1982 Flexion creep deformation and hysteresis in the lumbar vertebral column. Spine 7: 116–122

811. Twomey L, Taylor J 1985 Age changes in lumbar intervertebral discs. Acta Orthop Scand 56: 496–499

812. Twomey L T, Taylor J R 1983 Sagittal movements of the human lumbar vertebral column: a quantitative study of the role of the posterior vertebral elements. Arch Phys Med Rehabil 64: 322–325

813. Twomey L T, Taylor J R 1987 Age changes in lumbar vertebrae and intervertebral discs. Clin Orthop: 97–104

814. Twomey L T, Taylor J R, Taylor M M 1989 Unsuspected damage to lumbar zygapophyseal (facet) joints after motor-vehicle accidents. Med J Aust 151: 210–212, 215–217

815. Tyrrell A R, Reilly T, Troup J D 1985 Circadian variation in stature and the effects of spinal loading. Spine 10: 161–164

816. Umehara S, Tadano S, Abumi K et al. 1996 Effects of degeneration on the elastic modulus distribution in the lumbar intervertebral disc. Spine 21: 811–819; discussion 820

817. Urban J P 1994 The chondrocyte: a cell under pressure. Br J Rheumatol 33: 901–908

818. Urban J P, McMullin J F 1988 Swelling pressure of the lumbar intervertebral discs: influence of age, spinal level, composition, and degeneration. Spine 13: 179–187

819. Urban J P, Holm S, Maroudas A et al. 1977 Nutrition of the intervertebral disk. An in vivo study of solute transport. Clin Orthop: 101–114

820. Valli M, Leonardi L, Strocchi R et al. 1986 'In vitro' fibril formation of type I collagen from different sources: biochemical and morphological aspects. Connect Tissue Res 15: 235–244

821. Vanharanta H, Sachs B L, Spivey M A et al. 1987 The relationship of pain provocation to lumbar disc deterioration as seen by CT/discography. Spine 12: 295–298

822. Vascancelos D 1973 Compression fractures of the vertebra during major epileptic seizures. Epilepsia 14: 323–328

823. Vernon-Roberts B 1988 Disc pathology and disease states. In: Ghosh P (ed) The biology of the intervertebral disc. CRC Press, Boca Raton, Florida, Vol. 2: 73–119

824. Vernon-Roberts B, Pirie C J 1973 Healing trabecular microfractures in the bodies of lumbar vertebrae. Ann Rheum Dis 32: 406–412

825. Vernon-Roberts B, Fazzalari N L, Manthey B A 1997 Pathogenesis of tears of the annulus investigated by multiple-level transaxial analysis of the T12–L1 disc. Spine 22: 2641–2646

826. Verzijl N, DeGroot J, Thorpe S R et al. 2000 Effect of collagen turnover on the accumulation of advanced glycation end products. J Biol Chem 275: 39027–39031

827. Videman T, Battie M C 1999 The influence of occupation on lumbar degeneration. Spine 24: 1164–1168

828. Videman T, Nurminen M, Troup J D 1990 Lumbar spinal pathology in cadaveric material in relation to history of back pain, occupation, and physical loading. Spine 15: 728–740

829. Videman T, Battie M C, Gill K et al. 1995 Magnetic resonance imaging findings and their relationships in the thoracic and lumbar spine. Insights into the etipathogenesis of spinal degeneration. Spine 20: 928–935

830. Videman T, Sarna S, Battie M C et al. 1995 The long-term effects of physical loading and exercise lifestyles on back-related symptoms, disability, and spinal pathology among men. Spine 20: 699–709

831. Videman T, Leppavuori J, Kaprio J et al. 1998 Intragenic polymorphisms of the vitamin D receptor gene associated with intervertebral disc degeneration. Spine 23: 2477–2485

832. Vingard E, Nachemson A 2001 Work related influences on neck and low back pain. Swedish Council on Technology Assessment in Health Care. Lippincott, Stockholm/Philadelphia (English translation in press)

833. Virgin W J 1951 Experimental investigations into the physical properties of the intervertebral disc. J Bone Joint Surg [Br] 33: 607–611

834. Vleeming A, Volkers A C, Snijders C J et al. 1990 Relation between form and function in the sacroiliac joint. Part II: Biomechanical aspects. Spine 15: 133–136

835. Vleeming A, Stoeckart R, Volkers A C et al. 1990 Relation between form and function in the sacroiliac joint. Part I: Clinical anatomical aspects. Spine 15: 130–132

836. Vleeming A, Snijders C J, Stoeckart R et al. 1997 The role of the sacroiliac joints in coupling between spine, pelvis, legs and arms. In: Vleeming A et al. (eds) Movement, stability and low back pain. Churchill Livingstone, Edinburgh

837. Vleeming A, Pool-Goudzwaard A L, Stoeckart R et al. 1995 The posterior layer of the thoracolumbar fascia. Its function in load transfer from spine to legs. Spine 20: 753–758

838. Volinn E 1999 Do workplace interventions prevent low-back disorders? If so, why?: a methodologic commentary. Ergonomics 42: 258–272

839. Waddell G 1987 A new clinical model for the treatment of low-back pain. Spine 12: 632–644

840. Waddell G 1998 The back pain revolution. Churchill Livingstone, Edinburgh

841. Waddell G, Burton A K 2000 Occupational health guidelines for the management of low back pain at work – evidence review. Faculty of Occupational Medicine, London

842. Waddell G, Burton A K 2001 Occupational health guidelines for the management of low back pain at work: evidence review. Occup Med (Lond) 51: 124–135

843. Waddell G, Main C J, Morris E W et al. 1982 Normality and reliability in the clinical assessment of backache. Br Med J (Clin Res Ed) 284: 1519–1523

844. Walsh K, Cruddas M, Coggon D 1992 Low back pain in eight areas of Britain. J Epidemiol Community Health 46: 227–230

845. Walsh T R, Weinstein J N, Spratt K F et al. 1990 Lumbar discography in normal subjects. A controlled, prospective study. J Bone Joint Surg Am 72: 1081–1088

846. Wang M, Dumas G A 1998 Mechanical behavior of the female sacroiliac joint and influence of the anterior and posterior sacroiliac ligaments under sagittal loads. Clin Biomech 13: 293–299

847. Wassell J T, Gardner L I, Landsittel D P et al. 2000 A prospective study of back belts for prevention of back pain and injury. JAMA 284: 2727–2732

848. Watson P J, Booker C K, Main C J et al. 1997 Surface electromyography in the identification of chronic low back pain patients: the development of the flexion relaxation ratio. Clin Biomech 12: 165–171

849. Waxman R, Tennant A, Helliwell P 1998 Community survey of factors associated with consultation for low back pain. BMJ 317: 1564–1567

850. Weber H, Burton A K 1986 Rational treatment of low back trouble? Clin Biomech 1: 160–167

851. Weightman B 1976 Tensile fatigue of human articular cartilage. J Biomech 9: 193–200

852. Wenger K H, Schlegel J D 1997 Annular bulge contours from an axial photogammetric method. Clin Biomech 12: 438–444

853. Westacott C I, Webb G R, Warnock M G et al. 1997 Alteration of cartilage metabolism by cells from osteoarthritic bone. Arthritis Rheum 40: 1282–1291

854. Westgaard R H, Winkel J 1997 Ergonomic intervention research for improved musculoskeletal health: A critical review. Indust Ergonom 20: 463–500

855. Wiberg G 1947 Back pain in relation to the nerve supply of the intervertebral disc. Acta Orthop Scand 19: 211–221

856. Wilder D G, Pope M H 1996 Epidemiological and aetiological aspects of low back pain in vibration environments – an update. Clin Biomech 11: 61–73

857. Wilder D G, Aleksiev A R, Magnusson M L et al. 1996 Muscular response to sudden load. A tool to evaluate fatigue and rehabilitation. Spine 21: 2628–2639

858. Wilk V 1995 Pain arising from the interspinous and supraspinous ligaments. Australas Musculoskelet Med 1: 21–31

859. Wilke D R 1979 Institute of Biology, Studies in Biology No 11: Muscle, 2nd edn. Edward Arnold, London

860. Wilke H J, Claes L, Schmitt H et al. 1994 A universal spine tester for in vitro experiments with muscle force simulation. Eur Spine J 3: 91–97

861. Wilke H J, Wolf S, Claes L E et al. 1995 Stability increase of the lumbar spine with different muscle groups. A biomechanical in vitro study [see comments]. Spine 20: 192–198

862. Wilke H J, Neef P, Caimi M et al. 1999 New in vivo measurements of pressures in the intervertebral disc in daily life. Spine 24: 755–762

863. Williams I F, Craig A S, Parry D A D et al. 1985 Development of collagen fibril organization and collagen crimp patterns during tendon healing. Int J Biol Macromol 7: 275–282

864. Williams M, Solomonow M, Zhou B H et al. 2000 Multifidus spasms elicited by prolonged lumbar flexion. Spine 25: 2916–2924

865. Williams P, Watt P, Bicik V et al. 1986 Effect of stretch combined with electrical stimulation on the type of sarcomeres produced at the ends of muscle fibers. Exp Neurol 93: 500–509

866. Williams P E, Goldspink G 1971 Longitudinal growth of striated muscle fibres. J Cell Sci 9: 751–767

867. Williams P E, Goldspink G 1984 Connective tissue changes in immobilised muscle. J Anat 138: 343–350

868. Wilson A M, Goodship A E 1994 Exercise-induced hyperthermia as a possible mechanism for tendon degeneration. J Biomech 27: 899–905

869. Wiltse L L 1962 The etiology of spondylolisthesis. J Bone Joint Surg [Am] 44: 539–560

870. Winkelstein B A, Rutkowski M D, Weinstein J N et al. 2001 An in vivo approach to characterising local biomechanics in a radiculopathy model. Proceedings of the International Society for the Study of the Lumbar Spine. Edinburgh, UK

871. Wood D J 1987 Design and evaluation of a back injury prevention program within a geriatric hospital. Spine 12: 77–82

872. Wood K A, Standell C J, Adams M A et al. 1997 Exercise training to improve spinal mobility and back muscle fatigability: a possible prophylaxis for low back pain? Proceedings of the Physical Medicine Research Foundation Symposium, Prague

873. Wood P H N, Badley E M 1980 Epidemiology of back pain. In: Jayson M I V (ed) The lumbar spine and back pain, 2nd edn. Pitman Medical, Tunbridge Wells, 29–55

874. Wu H C, Yao R F 1976 Mechanical behavior of the human annulus fibrosus. J Biomech 9: 1–7

875. Yahia L H, Audet J, Drouin G 1991 Rheological properties of the human lumbar spine ligaments. J Biomed Eng 13: 399–406

876. Yamamoto I, Panjabi M M, Oxland T R et al. 1990 The role of the iliolumbar ligament in the lumbosacral junction. Spine 15: 1138–1141

877. Yamashita T, Minaki Y, Ozaktay A C et al. 1996 A morphological study of the fibrous capsule of the human lumbar facet joint. Spine 21: 538–543

878. Yang K H, King A I 1984 Mechanism of facet load transmission as a hypothesis for low-back pain. Spine 9: 557–565

879. Yao J Q, Seedhom B B 1993 Mechanical conditioning of articular cartilage to prevalent stresses. Br J Rheumatol 32: 956–965

880. Yasuma T, Arai K, Yamauchi Y 1993 The histology of lumbar intervertebral disc herniation. The significance of small blood vessels in the extruded tissue. Spine 18: 1761–1765

881. Yingling V R, Callaghan J P, McGill S M 1997 Dynamic loading affects the mechanical properties and failure site of porcine spines. Clin Biomech 12: 301–305

882. Yoganandan N, Myklebust J B, Wilson C R et al. 1988 Functional biomechanics of the thoracolumbar vertebral cortex. Clin Biomech 3: 11–18

883. Yoganandan N, Ray G, Pintar F A et al. 1989 Stiffness and strain energy criteria to evaluate the threshold of injury to an intervertebral joint [see comments]. J Biomech 22: 135–142

884. Yoganandan N, Larson S J, Gallagher M et al. 1994 Correlation of microtrauma in the lumbar spine with intraosseous pressures. Spine 19: 435–440

885. Yoshizawa H, O'Brien J P, Smith W T et al. 1980 The neuropathology of intervertebral discs removed for low-back pain. J Pathol 132: 95–104

886. Ziv I, Maroudas C, Robin G et al. 1993 Human facet cartilage: swelling and some physicochemical characteristics as a function of age. Part 2: Age changes in some biophysical parameters of human facet joint cartilage. Spine 18: 136–146

Index

Page numbers in **bold** indicate figures and tables. Numbers in *italic* indicate plates in the plate section at the beginning of the book.